ON CALL
CARDIOLOGY

Be ON CALL with confidence!

Successfully managing on-call situations requires a masterful combination of speed, skill, and knowledge. Rise to the occasion with **W.B. SAUNDERS' On Call Series!** These pocket-size resources provide you with immediate access to the vital, step-by-step information you need to succeed!

Other titles in the On Call Series

ON CALL
CARDIOLOGY
Second Edition

M Gabriel Khan, MD, FRCP (London),
FRCP(C), FACP, FACC
Associate Professor of Medicine
University of Ottawa Faculty of Medicine
Cardiologist, The Ottawa Hospital
Ottawa, Ontario, Canada

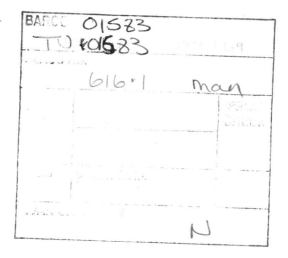
W.B. SAUNDERS COMPANY
A Harcourt Health Sciences Company
Philadelphia   London   New York   St. Louis   Sydney   Toronto

W.B. SAUNDERS COMPANY
A Harcourt Health Sciences Company

The Curtis Center
Independence Square West
Philadelphia, Pennsylvania 19106

Library of Congress Cataloging-in-Publication Data

On call cardiology / M. Gabriel Khan.

p.   cm.—(On call series)

ISBN 0–7216–9222–2

1. Cardiovascular system—Diseases.   2. Cardiology.   I. Title:
Cardiology.   II. Title.   III. Series.
[DNLM: 1. Cardiovascular Diseases—therapy.   2. Cardiovascular
Diseases—diagnosis.   3. Emergencies. WG 205 K45o 2001]

RC667.K48 2001   616.1—dc21   00–054787

Acquisitions Editor: William Schmitt
Manuscript Editor: Amy Norwitz
Production Manager: Frank Polizzano
Illustration Specialist: John Needles
Book Designer: Matt Andrews
Indexer: Dennis Dolan

ON CALL CARDIOLOGY   ISBN 0–7216–9222–2

Printed in the United States of America

Last digit is the print number: 9   8   7   6   5   4   3   2   1

PREFACE

On-call housestaff and medical students virtually run teaching hospitals at night and on weekends. They should be proud of their achievements. Their hard-earned competence results from being on call in hospitals that handle a wide variety of medical emergencies and admissions to wards.

The purpose of this book is to strengthen the reader's ability to deal with on-call problems in cardiology. The text emphasizes

- How to approach on-call problems with a relevant history and physical examination; coverage of cardiac bedside diagnosis is given in depth.
- How to define the problem accurately, with consideration of appropriate causes and the differential diagnosis.
- How to exclude mimics before ordering treatment that may be misguided by incorrect definition of the problem.

This second edition is a thoroughly revised text. Approximately 125 new pages have been added. **New features include**

- Expansion of major chapters to keep abreast of new diagnostic and therapeutic strategies.
- At the end of many chapters that deal with patient-related problems, *Study Sections* that will allow trainees to study the topic in greater detail when time permits.
- A new chapter: Evaluation and Treatment of Patients With Murmurs.
- In the Appendix: A Global Drug Table that gives the generic and trade names of cardiac drugs in the Untied States, Canada, UK, Europe, and Japan. This table should prove useful for all doctors and emergency physicians worldwide.

Cardiologic emergencies are a common scenario in the emergency room, in ICUs, and on wards. This is not surprising because more than one million individuals die from cardiovascular disease annually in North America. Over half a million heart attack patients survive and are discharged from hospitals in the United States and Canada each year. The management of acute heart attacks requires the differentiation of mimics of acute myocardial infarction, rapid confirmation of the diagnosis, and administration of thrombolytic therapy within 20 minutes of the patient's arrival at the emergency room.

Despite the advent of expensive and sophisticated cardiologic tests, the ECG remains the most reliable and inexpensive tool for the confirmation of acute myocardial infarction and ischemia. The results of this simple test, and not the CK-MB, echocardiogram, or SPECT or PET scan, dictate the rapid treatment with lifesaving thrombolytic agents. Thus, this book includes a detailed chapter that highlights the hallmarks of relevant electrocardiographic diagnoses. Also, the management of on-call cardiologic problems requires a thorough understanding of the pharmacologic actions, appropriate indications, and adverse effects of cardiovascular drugs; these topics are given appropriate coverage.

Coping with on-call situations requires an armamentarium that integrates

- A sound knowledge base
- The art of obtaining a relevant history rapidly
- The skills needed to perform a relevant physical examination
- Applied common sense
- A confident and pleasant bedside manner
- The thought process and the logic that bring about a clear definition of the problem and rapid evolution of a sound plan of management

I am confident that the expansion of the text from 343 pages to a second edition of 486 pages will allow students, interns, residents in internal medicine, and first-year residents in cardiology to use the text on the wards and in calmer domains of the hospital or at home as a study guide.

M Gabriel Khan

ACKNOWLEDGMENTS

Several electrocardiographic tracings were reproduced from *Electrocardiography in Clinical Practice* by the late Dr. Te-Chuan Chou and from *The ECG in Emergency Decision Making* by Dr. Hein JJ Wellens and Mary Conover. I am grateful to these authors for the loan of their instructive tracings. Amy Norwitz, Project Supervisor at WB Saunders, deserves a special thank-you for her assistance.

William Schmitt at W.B. Saunders had the foresight to provide students and housestaff with an *On Call* series and particularly a cardiology text that is now expanded to meet the needs of most trainees. His support has been greatly appreciated. I appreciate the freedom he has given me to add the Study Sections, which give depth to this book.

NOTICE

STRUCTURE OF THE BOOK

This book is divided into three main sections.

The first section, Introduction, covers introductory material in five chapters: (1) Approach to the Diagnosis and Management of On-Call Problems, (2) Documentation of On-Call Problems, (3) Examination for Extrathoracic Physical Signs of Heart Disease, (4) Examination of the Heart, and (5) Rapid Guide to Relevant ECG Diagnosis. Reference to these chapters is essential in the proper management of on-call problems.

The second section, Patient-Related Problems: The Common Calls, contains the common calls associated with patient-related problems. Each problem is approached from its inception, beginning with the relevant questions that should be asked over the phone, the temporary orders that should be given, and the major life-threatening problems to be considered as one approaches the bedside. The book uses the following format:

■ PHONE CALL

Questions

Pertinent questions to assess the urgency of the situation.

Orders

Urgent orders to be carried out before the housestaff arrives at the bedside.

Inform RN

RN to be informed of the time the housestaff anticipates arrival at the bedside.

■ ELEVATOR THOUGHTS

The differential diagnoses to be considered by the housestaff while on the way to assess the patient.

■ MAJOR THREAT TO LIFE

Identification of the major threat to life is essential in providing focus for the subsequent effective management of the patient.

■ BEDSIDE

Quick Look Test

The quick look test is a rapid visual assessment to place the patient into one of two categories: sick or critical. This helps determine the necessity of immediate intervention.

Vital Signs

Selective History and Chart Review

Selective Physical Examination

■ DIAGNOSTIC TESTING

■ MANAGEMENT

The third section, the Appendices, contains infusion pump charts; an SI units conversion table; a series of tables showing indications, dosages, adverse effects, and interaction of commonly prescribed drugs; and American Heart Association cardiac arrest protocols.

COMMONLY USED ABBREVIATIONS

$>$	greater than, more than, over
$\geq$	equal to or greater than
$<$	less than, fewer than, under
$\leq$	equal to or less than
$\uparrow$	increase
$\downarrow$	decrease
ABG	arterial blood gas
ACC-AHA	American College of Cardiology–American Heart Association
ACE	angiotensin-converting enzyme
APB	atrial premature beats
ASD	atrial septal defect
AST	aspartate transaminase
AV	atrioventricular
A-V	arteriovenous
AVNRT	atrioventricular nodal reentrant tachycardia
BP	blood pressure
BID	two times daily, twice daily
BUN	blood urea nitrogen
CABS	coronary artery bypass surgery
CBC	complete blood cell count
CCU	coronary care unit
CHD	coronary heart disease
CHF	congestive heart failure
CK-MB	creatine kinase, MB band
CO	cardiac output
COPD	chronic obstructive pulmonary disease

CPR	cardiopulmonary resuscitation
CT	computed tomography
CVS	cardiovascular system
D5W	5% dextrose in water
dl	deciliter
DVT	deep venous thrombosis
EC	ejection click
ECG	electrocardiography
EEG	electroencephalography
EF	ejection fraction
EP	electrophysiologic
ER	emergency room
ESD	end-systolic dimension
FUO	fever of unknown origin
GFR	glomerular filtration rate
Hb	hemoglobin
HCM	hypertrophic cardiomyopathy
HIT	heparin-induced thrombocytopenia
HR	heart rate
ICU	intensive care unit
IHD	ischemic heart disease
INR	International Normalized Ratio
IV	intravenous
JVP	jugular venous pressure
K+	potassium
L	liter
LAFB	left anterior fascicular block
LAH	left anterior hemiblock
LBBB	left bundle branch block
LDH	lactate dehydrogenase
LDL	low-density lipoproteins
LMWHs	low-molecular-weight heparins

LPFB	left posterior fascicular block
LPH	left posterior hemiblock
LV	left ventricular
LVF	left ventricular failure
LVH	left ventricular hypertrophy
MAT	multifocal atrial tachycardia
mEq	milliequivalent
mg	milligram
MI	myocardial infarction
mmol	millimole
MRI	magnetic resonance imaging
MSC	midsystolic click
MVP	mitral valve prolapse
Na$^+$	sodium
ng	nanogram
NSAID	nonsteroidal anti-inflammatory drug
O$_2$	oxygen
OS	opening snap
PAT	paroxysmal atrial tachycardia
PCWP	pulmonary capillary wedge pressure
PDA	patent ductus arteriosus
PE	pulmonary embolism
PET	positron emission tomography
PK	pericardial knock
PO	per os (by mouth)
PRN	as needed
PTCA	percutaneous transluminal coronary angio-plasty
PTT	partial thromboplastin time
q6h	every 6 hours
RBBB	right bundle branch block
RR	respiratory rate

RV	right ventricular
RVH	right ventricular hypertrophy
SA	sinoatrial
SBE	subacute bacterial endocarditis
SK	streptokinase
SOB	shortness of breath
SPECT	single photon emission computed tomography
stat	immediately
SVT	supraventricular tachycardia
TEE	transesophageal echocardiogram
TIA	transient ischemic attack
TKVO	to keep vein open
tPA	tissue plasminogen activator
TID	three times daily
U	units
VPBs	ventricular premature beats
VF	ventricular fibrillation
VSD	ventricular septal defect
VT	ventricular tachycardia
WHO	World Health Organization
WPW	Wolff-Parkinson-White syndrome
μg	microgram

CONTENTS

APPENDICES

INTRODUCTION

Approach to the Diagnosis and Management of On-Call Problems

Clinical decision making requires a skillful combination of art and science that integrates the following:

- Skills to obtain a selective history from all sources in a timely fashion
- Skills to perform a relevant physical examination
- A sound knowledge base
- The thought process and logic that brings about a clear definition of the problem

The problem-formulated approach is essential, in particular during the months of clinical exposure to inpatients, and is the forerunner to the implementation of a sound plan of management. The trainee soon recognizes that clinical decision making is a dynamic process that should be continuously modified based on the information he or she derives from all sources.

Virtually all patients present with problems that require a solution or remedy. In most situations, a relevant patient history is the most important link in clinical problem solving. Pertinent examples of major cardiac diagnoses that depend mainly on the history for an appropriate diagnosis include angina, acute myocardial infarction, and syncope; in these and other settings, the clinician must listen closely to the patient's description of the problem before posing specific questions. The diagnosis of angina depends on the clear description of the pain: its location in the chest; its localization to an area the size of a fingertip or size of the hand; its area of radiation; its character—whether it is crushing, tightness, or heaviness; its duration; and most important, what makes the discomfort worse and what makes it better. With angina, for instance, cessation of the precipitating activity brings relief within 1 to 5 minutes. In many instances, the typical diagnostic features must be drawn out from the patient by skillfully posing short questions that are understood by the patient, allowing the patient sufficient time to reply without prompting. In a similar manner, >40% of syncopal attacks are caused by a vasovagal faint. A thorough history usually resolves the diagnosis and allows for appropriate therapy with the avoidance of expensive and time-consuming tests such as Holter monitoring, electroencephalography (EEG), tilt testing, and electrophysiologic studies.

Taking the history of an inpatient usually requires a 30- to 60-

minute assessment depending on the patient's problems. Information should be gathered from all sources: the patient, the nurses, the nursing notes, the emergency room (ER) assessment, and the admission orders from the patient's physician or the emergency physician. Occasionally it is necessary to obtain information from a spouse, relative, or friend and to consult the previous files. Patients assessed in the ER, however, require rapid assessment of the presenting problem, and this should be achieved within a 5- to 10-minute period. The patient with chest pain suggestive of acute myocardial infarction (MI) requires only a 3-minute history and a few minutes of examination, which is followed by the electrocardiogram (ECG), and these three steps should be completed within 10 minutes of a patient's arrival. Thus, the patient could be administered thrombolytic therapy within 20 minutes of arrival in any ER.

On-call problems in the wards should be handled like calls to the ER, and thus, a selective history and relevant physical examination should not take more than 15 minutes. The basic rule is that the student should continuously choose between asking and listening, directing and following. These clinical skills can be mastered by exposure of students to many clinical problems and with feedback from a senior member of the team.

A sound knowledge base and a trusted pocket reference book are necessities. *On Call Cardiology* provides an invaluable source of information presented in a user-friendly style.

Because core knowledge and clinical skills are essential to obtaining a relevant history and the completion of the physical examination, early chapters in this text are devoted to examination of the heart and extrathoracic physical signs of heart disease. Also, the diagnostic process in most cardiologic on-call problems requires an ECG diagnosis; thus, an extensive chapter on this subject is provided. Readers are strongly advised to refer to Chapters 3, 4, and 5 during their assessment of cardiologic problems.

This book offers a structured, systematic approach that enhances clinical problem solving when on call. Chapters so related are divided into six parts, as follows:

1. Phone call
2. Elevator thoughts
3. Major threat to life
4. Bedside
5. Diagnostic testing
6. Management

■ PHONE CALL

The majority of problems confronting the student or resident on call are first communicated by telephone. It is necessary to assess the severity and urgency of the problem during discussion with the nurse. This section of each chapter is divided into the following three parts:

1. Questions
2. Orders
3. Inform RN

The orders are suggested to help expedite the investigation and immediate management. The registered nurse (RN) is informed of the student's or intern's anticipated time of arrival at the bedside.

■ ELEVATOR THOUGHTS

Elevator thoughts are entertained during the 3 to 10 minutes after the phone call before the student or intern reaches the bedside. During the time spent to reach the ward, it is advisable to consider a differential diagnosis of the problem and relevant causes of the underlying disease. This thinking should provoke a more relevant questioning at the bedside and a pertinent physical examination.

■ MAJOR THREAT TO LIFE

Several cardiac problems pose a threat to life, and the student or intern must make a rapid decision as to the risk of death or a serious event. He or she should think of the one or two most likely threats to life that are associated with the on-call problem. In cases in which threat to life exists, the problem should be discussed with the senior resident as soon as possible.

■ BEDSIDE

It is necessary to use a systematic approach:

1. Perform a quick look test.
2. Assess the airway and vital signs.
3. Take a selective history.
4. Complete a relevant physical examination.
5. Perform a quick review of the patient's chart (may be required in some situations).
6. Make a differential diagnosis or problem formulation.

The assessment at the bedside should begin with the quick look test, which usually enables the physician to categorize the patient's condition as

- Sick (uncomfortable or distressed) or
- Critical (about to die)

■ DIAGNOSIS

The road to accurate diagnosis and therapy is not straight. The following is a suggested approach that has been tested and used by many excellent clinicians. A structured approach is highly recommended: use a step 1, step 2, step 3 approach. Such steps are rapidly done by computers and good clinicians. Develop a computerized approach to diagnosis, investigation, and management. Your diagnosis should involve the use of probabilities and logic. Investigations should follow a logical sequence; each investigative step should test the hypotheses generated by your findings from the history and physical examination.

Step 1. Define the problem and exclude mimics.

Step 2. Provide a short differential diagnosis based on probabilities.

Step 3. Consider the causes that underlie the differential diagnoses.

Reassess by further questioning of the patient, and check for particular physical signs directed by hypotheses obtained from steps 2 and 3; narrow the differential diagnosis to two conditions.

Perform sequential investigation to confirm diagnosis 1 and to exclude diagnosis 2.

Example 1: In a patient suspected of having hemolytic anemia, most students and clinicians request a Coombs test, along with the complete blood count (CBC). Unfortunately, the Coombs test is not a test that establishes the *presence* of hemolytic anemia; it is a test that helps to define the *cause* of hemolytic anemia. The logical investigative steps are as follows: Prove or define the diagnosis by requesting hemoglobin, reticulocyte count, indirect bilirubin, lactate dehydrogenase (LDH), and urinary hemosiderin. These tests should confirm or exclude the diagnosis of hemolytic anemia. If hemolytic anemia is proved present, then request the tests to elucidate the cause of the hemolytic anemia, i.e., Coombs' and other tests.

Example 2: Congestive heart failure (CHF) is not a diagnosis. You should establish the cause of CHF; occasionally, treatment of the cause produces a cure. Mimics of CHF include cardiac tamponade. In both conditions, the patient is short of breath and the jugular venous pressure is high. The usual treatments for CHF, i.e., nitrates, diuretics, and angiotensin-converting enzyme (ACE) inhibitors, cause a decrease in preload, however, and are contraindicated in patients with cardiac tamponade.

Mimics: Assessment for mimics makes clinical medicine exciting and interesting, and students often enjoy increasing their medical detective skills. Examples of mimics include the following:

- ST segment elevation of acute MI: also consider the possibility of a normal variant, i.e., ST elevation, which may be a normal finding in blacks and other ethnic groups (see Chapter 5); also, left bundle branch block typically causes ST elevation.

- Inferior MI: a mimic may be caused by pseudo-Q waves found in some patients with Wolff-Parkinson-White (WPW) syndrome. Also, there are several conditions that may mimic the ECG findings of old myocardial infarction.

Another essential step in the diagnostic process is to think in terms of

- Primary causes
- Secondary causes

For example, when a patient presents with acute gout, it is advisable to consider primary gout as a likely diagnosis; but gout secondary to diuretics, renal failure, and even lead toxicity must be excluded. Consider hypertension as primary (essential) or as secondary due to renal or endocrine diseases, coarctation of the aorta, or many other conditions.

■ MANAGEMENT

The final goal of the student or resident is to accomplish an appropriate plan of management that will restore the patient to a normal or stable status. Management of the problem constitutes a vast area of applied therapeutics that involves the following:

- Nondrug therapy
- Drug therapy
- Interventional therapy

I feel that these areas of management are the weak link in teaching curricula, and this book deals with this topic in an in-depth manner.

2 | Documentation of On-Call Problems

A resident must provide an accurate account of the on-call problem by providing the following:

- A brief selective history
- Relevant physical findings
- A differential diagnosis or problem formulation
- A plan of management

Also, any discussions you may have had with your senior resident should be documented.

The note generally written on the patient's chart by the on-call resident is usually a few lines to a full page of clearly written material.

Record the date, the time of the examination, and who you are. State who called you and at what time you were called; then describe the history of the present illness. Record your observations at the time of examination. Clearly record the vital signs: e.g., blood pressure (BP) 120/80, heart rate (HR) 110/min, respiratory rate (RR) 30/min. Record cardiovascular system (CVS) findings: e.g., pulse rate 110/min, regular rhythm (apical rate if atrial fibrillation is present); jugular venous pressure (JVP) <2 cm, no murmur, gallop, rub, or click. A call for a cardiology problem necessitates examination of the heart and the lungs.

Clearly state your diagnostic impression. Your documentation should state the investigations and measures taken during the night. An electrocardiogram (ECG) and a chest x-ray are often required. Sharpen your skills in the interpretation of the ECG by consulting Chapter 5.

Finally, sign and print your name clearly so that staff members know whom to contact if necessary.

In most instances, this documentation of diagnosis and management should be rechecked by your senior resident. Appropriate discussion with your senior resident at the earliest time should serve to improve your clinical skills and is necessary in the assessment of your degree of accuracy; this feedback will increase your confidence and improve your clinical acumen.

3 | Examination for Extrathoracic Physical Signs of Heart Disease

During the recording of the vital signs, i.e., pulse rate, respiratory rate, and blood pressure, much can be gleaned from observing the patient's facies, the patient's reactions, and the patient's breathing pattern. The physical examination must be methodical.

This area of cardiovascular medicine provides an array of abnormal physical signs that may clinch the clinical diagnosis and allow urgent institution of therapy, before time-consuming and expensive tests are performed.

■ FACIES

The patient's face may reveal important clues to underlying diseases or associated conditions.

- Apprehensive facies produced by pain and anxiety is a feature of acute myocardial infarction, dissecting aneurysm, acute pulmonary edema, and pulmonary embolism. In the absence of these conditions, thyrotoxicosis should be considered, especially if exophthalmos, thyroid enlargement, and atrial fibrillation are present.
- The face tells the story of the patient's acute distress, caused by life-threatening conditions and heralded by severe chest pain, severe acute shortness of breath, orthopnea, and clouding of consciousness; e.g., the patient with sustained ventricular tachycardia (VT) commonly has a malignant tachycardia of >30 seconds' duration that is often accompanied by distress signals, i.e., shortness of breath, chest pain, or loss of consciousness.

The examination usually consists of **inspection, palpation, percussion,** and **auscultation.** Inspection must not be overlooked because important information can be derived from observation at the patient's bedside.

Head movement may show
1. **Head bobbing,** coincident with each heartbeat, which is caused by the ballistic forces of severe aortic regurgitation (de Musset's sign).

Cheeks may reflect
1. **A malar flush,** which is rosy malar prominences consisting of dilated venules in the peripherally cyanosed skin of pa-

tients with long-standing mitral stenosis. A rash across the nose and cheek may be a manifestation of systemic lupus erythematosus (SLE).

Skin color and texture may reveal

1. **Pigmentation,** indicating
   - Ethnic origin
   - Exposure to sunlight
   - Brown creases, including buccal pigmentation in Addison's disease, a cause of postural hypotension
   - Muddy bronze of hemochromatosis, a cause of heart muscle disease
   - Brick red color of polycythemia, which may cause hypertension, vascular thromboses, and myocardial infarction
   - Café au lait spots, which may indicate endocarditis
2. **Neurofibromas,** which may be associated with pheochromocytoma, pulmonary neurofibromas, emphysema, and scoliosis
3. **Coarseness and dryness** (associated with a husky voice and "hung-up" ankle jerks) in patients with myxedema, which is a cause of bradycardia, cardiac failure (rarely), pericardial effusion, and cardiac tamponade
4. **Hidebound skin,** i.e., shiny, thick, leathery, and tightly bound to the underlying tissue of the nose and forehead in scleroderma, which may cause accelerated systemic hypertension, pulmonary hypertension, heart muscle disease, and renal failure
5. **Flushing,** a chronic cyanotic hue and telangiectasia in the carcinoid syndrome, which may cause tricuspid and pulmonary stenosis
6. **Spider angiomas** (nevi), seen in patients with cirrhosis; some patients with cirrhosis may exhibit a long QT interval associated with sudden cardiac death; spider nevi are also seen with thyrotoxicosis and in pregnancy
7. **Fat distribution** characteristic of moon facies, which occurs in Cushing's disease or syndrome and is a cause of hypertension

Eyes and lids require careful scrutiny.

1. **Lids** may reveal
   - Xanthelasmas, which are yellowish plaques of cholesterol deposits seen in patients with hypercholesterolemia but also in patients with diabetes
   - Edema of the lids, which should provoke a differential diagnosis that includes the nephrotic syndrome, angioneurotic edema, allergies, myxedema, and superior vena cava syndrome
   - Ptosis (drooping eyelids), possibly indicating Horner's syndrome, myxedema, familial occurrence, Noonan's syndrome, myasthenia gravis, or neurosyphilis

- Lid retraction, which produces the typical stare of thyrotoxicosis
- Cutis laxa or looseness of the skin, which causes pendulous eyelids due to elastic tissue defects and which may be associated with aortic dissection and pulmonary artery dilatation

2. **Conjunctivae** may be hyperemic, indicating an inflammatory or an allergic response; may have purulent exudate, typical of conjunctivitis; may have pallor, indicating anemia; may be brick red, indicating polycythemia; or may have petechial hemorrhages with white centers, indicating endocarditis.

3. **Corneas** may show corneal arcus, also called arcus senilis, a light gray ring around the iris. When seen in whites younger than 50 years, an arcus indicates severe hyperlipidemia and premature coronary heart disease. The abnormal arcus begins inferiorly and leaves a rim of iris peripherally. In patients older than age 60, an arcus is a normal finding; the normal ring usually begins superiorly and extends to the rim of the iris. It may occur as a normal finding in blacks younger than age 60. The cornea may be clouded in Hurler's syndrome.

4. **Sclerae** may be yellow, indicating jaundice, which may occur with gallbladder disease, cirrhosis, cardiac cirrhosis, or severe tricuspid regurgitation. Blue sclerae may be seen with Marfan syndrome, osteogenesis imperfecta, and Ehlers-Danlos syndrome, which may manifest cardiac complications including aortic dissection, aortic regurgitation, and mitral valve prolapse. Osteogenesis imperfecta may have the above cardiac complications and atrial septal defect (ASD), or tetralogy of Fallot.

5. **Irises** may indicate tremulous iris, which is typical of dislocation of the lens, seen in Marfan syndrome. A circle of gray-white pigmented dots around the outer circumference occurs in Down syndrome.

6. **Lenses** may indicate subluxation in patients with Marfan syndrome and homocystinuria; premature cataracts may occur with myotonic dystrophy, which may be complicated by intraventricular conduction defects and complete heart block.

   Other causes of premature cataracts include Werner's syndrome, which may cause premature graying and coronary heart disease. Rubella syndrome is associated with patent ductus arteriosus, ASD, and pulmonary stenosis. Refsum's disease, hypocalcemia, galactosemia, and chronic corticosteroid use may also cause premature cataracts.

7. **Globes** of the eyes may exhibit exophthalmos and thyroid

stare in patients with thyrotoxicosis, who may manifest tachycardia, atrial fibrillation, and heart failure.

8. **Pupils** that react to accommodation and not to light are typical of the Argyll Robertson pupils of neurosyphilis; cardiovascular involvement includes aortic regurgitation and aortic disease with its typical linear calcification of the ascending aorta, visible on the chest radiograph.

Bony developmental abnormalities require careful scrutiny.

1. **A large head** may be seen in patients with Paget's disease, in which the presence of arteriovenous (AV) fistulas may cause congestive heart failure (CHF); also, calcification of the aortic valve produces the aortic systolic murmur of aortic sclerosis, and calcification of the conduction tissue may result in bradycardia and complete heart block.

2. **Acromegaly** with its typical lantern jaw may be complicated by hypertension and CHF.

3. **Chromosomal** anomalies or congenital disorders that may manifest cardiovascular derangements include
   - Down syndrome, which is associated with ASD or ventricular septal defect (VSD)
   - Hurler's gargoylism, which is associated with mitral regurgitation and arrhythmias
   - Noonan's syndrome, including hypertelorism (widely set eyes) and ptosis, which is associated with pulmonary stenosis
   - Marfan syndrome, which is characterized by a long, narrow face, tremulous iris with aortic regurgitation, aneurysms, aortic dissection, and mitral valve prolapse; also may manifest arachnodactyly, in which the thumbs protrude from the clenched fists (Fig. 3–1)
   - Williams syndrome, which is characterized by a small, elf-like forehead, turned-up nose, egg-shaped teeth, and low-set ears, and is associated with supravalvular aortic stenosis

■ CYANOSIS

This important sign is somewhat ignored because of emphasis on sophisticated instrumentation and high-tech investigations.

Cyanosis is a bluish discoloration of the mucous membranes and skin caused by a decreased amount of hemoglobin and blood flowing through these regions. Cyanosis is not apparent if the blood hemoglobin is <5 g/L. Therefore, cyanosis may not be apparent in severely anemic patients. In patients with congenital heart disease, cyanosis is usually observed when a right-to-left shunt is >25% of left ventricular output. In this situation, cyanosis becomes worse during exercise, because right-to-left shunting

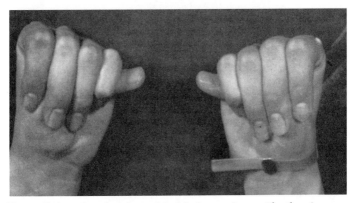

Figure 3–1 □ The "thumb sign" in Marfan syndrome. The thumbs protrude from the clenched fists of a 24-year-old man who presented with congestive heart failure due to severe chronic aortic regurgitation and left ventricular dysfunction. Arachnodactyly ("spider finger") and loose joints account for the ability to position the fingers in this way. The patient also had other skeletal features of Marfan syndrome, including pectus excavatum and a high-arched palate. (From Falk RH: Images in clinical medicine: The "thumb sign" in Marfan's syndrome. N Engl J Med 1995;333:430. Copyright © 1995 Massachusetts Medical Society. All rights reserved.)

is increased. Cyanosis caused by right-to-left shunts is not improved by inhalation of 100% oxygen.

Cyanosis commencing in infancy suggests a right-to-left shunt, but hereditary methemoglobinemia must be excluded. In patients with congenital heart disease, cyanosis developing between ages 5 and 20 years suggests the development of significant pulmonary arterial hypertension with reversal of the shunt, which is referred to as Eisenmenger's syndrome.

Observe and examine the tongue, lips, ear lobe, fingers, and toes in good light to ascertain the presence of the four types of cyanosis.

Central Cyanosis. When the oxygen content of arterial blood is low, usually <55 mm Hg, because of poor oxygenation in the lungs or congenital right-to-left shunts, the desaturated blood imparts a bluish tinge to the tongue and lips. The presence of central cyanosis therefore indicates a serious lack of arterial blood oxygen. In some patients cyanosis may not be detected until the partial pressure of oxygen (PO_2) is <45 mm Hg, a desperate situation, at which point the patient's life is being threatened. Because the entire blood supply is desaturated, the toes and fingers also appear blue; this feature does not imply that peripheral cyanosis is present. When the peripheries are blue, you should determine whether they are warm or cold. The peripheries

Table 3–1 □ CAUSES OF CYANOSIS

Causes	Comments
Left ventricular failure/ congestive heart failure	Peripheral cyanosis (always); central cyanosis (sometimes), with severe pulmonary edema
Superior vena cava obstruction	Peripheral cyanosis
Peripheral cutaneous vasoconstriction	Peripheral cyanosis induced by cold
Congenital cyanotic heart disease	Central cyanosis
Lung diseases, e.g., chronic bronchitis, emphysema, pneumonia, adult respiratory distress syndrome	Central cyanosis

will be warm in the presence of central cyanosis and become cold if peripheral cyanosis supervenes. The causes of cyanosis are given in Table 3–1.

Blue tongue, lips, mucous membranes, and extremities with warm peripheries indicates central cyanosis.

Peripheral Cyanosis.   Peripheral cyanosis results from a sluggish circulation in the peripheries, which allows a marked reduction in oxygenated hemoglobin to occur in the capillaries. This sluggish circulation causes the extremities to become cold, and they appear blue. Because the oxygen of the blood in the lungs is normal, the tongue is not blue. The most common cause of peripheral cyanosis is exposure to cold. Severe heart failure causes a low cardiac output and diminished circulation time and commonly causes peripheral cyanosis. Heart failure may add central cyanosis when severe pulmonary edema results in decreased arterial oxygenation in the lungs. Patients in the latter situation are often moribund. Cor pulmonale causes central cyanosis, but if severe heart failure occurs the peripheries become cold. The combination of central cyanosis and peripheral cyanosis thus carries a poor prognosis.

Differential Cyanosis.   Differential cyanosis nearly always indicates congenital heart disease that involves coarctation of the aorta and a patent ductus arteriosus in conjunction with another lesion. Usually, the lower limbs are cyanosed and the upper limbs appear pink. The feet are more cyanosed than the right hand, which may not show cyanosis. The situation is seen with patent ductus arteriosus with reversal of the left-to-right shunt; deoxygenated blood flows from the pulmonary artery through the ductus into the aorta distal to the region of the carotid and subclavian arteries. Because the left subclavian artery originates close to the ductus, some deoxygenated blood can enter the subclavian artery, resulting in mild cyanosis of the left hand.

Reversed Differential Cyanosis. Reversed differential cyanosis may be caused by transposition of the great vessels with coarctation of the aorta. Blood from the right ventricle ejected into the aorta reaches the head and upper limbs but cannot reach the lower limbs. Blood from the left ventricle ejected into the pulmonary artery flows through a patent ductus arteriosus to the descending aorta and reaches the legs, which are therefore less cyanotic.

■ BREATHING PATTERNS

Observe whether the patient is short of breath when lying flat, i.e., whether the patient is orthopneic or dyspneic on mild activities.

1. Is the patient using accessory muscles of respiration, i.e., the sternomastoids, the trapezius? This situation is seen with chronic obstructive pulmonary disease (COPD), asthma, severe pulmonary edema, and fulminant pneumonias.
2. Is the patient's breathlessness associated with audible wheezing, as may occur with asthma, COPD, or left ventricular (LV) failure?
3. Is stridor present, indicating upper airway obstruction and a life-threatening situation that requires immediate relief of the obstruction?
4. Is Cheyne-Stokes respiration present? In this condition, the patient is observed to stop breathing for a few seconds, the retention of carbon dioxide stimulates hyperventilation, and then when carbon dioxide is blown off, the respiratory drive decreases and there is cessation of breathing, apnea follows, and the pattern is repeated. Cheyne-Stokes respiration is observed occasionally during normal sleep in elderly people, after strokes, with CHF, with uremia, or with oversedation.

■ VITAL SIGNS

Assess the pulse rate, blood pressure, and respiratory rate. The normal respiratory rate is 12 to 20 breaths/min at rest, but individuals display normal variation outside these limits. A respiratory rate of >30 breaths/min is an ominous sign. If this is associated with a heart rate of >120 beats/min, check for pulsus paradoxus, which may be present in patients with life-threatening pericardial tamponade or asthma. If the high respiratory rate is associated with pyrexia, chills, and flared nostrils, assess for pneumonia. See the discussion under Pulse.

■ HANDS

1. **Tremor.** Ask the patient to stretch both arms and hands forward horizontally at shoulder level, and then observe for tremor. A fine tremor in the presence of warm hands may indicate thyrotoxicosis. (Tremor of anxiety is associated with cold, sweaty palms.)
2. **Clubbing** of the fingers. Look for obliteration of the normal lunular angle between the base of the nail and the proximal skin. Normally, there is a depression between the skin and the base of the nail producing approximately a 140-degree angle between the nail and cuticle. With true clubbing, this angle is lost; the skin and nail base form a straight line, because there is lifting of the root of the nail off its bed associated with thickening of the tissues at the base of the nail. Document the loss of nail angle and feel the loose end of the nail root (Fig. 3–2). Place the tip of your index finger or thumbnail on the nail that appears clubbed, and press the root of the patient's nail. Check for fluctuation or rocking of the nail bed. The floating nail bed feels fluctuant as you depress the root of the patient's nail. Note that your thumbnail should point in the same direction as the patient's nail. Other less reliable signs of clubbing are beaking of the nail

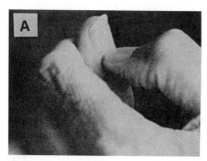
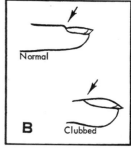

Figure 3–2 □ *A,* Method of testing for early clubbing. The examiner's thumbnail presses at the root of the patient's nail to detect elevation above the nail bed. *B,* Profiles of a normal and a clubbed finger and nail; note the lunular angle *(top arrow)* in normal, and loss of the lunular angle *(bottom arrow)* in the clubbed digit with increased curvature of the nail and increased anteroposterior diameter of the finger pad. (From Marriott HJL: Bedside Cardiology Diagnosis. Philadelphia, JB Lippincott Co., 1993, p 39.)

Table 3–2 □ CAUSES OF FINGER CLUBBING

Pulmonary
    Chronic suppurative lung disease, e.g., bronchiectasis, lung
        abscess, empyema, and cystic fibrosis
    Carcinoma of the lung
    Interstitial pulmonary fibrosis
    Pulmonary arteriovenous fistula
Cardiac
    Bacterial endocarditis
    Congenital cyanotic heart disease
Hepatic
    Cirrhosis
Gastrointestinal
    Celiac disease (tropical sprue)
    Crohn's disease
    Ulcerative colitis
Familial

and the terminal phalanx's appearing bulbous, like the end of a drumstick.

Causes of clubbing are given in Table 3–2. Clubbing takes more than 4 weeks to develop; therefore, it is seen in patients with subacute bacterial endocarditis and not in patients with the acute variety. Clubbing disappears about 6 weeks after cure of the underlying disease. In some patients the fingers may be normal but the toes are clubbed and cyanotic because of a reversed shunt through a patent ductus arteriosus, or there may be unilateral clubbing in association with differential cyanosis.

3. **Koilonychia,** or spoon-shaped nails. The normal convexity of the nail is replaced by concavity. This occurs with iron deficiency anemia and with Plummer-Vinson syndrome (iron deficiency, dysphagia, and esophageal web).

4. **Capillary pulsation** (Quincke's sign). A slight pressure on the nail beds reveals intermittent flushing in patients with a large pulse pressure or quick runoff from the arterial tree, which can be caused by aortic regurgitation or by vasodilation resulting from fevers, hot weather, thyrotoxicosis, pregnancy, and vasodilators.

5. **Splinter hemorrhages.** Hemorrhages under the base of the nails may be observed in a patient with bacterial endocarditis. Trauma or dwelling at high altitudes commonly causes splinter hemorrhages. It is advisable to count the number of hemorrhages; an increase in number over days of observation is an important clue to endocarditis. Other causes of splinter hemorrhages include acute glomerulonephritis and blood dyscrasia.

6. **Osler's nodes.** These nodes are 0.5- to 1-cm, reddish-brown subcutaneous papules that occur on the tips of the fingers or toes, along the palms of the hand, or on the plantar surface of the feet. They are painful and tender. These microemboli are observed in patients with bacterial endocarditis, and they disappear after 2 to 5 days. They may occur during a course of adequate therapy.

7. **Arachnodactyly.** Long, slender hands and fingers or "spider fingers" may be observed in Marfan syndrome. When the patient encircles the wrist with the thumb and the small finger using very light pressure, the thumb overlaps by at least 1 cm in most patients with Marfan syndrome because of a long thumb and lax joints (wrist sign). In patients with Marfan syndrome, when the fist is made over a clenched thumb, the thumb protrudes beyond the ulnar side of the hand (see Fig. 3–1). This may occur normally in 3% of children.

8. **Firm, taut, hidebound skin** proximal to the metacarpophalangeal (MCP) joints. This is the diagnostic criterion for systemic sclerosis (scleroderma). An experienced physician's touch is as diagnostically sensitive as a skin biopsy. Vascular obliteration in the skin occurs in concert with changes in small arteries and microvessels of the heart, kidneys, gastrointestinal tract, lungs, and connective tissue. If hidebound skin is confined to the fingers distal to the MCP joints, the condition is called sclerodactyly and is not diagnostic of systemic sclerosis. Raynaud's phenomenon is a common occurrence with scleroderma.

9. **Xanthomas.** These may be observed on the extensor tendons (xanthoma tendinosum) or palms (xanthoma planum); if these are present, assess the tuberosities for xanthoma tuberosum. These are features of familial hyperlipidemia.

■ PULSE

Determine the
1. Rate
2. Rhythm
3. Character
4. Symmetry

Feel both radial pulses and determine if the pulse is absent or much weaker on one side.

Examine the radial and carotid pulses. The other pulses, i.e., femoral, posterior tibial, and dorsalis pedis, are more conveniently palpated when completing the examination of the lower extremities after examining the neck veins and chest. Proceed from the face to the hands, the pulse, then the neck for jugular venous waves and jugular venous pressure (JVP), and then examine the chest (heart and lungs).

The pulse wave is a pressure wave that is propagated both forward and laterally by the incompressible blood by the propulsive force generated down the arterial system from the aortic root. It is the lateral, pulsatile movement that distends the elastic arterial walls and gives rise to the pulse wave.

Radial Pulse

This is the most convenient pulse to palpate and should be done before examining the carotid arteries. Although the carotid pulse gives the best indication of the arterial waveform, it is better not to palpate the patient's carotid arteries first, because patients feel uncomfortable during carotid palpation. It is best to start with palpating the radial pulse, which is always accessible, even when the patient is partly dressed.

Rate. Time the rate over 1 minute. When a rapid assessment is necessary, determine the rate over 15 seconds, multiply by 4, and record the number of beats per minute. Causes of sinus tachycardia are given in Table 3–3. The heart rate with sinus tachycardia occurring at rest commonly ranges from 100 to 140 beats/min. A resting heart rate of ≥140 beats/min is commonly caused by arrhythmias. Causes of sinus bradycardia, a heart rate of <60 beats/min, are shown in Table 3–4.

Table 3–3 □ CAUSES OF SINUS TACHYCARDIA

Exercise
Infancy and early childhood (normal)
Anxiety and reaction to stress, trauma, or surgery
Infections
Thyrotoxicosis
Hemorrhage
Acute fall in vascular volume due to hemorrhage, dehydration, burns
Acute myocardial infarction or ischemia
Pulmonary embolism
Congestive heart failure
Hypoxemia
Anemia
Drugs that directly or indirectly stimulate the sinus node
   Catecholamines (including cough and cold remedies)
   Beta agonists, e.g., albuterol (salbutamol), isoproterenol,
      dobutamine, and dopamine
   Atropine
   Nicotine
   Caffeine

Table 3–4 □ CAUSES OF SINUS BRADYCARDIA

↑ vagal or ↓ sympathetic tone
  Normal in well-trained athletes
  Normal during sleep, i.e., may fall to 40–50 beats/min
Hypothyroidism
Inferior myocardial infarction
↑ intracranial pressure
Hypothermia
Convalescence from influenza or typhoid fever
Drugs
  Beta blockers (including eye drops)
  Some calcium antagonists (verapamil and diltiazem)
  Amiodarone
  Lithium
  Reserpine
  Clonidine
  Propafenone
Sinus node disease

Rhythm. Determine whether the rhythm is regular or irregular. An irregular pulse has two varieties. In the first variety, the irregularity has a recurring pattern or has an otherwise regular rhythm but at times is interrupted by slight irregularities. The pulse in these settings is described as "regularly irregular," and this condition is commonly caused by premature atrial or ventricular beats or extrasystoles.

In the second variety of irregular pulse, the rhythm is found to be completely irregular ("irregularly irregular" rhythm) and is typical of atrial fibrillation; a rare cause is multifocal atrial tachycardia. In atrial fibrillation, the atrial rate is faster than 300 beats/min and the ventricular rate varies from 60 to 200 beats/min. In the presence of fast heart rates, the diastolic interval is short and may not allow sufficient time for ventricular filling. During systole there may be insufficient stroke volume to cause opening of the aortic valve, resulting in no pulse wave, and thus the ventricular response may be 150 beats/min, but the radial or carotid pulse rate may be 100 to 130 beats/min. With atrial fibrillation, the heart rate cannot be determined by assessing the radial or carotid pulse; auscultation at the apex of the heart is necessary. The apical rate minus the pulse rate equals the pulse deficit.

Character. Considerable data can be obtained from careful palpation of the pulse. The study of the carotid pulse, especially its waveform, is more accurate than that determined at the wrist. As mentioned earlier, palpation of the carotid is always uncomfortable for patients, and it is wise to assess the radial arteries first. Important information can be obtained by examination of the radial arteries before palpating the carotids. Assess the radial arteries for the presence of a collapsing, bounding pulse.

1. **Collapsing pulse.** Grasp the wrist firmly in the palm of the right hand. Lift the outstretched hand vertically toward the ceiling (Fig. 3–3); the normal pulse nearly completely disappears. In patients with a high pulse pressure, a bounding pulse, or hyperkinetic circulation, the pulse wave is felt as a prominent, slapping sensation against the firmly pressed palm or finger pads. This type of pulse, in which the wave disappears and then kicks in vigorously, has been termed collapsing, bounding, water-hammer, or Corrigan's pulse. Feel and confirm this rapid upstroke of the pulse wave and its disappearance by palpating the carotid artery in the neck. The underlying mechanism is a rapid rise in upstroke, followed by an abrupt collapse due to a quick runoff from the arterial tree during diastole. Conditions that cause a brisk runoff from the arterial tree and produce a collapsing pulse are given in Table 3–5. The blood pressure in these patients shows a large difference (pulse pressure) between systolic and diastolic, e.g., 150/50, and the dorsalis pedis pulse is bounding.

2. **Plateau pulse.** In this situation, the pulse wave is found to rise slowly. Occasionally, it is slow-rising with a notch; it is then termed an "anacrotic pulse."

Brachial Pulse

Palpate the right brachial arterial pulse with the thumb (Fig. 3–4).

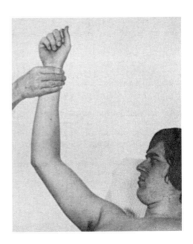

Figure 3–3 □ Method for palpation of Corrigan's (collapsing) pulse in the radial artery. (From Boucher ID, Morris J: Clinical Skills: A System of Clinical Examination, 2nd ed. London, WB Saunders Co., 1982, p 62.)

Table 3–5 □ CAUSES OF A COLLAPSING PULSE

Aortic regurgitation
Patent ductus arteriosus
Ruptured sinus of Valsalva
Arteriovenous fistulas
  Pregnancy
  Paget's disease of bone
High-output states with arterial vasodilatation
  Thyrotoxicosis
  Anemias
  Fevers
Vasodilator drugs

Carotid Pulse

Another method using the thumb to palpate is shown in Figure 3–4. Feel for the carotid artery by using the first two fingers applied to the groove just medial to the medial edge of the sternomastoid muscle and just lateral to the thyroid cartilage. With practice, the normal or abnormal arterial pulse wave is easily appreciated on palpation of the carotid artery. Findings are not accurate in the elderly because of a loss of elasticity, and abnormal waveforms are misleading and provide inaccurate data.

Abnormal rates of rise and fall of the pressure wave and notches may be detected after considerable practice. Severe aortic stenosis reduces ventricular ejection and stroke volume, resulting in a slow-rising pulse wave; this is appreciated as a plateau or a notch (anacrotic) before a delayed peak. A plateau or anacrotic pulse in patients younger than 70 years usually indicates significant aortic stenosis. A thrill may be imparted to the finger palpating the carotid artery in patients with aortic stenosis.

Jugular Venous Pulse Wave

A considerable amount of very important data concerning the hemodynamics of the right and left sides of the heart can be gleaned by examination of the jugular venous waves in the neck. The internal jugular vein, not the external, is used to assess the venous waves. The internal jugular vein is not usually visible because it is covered by the sternocleidomastoid muscle. Pulsations of the internal jugular vein transmitted to the skin overlying the sternomastoid muscle are easily visible if the patient is properly positioned and tangential light and shadow effects are used in observing the pulsations. Pulsations are usually visible at the root of the neck just lateral to the clavicular insertion of the sternocleidomastoid muscle.

Restrictive clothing should be removed and the patient should

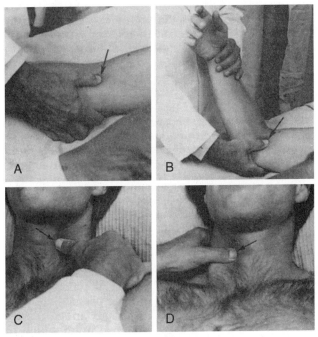

Figure 3-4 □ *A,* Palpation of the right brachial pulse with the thumb *(arrow)* while the patient's arm lies at the side with the palm up. *B,* Palpation of the right brachial pulse with the patient's elbow resting in the palm of the examiner's hand. The thumb explores the antecubital fossa *(arrow),* while the patient's forearm is passively raised and lowered to achieve maximum relaxation of muscles around the elbow. *C* and *D,* Palpation of the carotid pulse. The examiner places the right thumb *(arrow)* on the patient's left carotid artery *(C).* The left thumb *(arrow)* is then applied separately to the right carotid *(D).* (From Perloff JK: Physical Examination of the Heart and Circulation. Philadelphia, WB Saunders Co., 1990.)

lie comfortably, preferably with the legs slightly elevated. Start with the patient propped up comfortably at approximately a 15-degree angle to the horizontal with the head resting on a pillow. Keep the head, neck, and trunk in line. The neck must not be flexed or extended at a sharp angle from the trunk. If the sternomastoid muscles are taut, they prevent the transmission of venous pulsations. In some patients, pulsations may not be seen because the angle of inclination may be inappropriate. It may be necessary to put the patient at a near 90-degree inclination. In a patient with severe CHF, the internal jugular veins may be quite distended, and pulsations may not be visible because the upper level of pulsations is above the angle of the jaw; the very high pressure may cause the ear lobes to pulsate. It may be necessary to lower the patient to 30 degrees to observe pulsations at the root of the neck. In a patient with a low venous pressure, venous waves may not be visible until the patient is placed in the supine position with the legs elevated to increase venous return.

Keep the patient's head in the midline. Daylight or artificial light can be used to verify the pulsations. Look at the patient from the front rather than from one side. Pulsations will usually be seen at the root of the neck. Use the collar of the patient's shirt or pajamas, the chin, or the sternomastoid muscle to cast a shadow. The edge of the shadow moves with the pulsations. As an alternative, stand on the right side, lean over the left side of the patient's torso, and view the outline of the neck against the patient's pillow. Venous pulsations must be analyzed in relation to the events of the cardiac cycle (Figs. 3–5 and 3–6).

Genesis of the Venous Waves

Observation of the internal jugular pulsation should reveal two waves (A and V). Normally, these waves are of very low amplitude and only the A wave may be visible. The A wave is produced by right atrial contraction, which begins near the peak of the P wave of the electrocardiogram (see Figs. 3–5 and 3–6). The

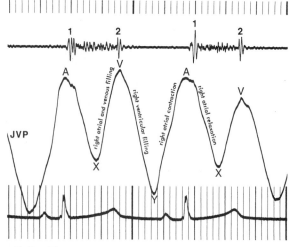

Figure 3–5 □ The two positive (A, V) and two negative (X, Y) waves in the jugular venous pulse (JVP) illustrating their relationship to the heart sounds and the electrocardiogram. 1 = first heart sound; 2 = second sound; A, X, V, Y = venous waves. (From Marriott HJL: Bedside Cardiology Diagnosis. Philadelphia, JB Lippincott Co., 1993, p 17.)

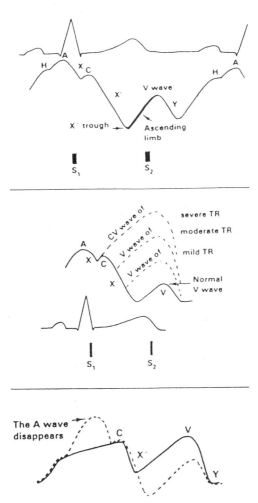

Figure 3–6 □ *Top,* Normal jugular venous pulse. The jugular V wave is built up during systole, and its height reflects the rate of filling and the elasticity of the right atrium. Between the bottom of the Y descent (Y trough) and the beginning of the A wave is the period of relatively slow filling of the "atrioventricle" or diastasis period. The wave built up during diastasis is the H wave. The H wave height also reflects the stiffness of the right atrium. S_1 and S_2 refer to the first and second heart sounds, respectively. *Center,* As the degree of tricuspid regurgitation (TR) increases, the X' descent is increasingly encroached on. With severe TR, no X' descent is seen, and the jugular pulse wave is said to be "ventricularized." *Bottom,* Effect of development of atrial fibrillation on the jugular venous pulse. The dominant descent in atrial fibrillation is almost always the y descent, i.e., it has the superficial appearance of the pulse wave of TR. (From Constant J: Bedside Cardiology, 3rd ed. Boston, Little, Brown & Co., 1995, pp 95, 105, and 108.)

A wave precedes ventricular systole and thus the first heart sound and carotid pulsation.

Because the abnormal A wave is a flicking wave that occurs appreciably earlier than the carotid (C) arterial pulse, the observer can say "AC" to time the A wave. In a similar manner, saying "CV" without a pause times the V wave.

Atrial relaxation or diastole produces the X descent just before ventricular contraction. The venous pulse wave then collapses rapidly during early right ventricular contraction, because the floor of the atrium at the base of the ventricle descends toward the apex, causing a fall in atrial pressure. This systolic collapse of the venous pulse is the deepest, most rapid collapsing movement that is visible on inspection of the neck veins.

During ventricular systole, the V wave of the venous pulse rises and blood continues to fill the right atrium against a closed tricuspid valve. Normally, the V wave is small and may be invisible to the observer, because the right atrium is distensible and does not allow its pressure to rise significantly when the tricuspid valve is closed. It is thus easy to visualize how severe tricuspid regurgitation causes a large regurgitant V wave.

When the tricuspid valve opens, there is a sudden, rapid inflow of blood into the right ventricle and thus a reduction in intra-atrial pressure, which causes the descending limb (Y descent) of the V wave (see Figs. 3–5 and 3–6).

Venous Versus Carotid Pulsation

Press a pencil or finger firmly across the root of the neck, about 1 cm above the right clavicle; venous pulsations will disappear, but carotid pulsations will remain.

1. Deep inspiration will usually decrease the upper limit of venous pulsations except in patients with constrictive pericarditis.
2. Sitting upright will decrease the upper limit of jugular venous pulsation.
3. The carotid pulse is easily palpable as a thrust, whereas venous pulsations cannot be palpated.
4. The carotid pulse is a single abrupt pulsation seen halfway up the neck, whereas venous pulsations are best seen at the root of the neck or over a 1- to 5-cm area when the venous pressure is high, and especially when CHF and tricuspid regurgitation cause prominent V waves.

Abnormalities of Venous Waves

1. **Giant A waves.** Giant A waves occur when right atrial workload is increased, e.g., when there is
   - Right atrial contraction against an obstructed tricuspid valve, in particular, stenosis, atresia, or myxoma
   - Increased atrial contraction in conditions in which the

resistance to right atrial emptying is increased, such as right ventricular hypertrophy, pulmonary stenosis, pulmonary arterial hypertension caused by recurrent pulmonary embolism, ASD, VSD, and Eisenmenger's syndrome
- Left ventricular hypertrophy, because a thickened septum interferes with right ventricular filling

2. **Cannon A waves.** If the atrium contracts against a closed tricuspid valve, as may occur in patients with AV dissociation, a huge A wave may be observed. In patients with complete heart block, the atrium may contract at 72 beats/min, and the ventricle at 28 beats/min; at some time, the atrium contracts against a closed tricuspid valve. It may be necessary to observe the neck pulsations for >2 minutes to observe a cannon wave in patients with complete heart block. Isolated cannon A waves are sometimes seen with atrial, ventricular, and junctional beats.

3. **Prominent V waves.** Prominent V waves are observed when there is
- Tricuspid regurgitation, which may cause movement of the ear lobes during systole; the V wave is visibly prominent because of a rapid Y descent consequent on the rapid fall of the very high atrial pressure
- ASD, causing right atrial diastolic overloading

4. **Rapid Y descent.** A rapid Y descent is seen in patients with very high atrial pressures and a normal tricuspid valve opening. This may be observed with severe right ventricular failure and is a typical feature of constrictive pericarditis, but pericardial tamponade does not cause a rapid Y descent.

5. **Absent Y descent.** In cardiac tamponade, the high atrial pressure cannot fill the ventricle, because the major restriction in movement occurs during diastole; thus, the Y descent is markedly attenuated and virtually invisible. A very high venous pressure with the presence of large V waves and Y descent is a valuable sign, because it signifies severe CHF and helps to exclude cardiac tamponade.

6. **Absent venous pulsation.** If the JVP is very high with absent pulsations and there is no change in the upper level of venous pressure with a change of posture, consider superior vena cava obstruction.

7. **Venous waves and arrhythmias.**
- The A wave is absent in patients with atrial fibrillation, because there is no atrial contraction, but in atrial flutter, multiple small A waves may be visible.
- Irregular, intermittently occurring cannon A waves occur with complete heart block or with ectopic beats, if contractions of the atrium occur against a closed tricuspid valve.

Jugular Venous Pressure

Because there are no valves between the right atrium, the superior vena cava, and the internal jugular vein, the internal jugular vein is more accurate than the external jugular for determination of JVP and observation of waveform. The patient's trunk is usually placed at an inclination of 45 degrees, with the head and trunk in a straight line without flexion of the neck. **At a 45-degree inclination, pulsations are not usually visible at the root of the neck if right atrial pressure is normal.** Venous pulsations just visible at the root of the neck, i.e., ≤2 cm above the sternal angle of Louis, indicate that the JVP is normal. Any filling or pulsations seen in the neck above this level, with the patient at a 45-degree inclination, indicate an elevated JVP. **It is thus convenient to start the examination for venous pressure measurement with the patient propped up at a 45-degree angle. It must be understood that the venous pressure would be the same regardless of the inclination of the patient.** Assessment of the venous waveform, however, requires the patient to be placed at a level of inclination at which pulsations are best seen (see earlier discussion).

The venous pressure, expressed as centimeters of blood, is measured as the vertical distance between a horizontal plane passing through the sternal angle of Louis (the junction of the manubrium and the sternum) and another horizontal plane drawn through the highest point of visible internal jugular venous pulsation, with the patient at any angle of inclination. The above stipulation can be made because the distance between the mid right atrium and the sternal angle of Louis is approximately the same regardless of the patient's position. If no venous pulsations are visible with the patient at a 45-degree angle, lowering the patient to 15 to 30 degrees usually causes the pulsations to become visible. The absence of pulsations may indicate a low venous pressure caused by hypovolemia. When the venous pressure is very high, as outlined earlier, the neck veins may be engorged and pulsations may not be found until the patient sits upright; the upper level of pulsations may then be observed at the angle of the jaw, or the ear lobes may be observed to pulsate. In this situation, the venous pressure is usually >10 cm.

The JVP normally falls slightly during inspiration. In patients with COPD, the venous pressure rises during expiration and falls during inspiration. The determination should be recorded during inspiration. Table 3–6 gives the causes of increased JVP.

Hepatojugular Reflux.   With the patient at a 45-degree inclination, the palm of the hand is placed on the abdomen, and gentle but sustained pressure is maintained for about 30 seconds with the patient breathing quietly. During this period, in normal individuals, the upper level of venous pulsation in the neck is not

Table 3–6 □ CAUSES OF INCREASED JUGULAR VENOUS PRESSURE

Congestive heart failure
Constrictive pericarditis
Cardiac tamponade
Superior vena cava obstruction
Tricuspid stenosis, atrial myxoma
Increase in intrathoracic pressure due to pleural effusion, chronic obstructive pulmonary disease, or Valsalva's maneuver; normal in singers and trumpet players
Increase in intra-abdominal pressure due to ascites, obesity, pregnancy, and straining
Blood volume overload due to pregnancy and excessive intravenous infusion

altered significantly. If a small rise in pressure occurs, it returns quickly to the baseline during inspiration when abdominal compression is continued. In patients with CHF, the top-level pulsation increases considerably in height. The test may give erroneous information in patients with COPD because a marked increase in intrathoracic pressure occurs. Note that it is not necessary to press on the liver; some physicians therefore call the test abdomino-jugular reflux. Hepatojugular reflux has been the term used for >100 years and is still used by most physicians.

■ INSPECTION

Although inspection and palpation of the chest are commonly done as one maneuver, inspection must not be hurried by the desire to palpate. Observation of the chest, with the physician standing at the foot and then at the side of the examining table or bed, is a necessary component of the cardiac examination. It is advisable to look across the chest tangentially while standing at the bedside and to look across the chest from above the patient's head. A light beam directed across the precordium may enhance subtle findings. Observation may reveal abnormal physical signs not detectable on palpation and auscultation or by radiologic and electrocardiographic (ECG) evaluation.

Respirations. Observe for the frequency, regularity, and depth; assess for difficulties, e.g., orthopnea (see Chapter 3).

Venous Dilatation. Veins on the anterior chest wall may be dilated and tortuous; caudal flow indicates obstruction of the superior vena cava; cranial flow suggests obstruction of the inferior vena cava.

Thoracic Cage Deformities

1. Pectus excavatum. The lower sternum may be depressed posteriorly; a left sternal, midsystolic murmur and prominence of the pulmonary artery may occur. The deformity is associated with Marfan syndrome, mitral valve prolapse (MVP), Ehlers-Danlos syndrome, Hunter-Hurler syndrome, Noonan's syndrome, and homocystinuria.
2. Pectus carinatum. Pectus carinatum (pigeon chest) may occur in some patients with Marfan syndrome.
3. Straight back syndrome. Straight back syndrome caused by loss of normal thoracic kyphosis may be associated with MVP or a bicuspid aortic valve. Expiratory splitting of the second heart sound (S_2) and a left parasternal, midsystolic murmur and enlargement of the pulmonary artery on chest x-ray may mimic an atrial septal defect (ASD).

Abnormal Pulsations. Observe for pulsations in the following regions:

1. **Cardiac apex.** A 2-cm, thrusting impulse may indicate left ventricular enlargement. A "double apical impulse" may be

seen when the left ventricle is abnormally stiff and left atrial contractions become forceful; the low-frequency vibrations of an S_4 gallop may be better appreciated on inspection and palpation than on auscultation. A double apical impulse requires augmented left atrial contraction, and thus sinus rhythm must be present. A third heart sound gallop may be visible. A triple rhythm and other pulsations may be enhanced by attaching a wand to the chest wall, or placing a cotton-tipped swab in the hole of a pediatric ECG suction electrode attached to the chest wall. The motion of the stethoscope, placed lightly over the left ventricular impulse, may show movement indicating abnormal cardiac pulsations and vibrations.

2. **Left parasternal region.** A left parasternal lift indicates right ventricular (RV) activity and often is better visualized than palpated. Usually there should be no lift except in apprehensive young patients with a thin chest wall. Motion of the RV caused by systolic overload is reflected by a sustained outward lift; RV diastolic overload caused by an ASD is reflected by a vigorous motion that may not be sustained. A parasternal lift is usually present when an ASD causes a left-to-right shunt >2:1. In patients with severe mitral regurgitation, expansion of the large left atrium during systole may displace the RV forward, and with it, the parasternal region lifts indirectly.

3. **Third left and second right intercostal spaces.** Abnormal pulsations may indicate enlargement of the pulmonary artery and aorta, respectively.

4. **A few centimeters superior to the apex beat.** A sustained bulge in this region may occur with a left ventricular aneurysm. Two distinct impulses a few centimeters apart may be caused by left ventricular dyskinesia or an aneurysm. These findings on inspection should be verified by palpation. Visible systolic pulsations of the right or left sternoclavicular joint, or in the region of the first or second right intercostal space and suprasternal notch, may occur with enlargement or aneurysm of the ascending aorta or aortic arch.

■ PALPATION

Apex Beat. The patient should be examined while in the supine, the sitting, and the left lateral decubitus positions. The apex beat is defined as the point farthest downward and laterally at which a definite cardiac impulse is imparted to the palpating finger. The normal apex beat can be felt in <50% of individuals older than 50 years while in the supine position, but it can be palpated in almost all individuals in the left lateral decubitus position. The point of maximal intensity is not considered the apex beat, because some conditions, such as left ventricular aneurysm, right ventricular enlargement, pulmonary artery dilatation, or aneurysm of the aorta, may cause pulsations that are stronger than that of the cardiac apex beat.

The normal apex beat is palpable as a brief outward impulse, medial and superior to the intersection of the left midclavicular line and the fifth intercostal space. The apex beat should not be more than 10 cm (4 in.) lateral to the midsternal line.

Conditions that cause a displacement of the apex beat include scoliosis, straight back syndrome, pectus excavatum, and high diaphragm, as in pregnancy, obesity, and ascites.

An apical impulse with a diameter >2 to 3 cm indicates left ventricular enlargement. A sustained palpable lift of the impulse lasting up to the S_2 is a strong indicator of left ventricular hypertrophy (LVH). Palpate for a double apical impulse caused by LVH and forceful left atrial contractions. The outward thrust of LVH may be associated with retraction of the left lower parasternal region; the rocking motion may be elicited by placing the index finger of one hand on the apical impulse and the index finger of the other hand on the lower left parasternal region. An S_3 or S_4 sometimes may be better appreciated on inspection and palpation than on auscultation.

Left Parasternal Lift.   In the absence of pectus excavatum and with the patient supine, a palpable anterior systolic movement in the left parasternal region that is sustained up to the S_2 indicates right ventricular hypertrophy. The left parasternal lift is best appreciated by the distal palm at the base of the fingers or with the fingertips. An alternative technique is to use the heel of the right hand, pressing firmly downward at the left sternal border. A presystolic impulse caused by augmented right atrial contraction may be seen and felt. A giant presystolic lift overshadowing the systolic lift may be observed with hypertrophic cardiomyopathy. In patients with hyperdynamic states and diastolic overloading in ASD, an appreciable brief left parasternal lift with normal contour may occur.

Other Areas
- Pulsations caused by dyskinetic areas or cardiac aneurysm may be observed and felt superior and medial to the cardiac apex.
- When pulsations or the apex beat cannot be located with the patient in the left lateral decubitus position, the examiner should assess for the presence of dextrocardia.
- Aneurysm of the abdominal aorta may cause abnormal epigastric pulsations; with severe tricuspid regurgitation, systolic hepatic pulsations may be observed maximally in the right hypochondrium.

■ AUSCULTATION

To become a reliable auscultator, the examiner must use discipline and a systematic approach that is consistently repetitive. The patient is examined in the supine and left lateral decubitus positions, then upright, sitting, and leaning forward with the breath held momentarily after a deep exhalation.

With firm pressure applied to the chest wall, the diaphragm of the stethoscope is used to detect high-frequency sounds such as those produced by S_1 and S_2, clicks, aortic regurgitation, mitral regurgitation, and rubs. The bell of the stethoscope lightly placed detects low-frequency vibrations caused by third and fourth heart sounds (S_3, S_4) and the diastolic murmur of mitral stenosis. The examiner must listen selectively with complete concentration given to the S_1 and then the S_2 followed by the systolic interval and then the diastolic interval.

It is good practice for students starting their cardiology physical diagnosis course to listen only to the variations of S_1 and S_2 during the first few sessions. Concentration on S_1 and S_2, to the exclusion of all other sounds, must be mastered before the student is exposed to systolic murmurs. Later sessions should concentrate on diastolic murmurs and, later, gallop rhythms and rubs; clicks can be appreciated at the same time as S_1 and S_2, or preferably at a later stage. Experienced clinicians have no difficulty moving within seconds from S_1 and S_2 to systolic, then diastolic, intervals. This experience requires discipline, which must be imparted very carefully to students during their first few sessions on auscultation. The timing of murmurs is more important than the point of maximal intensity. The timing of murmurs is crucial and depends on knowledge of S_1 and S_2. Several murmurs, however, cause such memorable vibrations and frequencies that the experienced clinician can never forget them. The murmur of aortic regurgitation is high-pitched, blowing, and decrescendo, whereas the diastolic murmur of mitral stenosis is a low-pitched rumble. The character of the murmur is often a telltale to its timing, which can be confirmed easily by reference to S_1 or S_2. The clinician who has mastered a systematic approach and has listened to several hundred patients with a variety of cardiac murmurs will not expose his or her patient to the expense of phonocardiography and uses the echocardiogram for confirmation of difficult problems, in particular in patients with congenital heart disease and cardiomyopathies. Thus, there can be considerable financial savings if phonocardiography is relegated to academics and if echocardiography is used only when absolutely necessary.

Four traditional terms—mitral, tricuspid, pulmonary, and aortic—do not accurately describe valve positions. A murmur heard in the mitral area is not necessarily of mitral origin; this observation applies to all other areas.

Areas to auscultate are as follows:

- The cardiac apex (mitral area). Murmurs originating from the mitral valve are best heard in this area, but aortic stenosis caused by calcification in elderly patients may be best heard at the apex. Severe tricuspid regurgitation may be best heard in this area if the right ventricle occupies the apex.
- The lower left parasternal area, fourth interspace. The murmur of aortic regurgitation is often best heard at the left sternal edge at the third or fourth intercostal space. When aortic regurgitation is due to aortic root dilatation or a luetic lesion, the murmur may be best heard in the second right intercostal space; rarely, the murmur is heard mainly in the midaxillary line.
- The upper left parasternal area, second interspace (pulmonary area).
- The second right intercostal space (aortic area). Most murmurs arising from the aortic valve are best heard in this position and radiate to the neck vessels, but as mentioned earlier, aortic stenosis caused by a sclerotic valve may be heard at the apex or along the left sternal border; the murmur caused by a flail posterior mitral leaflet may radiate to the base and simulate an aortic murmur.
- The lower sternal edge (tricuspid area).
- The left axilla, for the radiation of murmurs caused by mitral regurgitation.
- Over the carotids.
- Just above the sternoclavicular joint for a venous hum.
- The upper epigastrium. In patients with emphysema and with exacerbation of chronic obstructive pulmonary disease (COPD), the heart sounds may be difficult to auscultate in other areas, and the murmur of tricuspid regurgitation is best heard in this area.
- Below the left clavicle, where the continuous murmur of patent ductus arteriosus (PDA) is heard best.
- The posterior chest, for bruits caused by large bronchial collaterals in patients with coarctation of the aorta.
- Over the spinous processes C3 to L2; with a flail mitral valve, the murmur may be heard over the spinous processes.

First Heart Sound

The first heart sound (S_1) is produced by the closure of the mitral and tricuspid valves. Phonocardiographic, hemodynamic, and ECG correlates indicate that the sound appreciated as S_1 develops in an instant after the valve leaflets have coapted at the time of maximal tensing of the valvular apparatus. S_1 occurs just before the palpable upstroke of the carotid pulse.

- The intensity of S_1 is increased with tachycardia, mitral stenosis with pliable valves, left atrial myxoma, short PR interval, tricuspid stenosis, and hyperthyroidism. In patients with mitral stenosis, S_1 is loud and has a typical "slapping" character. The intensity of S_1 is increased in conditions that cause tachycardia, vigorous ventricular contraction, and events tending to hold the atrioventricular (AV) valves open. In mitral stenosis, diastolic filling is prolonged and the valves remain widely open up to the moment of ventricular contraction and thus close with greater velocity.

- The intensity of S_1 is diminished with fibrosis or calcification of the mitral valve, PR-interval prolongation, heart failure, cardiogenic shock, mitral regurgitation not due to prolapse, severe aortic regurgitation, and left bundle branch block (LBBB).
- The intensity of S_1 should be assessed with the patient holding the breath after a deep exhalation. Conditions that cause variation in intensity of the S_1 occur when there is a varying relationship of atrial to ventricular contraction or varying cycle lengths, i.e., AV dissociation, complete AV block, and ventricular tachycardia. A variable intensity of S_1 in a patient with a wide complex regular tachycardia indicates a ventricular origin.
- Wide splitting of S_1 may be observed with right bundle branch block (RBBB), tricuspid stenosis, and Ebstein's anomaly.
- If S_1 is louder at the left sternal border than at the apex, suspect ASD.

Second Heart Sound

The second heart sound (S_2) is best heard in the second right and left intercostal spaces along the sternal edge.

S_2 is produced by the abrupt deceleration of retrograde flow of the blood column in the aorta and pulmonary arteries when the elastic limits of the taut diaphragm created by closed compliant valves are met. This hemodynamic event causes vibrations that are appreciated as the aortic second sound (A_2) and the pulmonary second sound (P_2) and are heard immediately after closure of the aortic and pulmonary valves (Fig. 4–1).

Leatham appropriately termed S_2 the "key to auscultation of the heart." Clinicians recognize the importance of A_2 and P_2 and thus listen for these sounds in the aortic, pulmonary, and apical areas, and in particular, at the third left interspace at the sternal edge where the aortic and pulmonic areas overlap and both A_2 and P_2 are heard best. The examiner should listen intently, using the diaphragm of the stethoscope during quiet inspiration and expiration by the patient, and then with the patient holding the breath in deep exhalation, at all areas to determine the intensity of A_2 and P_2.

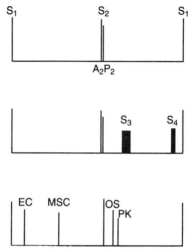

Figure 4–1 □ Sketches of normal first and second heart sounds (S_1, $S_2 = A_2P_2$) and extra sounds other than murmurs. Note the position of the ejection click (EC); midsystolic click (MSC); opening snap (OS); third and fourth heart sounds (S_3, S_4); and pericardial knock (PK).

The appreciation of abnormalities of A_2 and P_2 may assist with the clarification of several cardiac diagnoses.

- A marked increase in the intensity of P_2 occurs with pulmonary artery hypertension and dilatation of the pulmonary artery. (An increase in P_2 is not an uncommon finding in normal individuals younger than age 20.) Normally, only A_2 is heard on auscultation at the apex; P_2 heard in this area may indicate ASD or pulmonary hypertension, the many causes of which must be determined by the clinician.
- A_2 is increased with systemic hypertension. Both systemic and pulmonary hypertension alter a rate of change of the diastolic pressure gradient, which develops across the valves, and thus the force accelerating retrograde flow of the blood column into the base of these two great vessels.
- A_2 is decreased in intensity with severe aortic stenosis. In patients with calcific aortic stenosis, A_2 is soft or absent, but A_2 is relatively preserved in individuals with congenital aortic stenosis, because the valve is usually compliant.
- Normal physiologic splitting of the S_2 into components A_2 and P_2 occurs during inspiration and expiration; it is frequently heard in children and young adults and is uncommon after age 50. The aortic valve normally closes before the pulmonic because of higher aortic pressure. This short inter-

val of <30 msec during expiration cannot be appreciated with a stethoscope. During inspiration there is prolongation of right ventricular ejection and a concomitant decrease in left ventricular ejection, and the widened gap between A_2 and P_2 can be appreciated in most normal individuals. Splitting is best heard with the individual in a sitting position.

- Fixed splitting occurs in up to 70% of patients with ASD. In this condition, because of the increased output of the right ventricle, A_2 and P_2 are held abnormally apart during expiration; hence, during inspiration, A_2 and P_2 move about equally away from S_1 and thus remain the same distance from each other (Fig. 4–2). Some individuals appear to have fixed splitting of S_2 in the supine position that becomes single on standing. Other causes of fixed splitting include severe pulmonary stenosis, ventricular septal defect (VSD), anomalous pulmonary venous drainage, mitral regurgitation with severe right ventricular failure, and straight back syndrome.
- In RBBB there is exaggeration of normal physiologic splitting. Because of delayed right ventricular activation, P_2 occurs late; during inspiration P_2 separates further, and thus the splitting increases during inspiration (see Fig. 4–2).
- With LBBB during inspiration, splitting is decreased; paradoxical or reversed splitting occurs. In young patients with aortic stenosis in the absence of LBBB, paradoxical splitting indicates severe stenosis.
- Critical information regarding the timing of murmurs can be obtained by careful observation of the relationship of the murmur and S_2. Systolic murmur can be placed relative to the second heart sound as early, mid, or late. The timing of the murmur relative to S_2 may reflect the severity of mitral regurgitation; a systolic murmur in the apical area, which radiates to the axilla but with a clear gap between the murmur and S_2, is unlikely to be caused by severe chronic mitral regurgitation.
- The severity of aortic stenosis relates to the length of the murmur; a clear gap between the murmur and A_2 is not consistent with severe aortic stenosis. The peak of the murmur approaches midsystole, and A_2 decreases in intensity. A_2 heard clearly in the aortic area is not consistent with severe aortic stenosis except with congenital stenosis.
- The murmur of aortic regurgitation, heard best in the third left intercostal space, begins synchronously with S_2 as if it wraps the sound of S_2 into its vibrations. The clinician can imitate this decrescendo high-pitched murmur by replacing the usual-sounding second sound "Dub" with "Daww" (Fig. 4–3).
- S_2 marks the opening snap of mitral stenosis, and the distance between S_2 and the opening snap relates to severity.

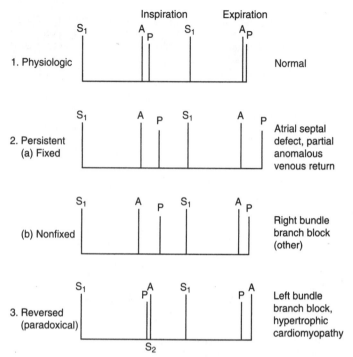

Figure 4–2 □ Splitting of the second heart sound (S_2). A = aortic; P = pulmonary components of the second heart sound.

- There is a clear auscultatory gap between a pericardial knock or a third heart sound gallop and S_2 (see Fig. 4–1).

Third Heart Sound

In up to 40% of adults younger than 40 years, a low-pitched third heart sound (S_3) is heard in early diastole after the second heart sound (see Fig. 4–1). The sound occurs during passive diastolic filling of the ventricle during the Y descent of the atrial pressure pulse. This normal S_3 disappears with advancing age, probably related to a decline of early ventricular filling. An S_3 is best heard at the apex with the patient recumbent in the left lateral position. In this position the apex beat is brought in close proximity to the chest wall. The low-pitched vibrations are best appreciated with the bell lightly placed at the cardiac apex.

The exact mechanism of production of S_3 remains controversial. The extra sound originates in the ventricle and requires rapid

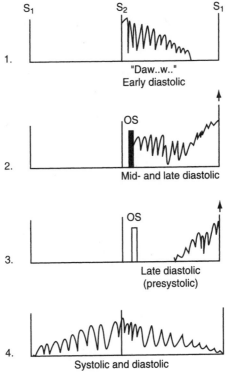

Figure 4–3 □ Patterns of diastolic and continuous murmurs.

1. Early diastolic murmur, high-pitched, decrescendo, maximal at the left sternal edge at the third or fourth intercostal space; typical of aortic regurgitation. Mimic by saying "Daw . . w;" the "D" replaces the S_2.
2. Mid- to late diastolic, low-pitched rumble with presystolic accentuation ending in a loud S_1; typical of mitral stenosis. OS = opening snap.
3. Late diastolic murmur, i.e., presystolic murmur ending in a loud S_1; indicates mitral stenosis. This murmur usually disappears if atrial fibrillation is present.
4. Systolic and diastolic continuous "machinery" murmur of patent ductus arteriosus; it is loudest at the time of S_2.

and unimpeded filling. The sound is believed to be caused by an early diastolic impact of the ventricle on the chest wall. Factors that enhance the production of an S_3 include

- An elevated atrial pressure
- Increase in the volume and velocity of blood flow across the mitral or tricuspid valves
- Proximity of the ventricle to the chest wall

- Incomplete ventricular relaxation; alteration of ventricular relaxation may allow the ventricle to produce a resonating sound at the moment of early diastolic filling and rapid deceleration of blood flow; the occurrence is usually 0.14 to 0.22 second after S_2

Because an S_3 can be heard in normal individuals younger than age 40, the sound is labeled an abnormal S_3 or S_3 gallop if it is accompanied by underlying disease known to produce an S_3. When an S_4 occurs along with an S_3 and the heart rate is increased, the two sounds, S_3 and S_4, may merge; the typical sound produced is termed a summation gallop. The summation gallop is often visible and palpable.

Causes of an S_3 include

- No cause: physiologic in some adults younger than age 40
- Severe mitral regurgitation
- In patients with valvular regurgitation an S_3 indicates severe regurgitation or ventricular failure, or both
- Severe tricuspid regurgitation
- Ventricular failure
- Dilated and hypertrophic cardiomyopathy
- Left ventricular dyskinesia or aneurysm caused by previous myocardial infarcts
- Restrictive left ventricular (LV) filling in some patients with normal systolic function (diastolic dysfunction)
- Hyperdynamic states, e.g., thyrotoxicosis and AV fistula
- Constrictive pericarditis. The added sound in early diastole, called a pericardial knock, is indeed a third heart sound (see Fig. 4–1). It occurs earlier than a normal or pathologic S_3, 0.09 to 0.12 second after S_2; it is loud, more widely transmitted, and has a higher pitch than the usual S_3 and thus can be heard with the diaphragm. The snapping quality and occurrence early in diastole may allow confusion with the early opening snap of mitral stenosis. In constrictive pericarditis a high atrial pressure empties rapidly across an unobstructed AV valve into a ventricle with markedly impaired compliance. The sound appears to be generated by the sudden arrest of ventricular filling when the noncompliant pericardium halts ventricular relaxation.

Fourth Heart Sound

An S_4 is rarely heard in individuals with normal hearts. An S_4 usually denotes a pathologic condition of the ventricle that has rendered it abnormally stiff and resulted in vigorous atrial contraction to propel blood across an unobstructed AV valve into the stiff ventricle. The S_4 is best heard with the bell lightly placed at the apex, or just medial to the apex, with the patient in the left lateral decubitus position. A right ventricular S_4 may be heard in the upper epigastric area; the S_4 is absent with atrial fibrillation.

Pathologic states associated with an S_4 gallop include

1. LVH due to hypertension or other causes, right ventricular hypertrophy, and conditions that cause pulmonary hypertension
2. Acute myocardial infarction; >60% of patients during the first few days after an acute myocardial infarct have an audible S_4 gallop; the infarcted area is dyskinetic or akinetic and causes loss of compliance
3. An attack of angina, during which ischemia causes a marked, decreased left ventricular stiffness, and an S_4 may become transient
4. Obstructive cardiomyopathy and dilated cardiomyopathy
5. Infiltration of the myocardium caused by specific heart muscle diseases
6. Significant aortic stenosis with a significant pressure gradient; a palpable S_4 usually indicates a gradient >75 mm Hg and a left ventricular end-diastolic pressure of about 12 mm Hg
7. Pulmonary stenosis

Occasionally, an S_4 merges with the S_1. Differentiation of the first heart sound can be reached by listening with the diaphragm and the bell. S_4 is best heard with the bell; sitting or standing by the patient may cause its disappearance. A split S_1 or ejection click remains unchanged. A split S_1 is heard best with the diaphragm, because the first component is higher pitched and is only narrowly separated from the second component. Firm pressure of the diaphragm usually eliminates an S_4 but not a split S_1 or an S_1 plus a click. Listening at sites distant from the apex decreases the intensity or eliminates an S_4. In patients older than 45 years an apparent reduplicated S_1 is more likely an atrial gallop.

Ejection Clicks

These early ejection sounds occurring immediately after S_1 are caused by the opening of stenotic but pliable semilunar valves or by the impact of increased blood flow into a dilated aorta or pulmonary artery. Ejection clicks are not usually heard in normal individuals. These high-pitched clicking sounds are heard best with the diaphragm. The click may sound louder than S_1 at the base; when S_1 appears louder at the base, the sound is likely caused by an ejection click. Loud ejection clicks may simulate S_1 or the second component of a split S_1. A split S_1 is heard best at the lower left sternal edge. The aortic ejection clicks are detected best at the apex but can be louder at the left sternal edge, and they are not affected by respiration. Pulmonary ejection clicks are detected best in the second or third left interspace at the sternal edge and may increase with deep exhalation.

Causes of ejection clicks include

1. Bicuspid aortic valve with or without stenosis. Uncomplicated coarctation does not cause a click; therefore, the presence of an ejection click in a patient with coarctation suggests an associated bicuspid valve.
2. Congenital aortic stenosis (acquired aortic stenosis if the valve is pliable)
3. Systemic hypertension
4. Coarctation of the aorta (often associated with bicuspid aortic valve)
5. Aortic regurgitation (increased flow)
6. Aneurysm of the aorta
7. Pulmonary stenosis (with pliable valve)
8. Pulmonary artery dilatation
9. Pulmonary hypertension
10. Eisenmenger's syndrome
11. Total anomalous pulmonary venous return

Mid- to Late Systolic Clicks

A mid- to late systolic click is commonly heard with MVP. These clicks may occur with or without the presence of a mid- to late systolic murmur. These sharp, high-pitched sounds are appreciated best with the diaphragm. They occur during maximum excursion of prolapsed mitral valve leaflets and elongated chordae; failure of the valve leaflets to coapt and prolapse of leaflets begin when the reduction of left ventricular volume in systole reaches a critical point. Other causes include atrial or ventricular aneurysms, LV free-wall aneurysms, and atrial myxomas.

Reduction in left ventricular volume by standing and Valsalva's maneuver make the click and murmur occur earlier; squatting and hand grip make them occur later. If left ventricular volume is increased by an increase in venous return, bradycardia, or a decrease in the myocardial contractility, the onset of the click and murmur is delayed. (This effect and control of arrhythmias may explain the salutary effects of beta blockers in the MVP syndrome.)

Opening Snap

The mitral opening snap is a sharp, high-pitched sound heard approximately 0.08 second after S_2 (see Fig. 4–1). It is caused by the opening of the stenotic but pliable mitral valve and is analogous to ejection clicks caused by opening of stenotic but pliable aortic and pulmonary valves. This short snapping sound coincides with the maximal opening of the anterior mitral valve leaflet. The mitral valve opening snap is heard best between the apex and the left sternal border but may be heard over a wide area including the base of the heart.

The high-pitched snap occurs much earlier in diastole than the third heart sound, which is a low-frequency "thud," heard best at the apex with the bell. The opening snap is a hallmark of mitral stenosis and, along with a loud S_1, is heard in >75% of patients with mitral stenosis. The opening snap softens and may disappear with severe calcification of the valve. Tricuspid stenosis may produce an opening snap heard best at the left lower sternal edge. An opening snap may be confused with P_2. The opening snap is often heard widely over the precordium including at the second right interspace. P_2 is loudest at the left upper sternal border and separates from A_2 on inspiration.

Pericardial Rub

Pericardial rub is discussed in Chapter 9.

Murmurs

The following observations are crucial to the diagnosis of cardiac murmurs:
1. The timing of the murmur relative to S_1, and in particular to S_2. This provides the most meaningful piece of information relating to its cause (see Fig. 4–3; Fig. 4–4). If the murmur is difficult to time, the observer should identify S_2 at the base, then slowly move the stethoscope down, from the base to the apex, fixing the cardiac cycle with S_2 as the reference point.
2. The point of maximal intensity. This provides information that is not always accurate. For example, the systolic murmur of aortic valve sclerosis may be best heard in the apical area. Nevertheless, the point of maximal intensity is sufficiently helpful and should be rigorously applied.
3. The character or quality of the murmur. Some aspects of quality are particularly helpful; ascertain whether the murmur is high pitched, low pitched, rumbling, only crescendo, only decrescendo, or crescendo–decrescendo. These features are so distinctive to the trained ear that most experienced clinicians can rapidly discern the difference between the early, high-pitched blowing diastolic murmur of aortic regurgitation and the rumbling, low-pitched diastolic murmur of mitral stenosis. Timing hardly enters the equation. Some aspects of quality are not as distinctive but should be recorded, e.g., harsh, rough, creaky, musical.

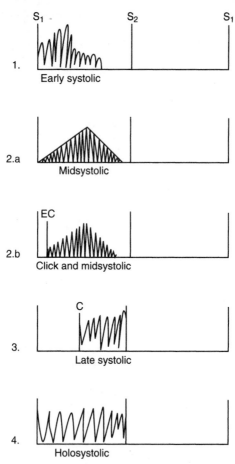

Figure 4–4 □ Patterns of systolic murmurs. Timing of the murmur can be diagnostic.

1. Early systolic murmur at apex and left lower sternal border caused by acute mitral or tricuspid regurgitation; by regurgitation into a normal-sized atrium; or by a very small ventricular septal defect with late shunting abolished.
2. (a) Midsystolic murmur at left sternal border and aortic area; is not always aortic stenosis—consider increased flow, high-output states, some forms of mitral regurgitation, and innocent murmurs.
   (b) Midsystolic murmur preceded by an ejection click (EC) is typical of congenital aortic stenosis. The click is absent in rheumatic calcific stenosis or nonpliable valves.
3. Late systolic murmur typical of mitral valve prolapse (C = click); one or more clicks may be heard.
4. Holosystolic murmur typical of chronic mitral or tricuspid regurgitation or ventricular septal defect.

4. Intensity of the murmur. Traditionally, the intensity of murmurs is graded as follows:
   - Grade 1: A very soft murmur that is faintly heard; the murmur may be missed during the initial examination
   - Grade 2: A soft murmur that is readily heard
   - Grade 3: A loud murmur with no thrill present
   - Grade 4: A loud murmur with a thrill present
   - Grade 5: A very loud murmur heard when the edge of the stethoscope is applied to the area of maximal intensity
   - Grade 6: The loudest murmur, audible with the stethoscope removed from the chest wall

It is worth recalling that aortic regurgitation causes a diastolic murmur and that when the underlying disease is due to syphilitic aortitis, aortic stenosis never occurs; yet, a very loud grade 4 systolic murmur may be heard because of increased blood flow into a dilated aortic root. A murmur of severe aortic stenosis may soften to grade 1 or grade 2 in patients with low cardiac output and heart failure. The intensity of systolic murmurs does not always relate to the severity of the lesion. The intensity may prove useful if the examiner considers the volume and velocity of blood flow and dilatation of the aortic root in the given individual.

Murmurs are classified as follows:
1. Systolic, beginning after S_1 and ending at or before A_2 or P
2. Diastolic, beginning with or after S_2 and ending just before S_1
3. Continuous, beginning in systole and continuing through S_2 into part or all of diastole

Systolic Murmurs

Systolic murmurs of no clinical significance are common; they can be heard in >60% of children. The systolic murmur of aortic valve sclerosis without stenosis is heard in >50% of individuals older than 50 years.

Systolic murmurs (see Fig. 4–4) can be classified as one of the following:
1. Early systolic
2. Midsystolic ("ejection")
3. Late systolic
4. Holosystolic (pansystolic)

Early Systolic Murmurs. These murmurs begin with S_1 and decrease with a decrescendo effect ending in midsystole. Causes of early systolic murmurs include
1. Acute severe mitral regurgitation. A large volume of blood regurgitates into a normal left atrium that has not become fibrosed or enlarged; the resistance in the normal left atrium halts blood flow during midsystole.
2. Acute tricuspid regurgitation.
3. A small VSD of the muscular septum can cause a short early

systolic murmur. The murmur may be heard best at the left sternal edge; it begins at the onset of ventricular systole, but as the ventricular size decreases, the small defect is temporarily sealed in midsystole and the murmur stops abruptly.

Midsystolic Murmurs. These murmurs begin after S_1 and end well before S_2; i.e., there is a clear gap between the end of the murmur and S_2. The murmur starts with ejection, increases to crescendo, and decreases in decrescendo as ejection decreases (see Fig. 4–4). Midsystolic murmurs occur when there is

1. Obstruction to ventricular flow as observed with aortic or pulmonary valve stenosis; with severe stenosis, the murmur becomes longer and peaks in midsystole, and S_2 becomes softer or absent (see Chapter 27).
2. Dilatation of the aorta or pulmonary trunk.
3. Accelerated and increased blood flow into the aorta; this is a common occurrence with severe aortic regurgitation. Other causes of increased blood flow include anemia, thyrotoxicosis, pregnancy, fevers, and heart block.

Soft, short, midsystolic murmurs of no clinical significance commonly occur. The absence of abnormal clinical cardiac findings with normal ECG and chest x-ray should suffice to define innocent murmurs, but occasionally echocardiography is required. So-called innocent murmurs are mainly midsystolic; they are of very short duration and are heard mainly at the left sternal border, and some have a musical "twangy" component. There is often no diagnostic difference between the characters of innocent and of organic murmurs. The physician must analyze the murmur in relation to "the company the murmur keeps."

- A midsystolic murmur may be produced by mitral regurgitation caused by abnormal left ventricular regional wall motion abnormalities. This midsystolic murmur is not an ejection murmur; thus, not all midsystolic murmurs can be labeled as ejection.

Late Systolic Murmurs. The murmur starts in mid- to late systole and extends to S_2 (see Fig. 4–4 and Chapter 27). They are usually caused by mitral and tricuspid valve prolapse and derangements of the papillary muscles. The typical late systolic murmur of MVP may be accompanied by a midsystolic click (see earlier discussion). The timing of the murmur and its intensity may vary with alteration in left ventricular volume; the murmur may, without provocation, change to a whoop or honk.

Mid- to late systolic murmurs are caused by

1. MVP (myxomatous)
2. Tricuspid valve prolapse
3. Rheumatic heart disease

4. Papillary muscle dysfunction caused by ischemic heart disease or cardiomyopathy

Holosystolic Murmurs. The murmur begins with S_1 and continues throughout systole up to S_2 (see Figs. 4–3 and 4–4). The murmur is caused by blood flow from a chamber or a vessel with a higher pressure and resistance than the receiving chamber or vessel. Holosystolic murmurs are often regurgitant, but there are exceptions.

Causes of holosystolic murmurs include the following:

1. Mitral regurgitation. The murmur is usually best heard at the apex, and it radiates into the posterior axilla. Depending on the part of the mitral apparatus that is affected, the murmur can radiate anteriorly to the aortic area or posteriorly to the back or spine.
2. Tricuspid regurgitation.
3. VSD. The murmur is maximal at the left sternal edge and radiates like the spokes in a wheel.
4. Aortopulmonary window or PDA. The murmur is heard when vascular resistance eliminates the diastolic components.

Innocent Systolic Murmurs. Innocent or functional murmurs are commonly heard in children and individuals younger than age 20. They occur during early LV or right ventricular ejection; are soft, grade 2 or less; are short, never pansystolic; and must be associated with no abnormal cardiac findings.

Diastolic Murmurs

These are classified as one of the following:

1. Early diastolic
2. Mid-diastolic
3. Late diastolic

Early Diastolic Murmurs. The most common early diastolic murmur is that of aortic valve regurgitation (see Fig. 4–3 and Chapter 27). The murmur begins with S_2 and, because there is a progressive decline in volume and rate of the regurgitant flow into the ventricle, the murmur is usually decrescendo. This murmur is best heard with the diaphragm firmly pressed against the chest wall, along the left sternal edge at the third or fourth intercostal space, with the patient sitting up at the side of the bed with the breath held after a full exhalation (Fig. 4–5). The point of maximal intensity is often the third left interspace but may be at the right second interspace in patients with aortic root dilatation (Marfan syndrome and luetic aortic incompetence); rarely, the murmur is heard mainly in the midaxilla.

As discussed earlier, this high-pitched, blowing decrescendo murmur has typical characteristics; imitate as "Daw . . . w" be-

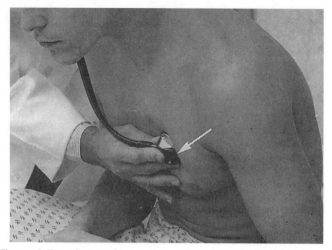

Figure 4–5 □ The soft, high-frequency early diastolic murmur of aortic regurgitation or pulmonary hypertensive regurgitation is best elicited by applying the diaphragm of the stethoscope very firmly to the mid-left sternal edge *(arrow)* as the patient sits and leans forward with breath held in full exhalation. (From Braunwald E: Heart Disease, 5th ed. Philadelphia, WB Saunders Co., 1997, p 48.)

cause the "Da" replaces the "Dup" that is normally caused by S_2 (see Fig. 4–3). Once this sound has been heard and documented, the observer will never mistake it for the soft, low-pitched, mid-diastolic rumbling murmur of mitral stenosis. Pulmonary valve incompetence or severe pulmonary hypertension is an uncommon cause of an early, high-pitched decrescendo murmur at the third interspace at the left sternal edge. The murmur starts with a loud pulmonic component of S_2.

Mid-diastolic Murmurs. The most common cause of a mid-diastolic murmur is mitral stenosis (see Fig. 4–3). There is a clear gap between the S_2 and the beginning of the murmur, or the murmur is ushered in by an opening snap. The murmur occurs during the rapid diastolic filling phase as blood flows across the partially obstructed and deformed mitral valve. The murmur is often accompanied by a very loud "slapping" S_1. The murmur may be difficult to detect, and the typical S_1 sound and opening snap may be the tip-off to its detection. If the murmur is not readily heard, the patient should sit up and touch his or her toes several times or stand and jog on the spot for 10 to 20 seconds. The patient must be warned to get into the ready position for the listening process. Immediately after the exercise, the patient lies in the left lateral position. The bell is placed lightly over the previously defined apex beat. The murmur is often confined to the apex, but occasionally it is heard at the apex and the left sternal edge.

Other causes of mid-diastolic murmurs include
1. Tricuspid stenosis
2. Atrial myxomas
3. High diastolic flow across an AV valve: severe mitral regurgitation, large left-to-right shunts, and complete AV block

Late Diastolic Murmurs. The only late diastolic murmur of clinical significance is that produced by mitral stenosis with the patient in sinus rhythm. The rough low-pitched murmur occurs during late ventricular filling generated by augmented atrial contraction. Thus, it is often referred to as presystolic accentuation of a mid-diastolic murmur. The rough, low-pitched, rumbling mid-diastolic murmur of mitral stenosis increases in intensity and, with a crescendo, ends in an almost-deafening loud S_1.

Continuous Murmurs

These murmurs begin in systole and continue throughout S_2 into part or all of diastole (see Fig. 4–3). The murmur is loudest at the time of the second heart sound. The most common cause of a continuous murmur is a PDA. The typical machinery-like murmur that occupies systole and diastole is heard best in the left infraclavicular area. The quick runoff of blood from the systemic arterial tree causes a collapsing pulse (see Fig. 3–3 and Table 3–5); palpation of the dorsalis pedis usually reveals a bounding pulse.

Prosthetic Valve Murmurs

Mechanical valves produce metallic closure sounds that diminish in intensity if there is tissue ingrowth or thrombosis around the valve. Some Starr-Edwards ball valves have opening sounds; aortic prostheses cause turbulence that produces a grade 1 to 2 ejection systolic murmur; a sudden increase in the systolic murmur may reflect obstruction by thrombus, but severe obstruction can cause a low cardiac output, and the murmur becomes softer or absent. A diastolic murmur is usually abnormal and suggests a perivalvular leak. **Bioprosthetic valves** normally produce no sounds; when they degenerate, systolic murmurs emerge. Musical murmurs suggest a tear of a leaflet.

5 | Rapid Guide to Relevant ECG Diagnosis

Despite the advent of sophisticated and expensive cardiologic tests, the electrocardiogram (ECG) remains the most reliable and inexpensive tool for the confirmation of acute myocardial infarction (MI). The results of this simple test, and not the creatine kinase MB (CK-MB), the echocardiogram, the single-photon emission computed tomography (SPECT) scan, or the positron emission tomography (PET) scan, dictate the rapid treatment with life-saving thrombolytic agents. The clinical diagnosis of pericarditis or myocardial ischemia can be confirmed only by ECG findings. The ECG has no rival for the diagnosis of arrhythmia, which is one of the most common on-call problems in cardiology. The ECG provides information not readily obtained by other methods. Thus, the correct interpretation of the ECG is vital to therapeutic decision making.

Because the electrical axis and the T waves of the ECG have little effect on diagnosis and do not alter therapeutic decisions, discussions of these topics are given later in this chapter, and abnormalities that can be confirmed from the ECG tracing are discussed first.

To obtain a clear understanding of the ECG diagnosis, the trainee must become familiar with

- The genesis of the normal QRS complex. From this, the trainee can ascertain the presence of acute or previous MI, right bundle branch block (RBBB) or left bundle branch block (LBBB), fascicular blocks (hemiblocks), hypertrophy of cardiac chambers, and other conditions.
- The status of the ST segment.
- Abnormal heart rhythms. Arrhythmia diagnosis is dealt with later in this chapter.

■ GENESIS OF THE QRS COMPLEX

The ECG picks up the heart's electrical impulses that stimulate the heart to contract. These impulses originate from the sinoatrial (SA) node. The spread through both atria produces the P wave of the ECG (Fig. 5–1). The impulse is slowed briefly in the atrioventricular (AV) node and then progresses rapidly down the His bundle, the left and right bundle branches, and Purkinje fibers of the ventricular myocardium. The passage of the impulses causes

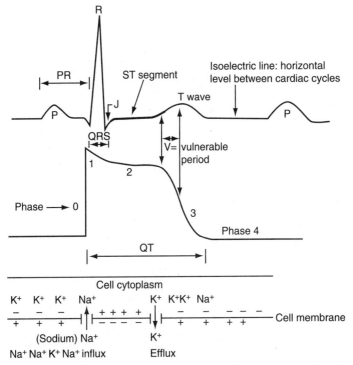

Figure 5–1 □ Sodium influx, potassium efflux, the action potential, and the electrocardiogram.

depolarization of the myocardial cells. The QRS complex is caused by spread of the electrical impulses through the ventricular muscle, i.e., depolarization or activation of the ventricular muscle, and coincides with the beginning of ventricular contraction. Depolarization spreads down the septum toward the apex of the heart, along the free wall of the left ventricle (LV) from endocardium to pericardium. The ECG picks up the depolarization sequence recorded as the QRS complex (see Fig. 5–1). The T wave represents ventricular repolarization. Figure 5–2 shows a normal ECG, and Table 5–1 gives important normal ECG intervals and parameters.

Except for arrhythmia diagnoses in which P waves give vital information, the QRS complex and ST segment are the two most important diagnostic components of the ECG. Knowledge of the normal sequence of depolarization or activation of the ventricles is crucial to the understanding of normal and abnormal QRS

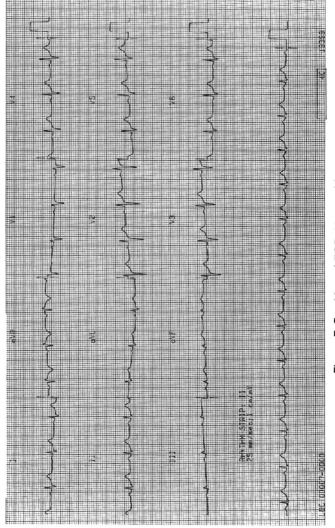

Figure 5-2 □ Normal ECG, 44-year-old man.

Table 5–1 □ **IMPORTANT ECG INTERVALS AND PARAMETERS***

PR interval	0.12–0.20 second (rarely up to 0.24 second)
P waves	<3 small squares in duration and amplitude; upright lead I, inverted lead aVR (if opposite, suspect reversed arm leads or dextrocardia)
QRS complex	0.04–0.10 second
Q waves	Normal in lead aVR Often lead III: should be ≤0.04 second in duration and ≤7 mm deep Other leads: <0.04 second in duration and ≤3 mm deep; up to 5 mm deep in individuals younger than age 25
R waves	V_1: 0–7 mm, age 20–70 yr V_2: 0.2–10 mm V_3: 2–20 mm
ST segment	Isoelectric or <1-mm elevation in limb leads; <2 mm in precordial leads except for normal variant
T wave	Inverted lead aVR; upright in leads I, II, and V_3 to V_6; variable in leads III, aVF, aVL, V_1, and V_2
Axis	0–110 degrees, age <40 yr −30 to 90 degrees, age >40 yr
QT interval	0.36–0.46 second, heart rate 45–65 beats/min 0.33–0.43 second, heart rate 66–100 beats/min <0.33 second, heart rate >100 beats/min

*ECG paper speed of 25 mm/sec.
ECG = electrocardiographic.

complexes. Understanding the genesis of the QRS complex and focusing on the ST segment are the keys to the recognition of

- The most important components of the normal ECG
- Normal variants
- Abnormalities caused by conditions such as MI, ischemia, conduction disturbances, and ventricular hypertrophy

Vector Forces

Each activated area of the heart can be represented by a vector force. The direction of the resultant force can be represented by an arrow, the length of which represents the magnitude of the force. The term "vector" does not imply vectorcardiography; the term explains how the QRS complex is produced and thus helps explain abnormalities of the QRS complex. The correct diagnosis of acute and previous MI, LBBB and RBBB, hemiblocks, and ventricular hypertrophy depends on knowing the resultant vectors contributing to the components of the QRS complex. Simply, a vector describes a force in terms of its duration and magnitude.

The following two caveats apply:
1. An electrical impulse traveling toward an electrode produces a positive deflection or R wave (Fig. 5–3).
2. When the impulse is traveling away from the electrode, a negative deflection is produced and is recorded as a small q wave or an S wave.

Three resultant vectors dictate the inscription of the QRS complex:

Vector I. The ventricular septum is stimulated from left to right. Thus, an electrode or lead positioned over the right ventricle (V_1) faces the wave of excitation and records a positive R wave (see Fig. 5–3). Because the force of the excitation wave is small, the positive deflection is small. The R wave recorded in leads V_1 and V_2 of a normal ECG is small and ranges from 1 to 4 mm in lead V_1 to 1 to 7 mm in lead V_2. The excitation wave or current flowing away from leads V_5 and V_6 results in a small negative deflection and a q wave in leads V_5 and V_6 and may be observed in lead I.

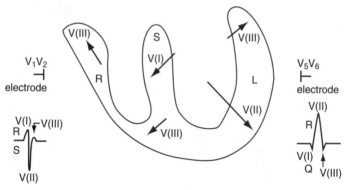

Figure 5–3 □ Vectors I, II, and III underlie the genesis of the QRS complex.

V(I)	= vector I produces a small r wave in leads V_1 and V_2 and a small Q wave in leads V_5 and V_6.
V(II)	= vector II produces an S wave in lead V_1 and an R wave in lead V_5 or V_6.
V(III)	= vector III produces the terminal S in leads V_5 and V_6 and the terminal r or r′ in leads V_1, V_2, and aVR.
V_1	= lead V_1 electrode.
V_6	= lead V_6 electrode.
R	= right ventricle muscle mass.
L	= left ventricle muscle mass.
S	= septum.

Vector II.   After septal activation, both ventricular walls are activated simultaneously. The electrical force rapidly activates the thin-walled right ventricle, but the magnitude of the forces is small in comparison with the forces in the thick left ventricular free wall. Thus, the resultant force, vector II, is directed through the center of the left ventricular free wall (see Fig. 5–3). The resultant force can be represented by an arrow directed toward the left, either upward or downward, depending on the position of the heart. An electrode positioned over the LV (V_5 and V_6) records a positive wave, i.e., an R wave caused by the resultant electrical force, which is represented as vector II, and is directed to the left toward the electrode over the LV. Simultaneously, the force travels away from the electrode overlying the right ventricle (V_1, V_2) and records a negative deflection, an S wave in V_1 and V_2. Thus, the larger the left ventricular muscle, the taller the R wave in leads V_5 and V_6, and the S wave in leads V_1 and V_2 becomes deeper. Vector II is reflected by a positive deflection, an R wave in leads I and II.

Vector III.   Vector III represents activation of the posterobasal right and left ventricular free walls and the basal right septal mass including the crista supraventricularis (see Fig. 5–3). The resultant force is therefore directed to the right, is small in magnitude, and may produce a small S wave in leads V_5 and V_6 and a terminal r^1 or R^1 in lead V_1 or V_2.

■ QRS NORMAL VARIANTS AND ABNORMALITIES

Variations in the normal QRS configuration are depicted in Figure 5–4. If the heart undergoes strong clockwise or counterclockwise rotation, marked changes in QRS morphology may occur. Failure to recognize these normal variants may result in the incorrect interpretation of the ECG.

With clockwise rotation, the lead V_1 electrode, like the aVR, faces the cavity of the ventricle and records a QS complex; thus, a deep Q wave can be a normal finding if there is extreme clockwise rotation of the heart (see Fig. 5–4). Also, there will be no initial small q wave in lead V_6; the resultant force of the initial vector I is no longer traveling toward the lead V_1 electrode. In a similar manner, if part of the interventricular septum is destroyed by an anteroseptal infarct or replaced by a tumor, the R wave in leads V_1, V_2, and V_3 disappears (a loss of R), resulting in a QS complex in leads V_1, V_2, and V_3.

Myocardial Infarction

An infarct is defined as an area of necrotic cells caused by a cutting off of blood supply to the area of cells. Infarction of the heart muscle denotes an area of necrosis.

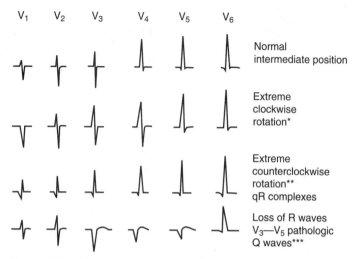

V₁   V₂   V₃   V₄   V₅   V₆

Normal
intermediate position

Extreme
clockwise
rotation*

Extreme
counterclockwise
rotation**
qR complexes

Loss of R waves
V₃—V₅ pathologic
Q waves***

Figure 5–4 □ Variation in the normal precordial QRS configuration and correlation with abnormal presentations.

*   = with clockwise rotation, the V_1 electrode, like aVR, faces the cavity of the heart and records a QS complex; no initial q in lead V_6.

** = qR complexes; q <0.04 second, <3 mm deep, therefore not pathologic Q waves.

*** = loss of R wave, V_3 to V_5 pathologic Q waves; signifies anterior myocardial infarction (see Fig. 5–5).

- If there is necrosis of the left ventricular muscle facing the lead V_4, V_5, and V_6 electrodes, no R waves—i.e., Q waves—will be produced (see Fig. 5–4), or the R in leads V_4 and V_5 may be considerably decreased (poor R wave progression) (Fig. 5–5). Loss of the R wave or a very poor R wave progression in leads V_3 to V_5 is typical of anterior MI. Because of the presence of R waves in leads V_1 and V_2 and a small R in lead V_3, the loss of R waves in leads V_4, V_5, and V_6 is diagnostic of anterolateral MI (see Fig. 5–5). Note that with dextrocardia the R wave is lost in leads V_4 to V_6, but the P wave will be inverted in lead I and upright in lead aVR.
- Infarction of the ventricular septum causes the loss of vector I; thus, there is a loss of the normal R wave in leads V_1, V_2, and V_3. The resulting wave is called a pathologic Q wave (see Fig. 5–4; Fig. 5–6).
- These pathologic Q waves are deep and wide. Normal Q waves are usually <0.04 second in duration, are <3 mm deep, and occur because the activation current is traveling away from the electrode and produces a small q wave. Small

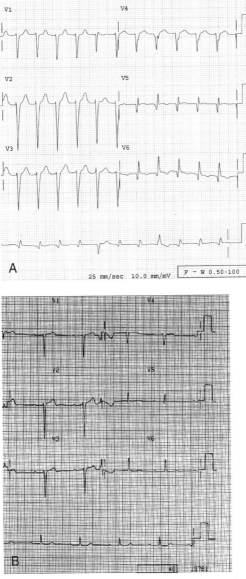

Figure 5–5 □ *A,* Loss of R wave V_4 to V_6: anterolateral infarction. *B,* Tracing from a 75-year-old man with a large anterior infarct at age 56; deep Q waves in leads V_2 to V_5. Recent ECG shows poor R wave progression in leads V_3 and V_4, and indicates a definite old anterior infarction.

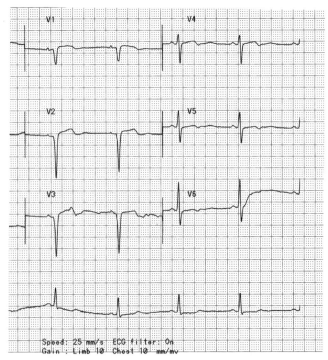

Figure 5–6 □ Loss of R waves in leads V_1 to V_3 signifies anteroseptal myocardial infarction (Q waves or QS in leads V_1 to V_3).

q waves are found in normal ECGs in leads V_5 and V_6 and lead I; normal changes in the position of the heart may cause small q waves in leads 3, aVF, and aVL, and with extreme counterclockwise rotation, q waves may occur in leads V_1 to V_6 (see Fig. 5–4).

Other Causes of Q Waves

1. If the septum is hypertrophied, q waves increase in depth. This situation is seen with hypertrophic cardiomyopathy (HCM), and the resulting deep Q waves may mimic MI (Fig. 5–7).
2. As outlined earlier, with extreme clockwise rotation, lead V_1 faces the ventricular cavity and the usual R wave may disappear, resulting in a QS complex (see Fig. 5–4).
3. All precordial leads may show q waves at extreme counterclockwise rotation, and thus, small q–large R (qR) complexes occur (see Fig. 5–4).

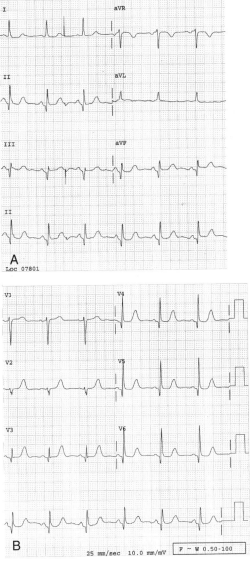

Figure 5–7 □ *A,* ECG limb leads from a 68-year-old woman with mild hypertrophic cardiomyopathy, simulating inferolateral infarction. *B,* ECG V leads in the same patient. Note the R wave in leads V_1 and V_2, then loss of the R wave; Q waves in leads V_3 to V_6 simulate anterolateral infarction.

4. Q waves may be observed in leads II, III, and aVF when the arm leads are placed on the legs; presence of virtually no ECG deflections (R or S waves) in lead I is the clue to this technical error.

5. Understanding vector forces and the position of the heart is important before deciding that the loss of an R wave is caused by infarction. Loss of R waves and the presence of Q waves may be caused by replacement of ventricular muscle by tumor, fibrosis, sarcoidosis, or other granuloma.

6. Large Q waves or QS complexes are normally observed in lead aVR, because lead aVR looks into the cavity of the ventricle and faces the endocardial surface. Because ventricular activation proceeds from the endocardium to the epicardium, the current or impulse travels away from lead aVR, and therefore, lead aVR shows a negative QRS complex.

7. A Q wave may be found in leads III and aVL, and this can be up to 6 mm deep. In lead III the Q wave can be ≤0.04 second wide. In all other leads, the Q wave should be <0.04 second's duration. Q waves in lead III occur often in normal individuals. If there are no Q waves in leads II or aVF, the Q wave in lead III should be ignored (see Table 5–1).

■ THE ST SEGMENT

The ST segment starts after the final deflection of the QRS complex, whether it is an R or an S wave, and ends imperceptibly with the ascending limb of the T wave (see Figs. 5–1 and 5–2). The ST segment curves gently into the T wave. The point at which the ST segment takes off from the QRS complex is called the junction (J)-point. The ST segment represents the period of time when all parts of the ventricular myocardium are in the activated or depolarized state.

Several features of the normal ST segment deserve critical appraisal. Knowledge of normal variants allows the clinician to recognize correctly the various abnormalities of the ST segment.

- The early diagnosis of acute MI is based on abnormalities of the ST segment.
- Because pathologic Q waves occur several hours after the onset of symptoms, diagnosis of acute MI based on Q waves does not allow for the early intervention of thrombolytic therapy. Most textbooks on ECG stress the recognition of Q waves and devote little attention to the ST segment.

ST Segment Elevation

- The horizontal level between cardiac cycles indicates the iso-electric line (see Fig. 5–1). The start of the ST segment is usually at the same horizontal level as the TP (the isoelectric interval). When the heart rate is >90 beats/min, the P wave may merge with the end of the T wave; thus, the TP interval can be difficult to recognize and often cannot be used to assess ST segment elevation; the PR and the ST segments are in close proximity. Thus, the PR segment is commonly used to judge the degree of ST segment elevation or depression.

- Occasionally, the ST segment may show up to a 1-mm elevation in limb leads I, II, III, and aVF and up to a 4-mm elevation in the precordial leads as a normal variant. This normal variant is not uncommon in blacks and other ethnic groups; when this occurs, the origin of the ST segment may have a curious "fishhook" appearance (Fig. 5–8) or may retain its normal concave contour. This normally occurring elevation of the ST segment is commonly (incorrectly) termed "early repolarization pattern." See the discussion under Mimics of Acute Myocardial Infarction.

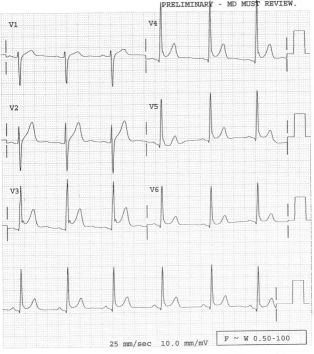

Figure 5–8 □ ST segment elevation in a normal 25-year-old: normal variant; note the notched J-point "fishhook" appearance in lead V_3.

- The ST segment is usually well defined in leads V_4, V_5, and V_6. Thus, abnormal elevations can be accurately assessed. In leads V_2 and V_3 the QRS may pass straight into the takeoff for the T wave without a discrete ST segment; thus, concluding that ST segment elevation in leads V_2 and V_3 is abnormal should be done cautiously. Abnormal ST segment elevation is never confined to one lead.
- The ST segment is elevated when there is an altered sequence of activation, as with conduction defects, in particular, LBBB (see later discussion of LBBB).

Abnormal ST segment elevation is a hallmark of
1. Acute MI; the ST segment is caused by a current of injury (see discussion under Acute Myocardial Infarction)
2. Coronary artery spasm (during the pain)
3. Left ventricular aneurysm
4. Acute pericarditis; the ST segment retains its concave shape
5. LBBB

The Shape of the ST Segment

- The shape of the ST segment can give crucial diagnostic information. The ST segment curves imperceptively into the early part of the T wave.
- The ST segment usually has a mild *concave* shape and should not form a sharp angle with the ascending limb of the T wave.
- A *convex* elevation of the ST segment is typical of acute MI (see discussion under Acute Myocardial Infarction).
- A horizontal ST segment is usually abnormal.

ST Segment Depression

- The ST segment is rarely depressed >0.5 mm in normal individuals. Often a wandering baseline is interpreted incorrectly as ST depression. ST segment depression that is >1 mm, horizontal, or downsloping is significant for ischemia, but upsloping depression is nonsignificant (see Fig. 5–49).
- The ST segment may be slightly depressed or slurred downward in lead III.

■ THE P WAVE

The P wave represents spread of electrical activity through both atria (see Fig. 5–1).
- The P wave is usually <0.12 second in duration (see Table 5–1).

- The P wave is normally inverted in lead aVR.
- The P wave is usually upright in leads I, II, and aVF and in the precordial leads V_4 to V_6.
- The P wave is variable in leads III, aVL, and V_1 to V_3.

P Wave Abnormalities

- Inversion of the P wave in leads I, II, aVF, or V_4 to V_6 but an upright position in lead aVR. This usually occurs when there is abnormal propagation of the electrical impulse through the atria, as occurs in atrial and AV junctional rhythms.
- Inversion of the P wave in lead I and a positive P wave in aVR, with lead I being the mirror image of normal lead I. This may occur when the arm leads are reversed or in dextrocardia, but in true dextrocardia there is a loss of R waves in leads V_4 to V_6.
- Increased duration of ≥ 0.12 second (3 mm) observed mainly in lead II. This occurs in left atrial enlargement (Figs. 5–9 and 5–10). P waves are seen best in leads II and V_1, and thus,

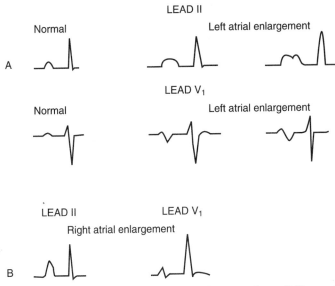

Figure 5–9 □ *A*, Left atrial enlargement: P duration ≥ 3 mm (0.12 second) in lead II; in lead V_1 the negative component of the P wave occupies at least one small box = 1 mm $\times$ 0.04 = P terminal force >0.04 mm/sec (see Fig. 5–10). *B*, Right atrial enlargement: lead II shows P amplitude ≥ 3 mm; in lead V_1, the first half of the P wave is positive and >1 mm wide.

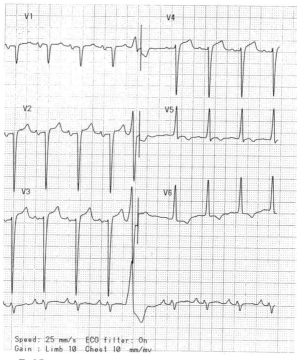

Figure 5–10 □ Left atrial enlargement observed in lead V₁ in a patient with left ventricular hypertrophy.

these two leads are used for rhythm strips and arrhythmia monitoring.

- Notching of a wide P wave in lead II. The distance between peaks of >0.04 second is in keeping with left atrial enlargement.
- Biphasic wave. The P wave in lead V₁ has a dominant negative and wide component (see Figs. 5–9 and 5–10). The depth of the inversion times, the width, represents the P-terminal force; if this is >0.04 mm/sec, it indicates left atrial enlargement.
- Increased amplitude: peaking; tall, pointed P waves, taller in lead III than in lead I. An increased amplitude of ≥3 mm (3 little boxes = 3 mm) in lead II, III, or aVF indicates right atrial enlargement and is not uncommon in patients with right ventricular hypertrophy (RVH), cor pulmonale, pulmonary hypertension, and pulmonary and tricuspid stenosis (see Fig. 5–9).
- Absent P waves. This may occur with SA block and AV junctional rhythms.

Summary.   The P wave results from overlapping right and left atrial depolarization and is a smooth, rounded wave. The total duration of a normal P wave is <0.12 second (3 mm) and its height is usually <3 mm.

■ THE T WAVE

The T wave represents repolarization, the recovery period of the ventricle. Assess the T wave's *direction, shape,* and *amplitude.*

- The T wave should be upright in leads I, II, and V_4 to V_6. The T wave is normally upright in leads aVL and aVF if the QRS is >5 mm tall, but it can be inverted if the R waves are small. The T wave is very variable in lead III.
- The T wave is always inverted in lead aVR (see Fig. 5–2; Fig. 5–11).
- The T wave in lead V_1 is often inverted (see Fig. 5–11). If the T wave is upright in lead V_1, it is usually not as tall as the T wave in lead V_6. In patients with true posterior infarction, the T wave is expected to be upright in leads V_1 and V_2. This finding is not diagnostic but supports the diagnosis of true posterior infarction if it is accompanied by a tall R wave in leads V_1 and V_2 and signs of inferior infarction.
- The T wave in lead II is often upright and in rare cases is flat or diphasic in lead V_3 or in women with the juvenile pattern, and inverted in leads V_1 to V_3.
- Inverted T waves in leads where they are usually upright (leads I, II, aVF, and V_3 to V_6) may occur in several conditions and are a nonspecific finding. The ECG interpretation "nonspecific ST-T wave changes" is a common occurrence.

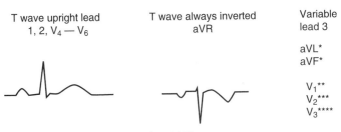

T wave upright lead 1, 2, V_4 — V_6	T wave always inverted aVR	Variable lead 3
		aVL* aVF*
		V_1** V_2*** V_3****

Figure 5–11 □ T wave, normal variability.

*   = usually upright; can be inverted if R wave <5 mm.
**   = inverted in >50% of women, <20% men >age 30.
***   = usually upright; can be inverted with juvenile pattern.
**** = usually upright, rarely flat or disphasic in women or with juvenile pattern.

- Deep T wave inversion without ST segment shifts is not diagnostic but may be associated with myocardial ischemia, post-MI conditions, apical cardiomyopathy, fibrosis, resolving myocarditis or pericarditis, alcohol-abuse electrolyte abnormalities, and other conditions (Figs. 5–12 and 5–13).
- Asymmetric T wave inversion in leads V_5 and V_6 may be observed in left ventricular hypertrophy (LVH) (see discussion under this topic).

■ HEART RATE AND INTERVALS

Heart Rate

If the ECG has markers at 3-second intervals, count the number of QRS complexes in two of these 3-second periods and multiply by 10 (Table 5–2, *top*). For 2½-second markers, multiply by 12. For an alternative method, see Table 5–2, *bottom*.

PR Interval

The PR interval varies from 0.12 to 0.20 second (see Table 5–1); some healthy adults have a PR interval of up to 0.24 second. A prolonged PR interval may be
1. A normal variant
2. Caused by first-degree AV block, due to ischemic heart disease, rheumatic heart disease, or other heart disease
3. Caused by drugs, e.g., digoxin, verapamil, and diltiazem, rarely beta blockers or amiodarone
4. Caused rarely by hyperthyroidism

A short PR interval of <0.12 second may be
1. Caused by low atrial or upper AV junctional rhythms
2. Caused by Wolff-Parkinson-White (WPW) syndrome
3. A normal variant
4. Caused by accelerated AV conduction
5. Caused by pheochromocytoma
6. Caused by glycogen storage disease
7. Caused by Fabry's disease

QRS Duration

This is usually 0.04 to 0.10 second (> one square, < three squares measured in the limb leads). A QRS duration of >0.10 second denotes an intraventricular conduction delay in the left or right bundle branches. The presence of a delta wave in WPW syndrome may increase the QRS duration. Table 5–1 gives a summary of important normal intervals and parameters.

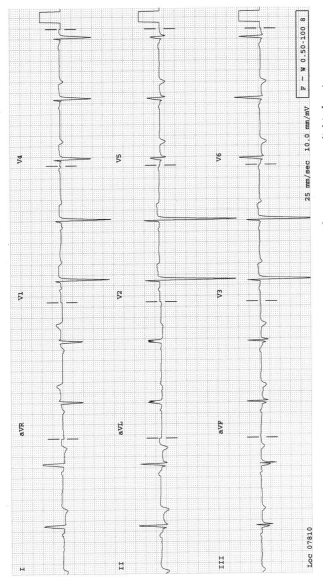

Figure 5–12 □ Abnormal T wave inversion in a patient with proven myocardial ischemia.

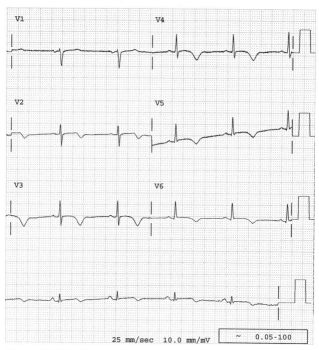

Figure 5–13 □ T wave inversion; probable anterolateral ischemia.

QT Interval

The QT interval should be less than one-half the preceding RR interval at heart rates of 60 to 100 beats/min. The QT interval varies with heart rate, and several formulas have been used to provide a corrected QT interval (QTc interval). The QTc interval also has limitations because of difficulties with exact measurement. Because it is sometimes difficult to define the end of the T wave, the measurement is often inaccurate, in particular when a U wave merges with the T wave. Thus, in clinical practice the QT interval should be assessed mainly for excessive prolongation; see Table 5–1 for a clinically useful approximation of QT intervals.

The QT interval indicates the total duration of ventricular systole. A prolonged QT interval represents delayed repolarization of the ventricles and predisposes to reentrant arrhythmias. Torsades de pointes may occur in patients with a long QT interval (see later discussion under Torsades de Pointes).

Causes of Prolonged QT Interval
1. Drugs, such as class 1 antiarrhythmics—disopyramide, quinidine, and procainamide; class 3 antiarrhythmics—

Table 5–2 □ DETERMINATION OF HEART RATE

Method One

Number of QRS Complexes in 6 Seconds*	Heart Rate per Minute
5 × 10	50
6	60
7	70
10	100
15	150
20	200

Method Two

Count Number of Large Squares (Bold Boxes in One RR Interval)	Heart Rate per Minute
1†	300
1.5	200
2	150
3	100
4	75
5	60
6	50
7	42
8	38
9	33
10	30

*If the ECG paper has markers at 3-second intervals, count the number of QRS complexes in two of these 3-second periods and multiply by 10. For markers at 2½-second intervals, multiply by 12.

†Normal paper speed 25 mm/sec. One large box or 5 small squares = 300/min.

For regular rhythm: start with a complex that lies on a bold vertical grid line.

Rate = 300 ÷ number of large boxes (fifths of a second). Normal rate between 60–100/min = 3–5 large squares; therefore, no need to calculate exact rate.

or rate = 1500 ÷ number of small (1-mm) squares

amiodarone and sotalol; tricyclic antidepressants—phenothiazines, astemizole, and other histamine H_1 antagonists
2. Ischemic heart disease
3. Cerebrovascular disease
4. Rheumatic fever
5. Myocarditis
6. Mitral valve prolapse (MVP)
7. Electrolyte abnormalities
8. Hypothyroidism
9. Liquid protein diets
10. Congenital prolonged QT syndrome

Causes of Short QT Interval. A short QT interval is not of great concern and occurs rarely with the following:

1. Hypercalcemia (a feature of malignancy and hyperparathyroidism)
2. Hyperkalemia
3. Digitalis intoxication

■ BUNDLE BRANCH BLOCK

The genesis of the QRS complex has been described earlier in this chapter. A clear understanding of the genesis of the QRS complex is the basis of a sound appreciation of the ECG pattern in RBBB and LBBB.

Right Bundle Branch Block

In RBBB, the initial impulse depolarizes the septum normally from left to right. Thus, vector I remains intact; the impulse traveling toward the lead V_1 electrode registers an initial r wave in leads V_1 and V_2 (Fig. 5–14). Because the right bundle branch does not conduct the electrical impulse, vector II traverses leftward and activates the LV and registers an S wave in lead V_1 or V_2. Because right ventricular depolarization occurs late, unopposed by left ventricular activation, the resultant force, vector III, produces a large R wave, termed R', in lead V_1 or V_2. The deflection of the R' wave may be greater than the amplitude of the small r wave produced by vector I septal depolarization. This unopposed late activation of the right ventricle produces the R' wave in lead V_1 or V_2 and is recorded as a slurred S wave by the electrodes facing the left ventricular free wall (leads V_5, V_6, and I) (see Fig. 5–14; Figs. 5–15 and 5–16).

The QRS complexes in leads V_1 and V_2 are therefore typically M-shaped. The QRS complexes vary in morphology, i.e., rsR', RSR', and Rsr'. The QRS duration is increased to 0.11 second or more.

Causes of RBBB

1. Normal variant in the heart of young adults
2. Coronary artery disease
3. Hypertension
4. Rheumatic heart disease
5. Congenital heart disease, in particular in association with atrial septal defect (ASD), ventricular septal defect (VSD), and Fallot's tetralogy (in secundum ASD, >90% of individuals have incomplete RBBB; see Fig. 5–16).
6. Pericarditis or myocarditis
7. Pulmonary embolism

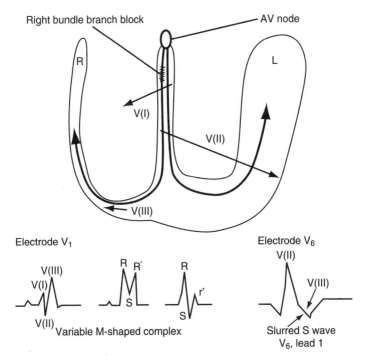

Figure 5-14 □ The contribution of vectors I, II, and III [labeled V(I), V(II), and V(III)] to the genesis of right bundle branch block.

8. Cor pulmonale
9. Cardiomyopathy
10. Chagas' disease
11. Endomyocardial fibrosis
12. Other conditions

The diagnosis of acute MI in the presence of RBBB is sometimes difficult but often can be made. In patients with acute anterior infarction, pathologic Q waves develop in leads V_1, V_2, V_3, and V_4; inferior infarction should be considered only if there are abnormal Q waves in leads II, III, and aVF. Q waves in leads III and aVF are not diagnostic. Because the right bundle branch and the interventricular septum share the same blood supply, an anteroseptal infarct may be associated with RBBB. RBBB can be associated with a normal axis or with right or left axis deviation. A common association is left anterior fascicular block (see later discussion).

Incomplete RBBB is not uncommon; patients with a secundum ASD commonly show incomplete RBBB (see Fig. 5-16); note the

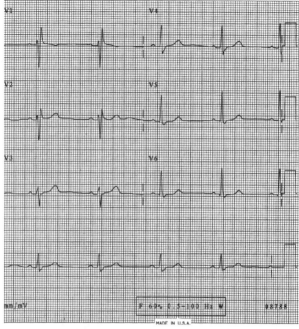

Figure 5–15 □ ECG shows right bundle branch block: M-shaped complex in lead V_1, slurred S in lead V_6.

RSr' in V_1 and slurred S wave in leads I, V_5, and V_6. The QRS duration should be 0.09 to 0.10 second. The incidence of RBBB is similar to that of LBBB.

Approximately 5% of normal individuals show an RSr' in lead V_1 or V_2. If the QRS duration is ≥0.08 second, accompanied by a slurred S wave in lead I and lead V_5 or V_6, a diagnosis of incomplete RBBB is made. In the absence of a slurred S wave and a QRS duration of <0.08 second, a diagnosis of RSr' is made as an observation.

CAUSES OF RSr' VARIANT
1. None—Approximately 5% of normal individuals show an RSR' or RSr'
2. Recording artifacts
3. Chest deformities, e.g., straight back syndrome and pectus excavatum (R' is usually small)
4. Congenital heart disease, i.e., ASD and rarely VSD and coarctation of the aorta
5. Acquired heart disease, e.g., mitral stenosis
6. Right ventricular hypertrophy

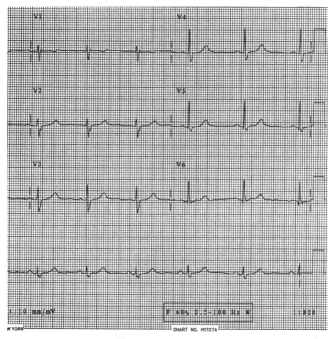

Figure 5–16 □ Incomplete right bundle branch block: Rsr' complex in lead V_1, slurred S in leads V_5 and V_6 in a 45-year-old woman with a large secundum atrial septal defect. This ECG postsurgical correction is similar to that recorded 2 years earlier.

7. Right ventricular diastolic or volume overload
8. Cor pulmonale
9. Pulmonary embolism
10. WPW syndrome
11. AV nodal reentrant tachycardia (AVNRT); a pseudo-S wave should be present in leads II, III, and aVF (see discussion under Atrioventricular Nodal Reentrant Tachycardia)
12. Duchenne's muscular dystrophy
13. A secondary R wave, which may occur due to late activation of the outflow tract of the right ventricle, i.e., the crista supraventricularis (see Fig. 5–3)

Whereas an RSR' pattern is observed in approximately 5% of normal individuals, incomplete RBBB occurs in <1%, and about 1% of these cases of incomplete RBBB progress to complete RBBB.

Left Bundle Branch Block

Activation of the LV is delayed; the QRS duration is ≥0.12 second, and the septum and LV are depolarized by the impulse from the right bundle. The normal direction of septal activation from left to right is reversed (see Fig. 5–3). Vector I flows from right to left through the lower septum. Therefore, an electrode over the LV causes an R wave in leads V_6 and I and a QS wave in lead V_1 (Figs. 5–17 and 5–18). Vector II travels from left to right through the right ventricular mass and may create a slur or notch in the R wave of lead V_6, marked "vector II" in Figure 5–17. Vector III travels right to left and causes an R' wave in lead V_6 (marked "III" in Figure 5–17). The notched R and R' waves may result in an M-shaped complex in lead I, V_5, or V_6 (see Figs. 5–17 and 5–18; Fig. 5–19).

In leads facing the right ventricle, e.g., in lead V_1, vectors I, II, and III usually cause a QS complex. In <50% of cases of LBBB, there is a small r wave in V_1, because right ventricular activation occurs more rapidly than septal activation (see Fig. 5–18); occasionally, the small r wave may be due to septal depolarization from left to right from a branch of the left bundle proximal to the block in the main left bundle branch.

Because of altered depolarization, the ST segment in leads V_1

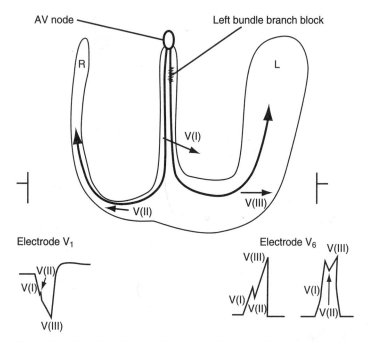

Figure 5–17 □ Contribution of vectors I, II, and III [labeled V(I), V(II), and V(III)] to the genesis of left bundle branch block.

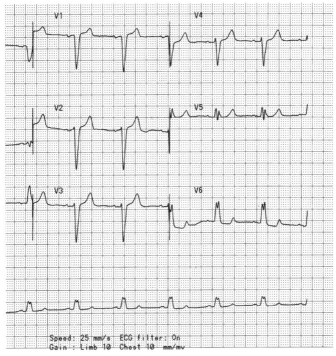

Figure 5–18 □ Left bundle branch block: QRS >0.12; poor R wave progression in leads V_1 to V_5; ST elevation, R wave notched in lead V_6.

to V_4 is commonly elevated and the ST and T waves are opposite in direction to the terminal QRS direction.

Because LBBB causes a derangement of normal vector forces, the diagnosis of LVH cannot be made; the ST elevation and poor R wave progression do not indicate myocardial injury or infarction, and the diagnosis of MI in the presence of LBBB is difficult (see later discussion).

LBBB can occur in normal hearts, but it is commonly caused by LVH and occurs in patients with coronary heart disease (CHD), cardiomyopathies, and degenerative diseases. Patients with CHD and LBBB have a high incidence of LV dysfunction and congestive heart failure (CHF). Rarely, no organic disease exists and prognosis is favorable. The diagnosis of acute MI in the presence of RBBB and LBBB is discussed later under Acute Myocardial Infarction.

■ FASCICULAR BLOCK (HEMIBLOCK)

The left bundle branch divides into anterior and posterior fascicles. The anterior fascicle takes an anterosuperior course and

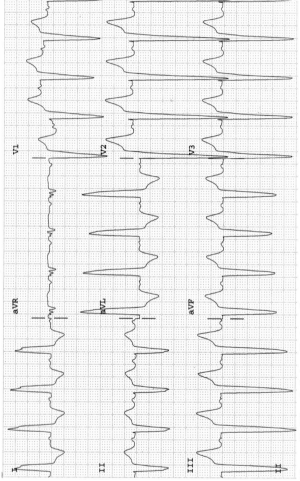

Figure 5-19 □ Left bundle branch block: QRS ≥ 0.12; R is notched in lead I, poor R wave progression and deep S in leads V₁ to V₃ with ST elevation typical of left bundle branch block; simulates infarction and left ventricular hypertrophy.

terminates at the base of the anterior papillary muscle (Fig. 5–20). Because the anterior fascicle is thin and long and has a single blood supply, it is commonly damaged, resulting in left anterior fascicular block (LAFB) or, as Rosenbaum initially called the block, *left anterior hemiblock* (LAH). LAFB is not uncommon and was observed in approximately 1.5% of a series of 8000 men, aged 45 to 69 years. The posterior fascicle is thick and short, has a double blood supply, runs inferiorly toward the base of the posterior papillary muscle, and is not commonly damaged. Thus, left posterior fascicular block is rare, and the ECG criteria are inaccurate for this diagnosis.

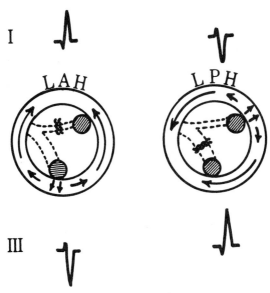

Figure 5–20 □ Diagrams illustrating the hemiblock pattern in the limb leads: left anterior hemiblock (LAH) and left posterior hemiblock (LPH). The "anterior" papillary muscle is above and lateral to the "posterior" papillary muscle, and the two divisions of the left bundle branch course toward their respective papillary muscles. Thus, if the anterior division is blocked, initial electromotive forces are directed downward and to the right, inscribing a small q wave in leads I and aVL and a small r wave in leads II, III, and aVF. The subsequent forces are directed mainly upward and to the left, writing an R wave in leads I and aVL and an S wave in leads II, III, and aVF, to produce a left axis deviation. In LPH, the initial forces spread upward and to the left, writing a small R wave in leads I and aVL and a small q wave in leads II, III, and aVF, and subsequent forces are directed downward and to the right to produce right axis deviation. (From Marriott HJL: Practical Electrocardiography, 8th ed. Baltimore, Williams & Wilkins, 1988, p 90.)

Left Anterior Fascicular Block (Hemiblock).   Block of the anterior fascicle causes activation to proceed from the posterior papillary muscle and inferior wall (see Fig. 5–20). Because the entire left ventricular muscle mass is above, the activating impulse is directed upward to the left. Thus, a left axis of −45 to −90 degrees must be present to consider the diagnosis of LAFB. The impulse from the posterior papillary muscle travels initially downward from the endocardium to the epicardium; this is a small force and registers a small r wave of <4 mm in lead III. This small impulse produces a small q wave in lead I. The activating impulse then travels upward and to the left, causing an R wave in lead I (Fig. 5–21); an S wave is recorded in lead III, because the wave of excitation is traveling away from the inferior lead.

CRITERIA FOR THE DIAGNOSIS OF LAFB (HEMIBLOCK)

- A left axis deviation of −45 to −90 degrees (an axis of −40 degrees is insufficient to make the diagnosis)
- A small q wave, 1 to 4 mm deep in lead I

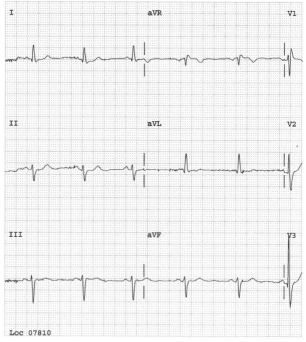

Loc 07810

Figure 5–21 □ Left anterior fascicular block (hemiblock): left axis, small q wave in lead I, small r wave in lead III.

- A small r wave, 1 to 4 mm tall in lead III (see Fig. 5–21)
- A normal QRS duration, provided that RBBB is absent

Because other fascicles conduct normally, the sequence of activation of the heart muscle is not delayed and the QRS duration remains within normal limits. LAFB lowers the QRS voltage in the left-side chest leads and may mask the findings of LVH.

LAFB and RBBB, i.e., bifascicular block, is a common occurrence (Fig. 5–22). This diagnosis does not indicate an unfavorable prognosis. Because the diagnosis of LAFB is commonly made, the clinician needs to know its significance and causes.

CAUSES OF LAFB (HEMIBLOCK)

1. Acute or previous MI. LAFB in the clinical setting of acute MI rarely progresses to serious heart block, and temporary or permanent pacing is not required. When LAFB is associated with RBBB, progression to more severe heart block is rare in the presence of acute infarction. When LAFB occurs during inferior infarction, the initial small r wave produced by LAFB in lead III may mask the Q wave of infarction
2. Ischemic heart disease without infarction (which is the most common cause)
3. Cardiomyopathy
4. Chagas' disease (which commonly causes LAFB and RBBB)

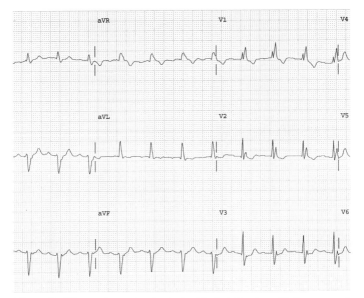

Figure 5–22 □ Left anterior fascicular block: left axis, −90-degree small q wave in lead I, small r wave in lead III, and commonly associated right bundle branch block.

Left Posterior Fascicular Block (LPFB). Left posterior fascicular block or *left posterior hemiblock (LPH)* is uncommon, because the posterior fascicle is short and thick and has a double supply. Because the criteria for the diagnosis of LPFB are based on very inaccurate parameters, it is wise not to consider making this diagnosis. The diagnosis should not be entertained unless RVH and cor pulmonale can be confidently excluded.

CRITERIA FOR THE DIAGNOSIS OF **LPFB**

- A right axis deviation, usually +120 to +180 degrees
- A small r wave (<5 mm) in lead I and a small q wave in leads III and aVF
- A normal QRS duration
- Exclusion of RVH and cor pulmonale before considering the diagnosis of LPFB

Trifascicular Block. Trifascicular block can be assumed to occur if RBBB plus LAFB and first- or second-degree AV block are present.

■ LEFT VENTRICULAR HYPERTROPHY

The ECG is an important and inexpensive tool for the diagnosis of LVH (refer to the earlier section, Genesis of the QRS Complex; see Fig. 5–3). Vector II is responsible for the S wave in leads V_1 and V_2 and the R wave in leads V_5 and V_6 (Fig. 5–23). The activating impulse must traverse the large muscle mass of the hypertrophied LV, and thus, the S wave in leads V_1 and V_2 is deep and the R wave in leads V_5 and V_6 is tall (Figs. 5–24, 5–25, and 5–26).

In LVH, the left atrium becomes hypertrophied to assist the decreased compliance of the compromised LV. Thus, left atrial enlargement is an early ECG sign of LVH.

ECG Criteria for the Diagnosis of LVH

1. The Sokolow/Lyon criterion for LVH is as follows:
   - An S wave in lead V_1 or V_2 plus an R wave in lead V_5 or V_6 of >35 mm; specificity = 98%, sensitivity = 25% (see Figs. 5–24, 5–25, and 5–26)
2. The Romhilt/Estes scoring system is as follows:
   - An R wave in limb leads of >20 mm, an S wave in lead V_1 or V_2 of >30 mm, or an R wave in lead V_5 or V_6 of >30 mm = 3 points
   - A P-terminal force in lead V_1 of ≥0.04 mm/sec = 3 points
   - ST-T wave changes (if not taking digoxin) = 3 points (taking digoxin = 1 point)
   - A left axis = 2 points
   - A score of 4 points indicates probable LVH and a score of

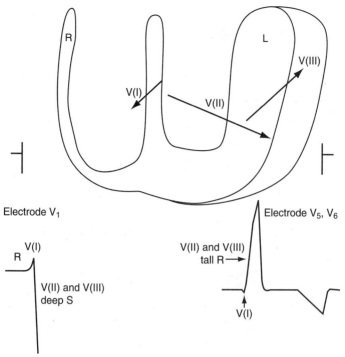

Figure 5–23 □ The contribution of vector II to the ECG features of left ventricular hypertrophy. The thicker the left ventricular muscle, the greater the magnitude of vector II, and therefore, the deep S in lead V_1, and tall R wave in leads V_5 and V_6. Note that the T wave has a gradual descending and a steep ascending limb "strain pattern."

      5 or more points indicates LVH; specificity = 94%, sensitivity = 32%

3. The Cornell voltage criteria are as follows:
  - An S wave in lead V_3 plus an R wave in lead aVL of >28 mm (men) or of ≥20 mm (women); specificity = 96%, sensitivity = 42% (see Figs. 5–24, 5–25, and 5–26)

4. Because the ECG criteria are not sufficiently sensitive at only <42%, I prefer the following:
  - An S wave in lead V_1 or V_2 plus an R wave in lead V_5 or V_6 of ≥35 mm = 1 point
  - An R wave in lead aVL and an S wave in lead V_3 of >24 mm (men) or >18 mm (women) = 1 point = LVH
  - The presence of left atrial enlargement and an ST-T wave "strain pattern" in lead V_5 or V_6 increases the specificity and sensitivity and indicates LVH if the voltage is border-

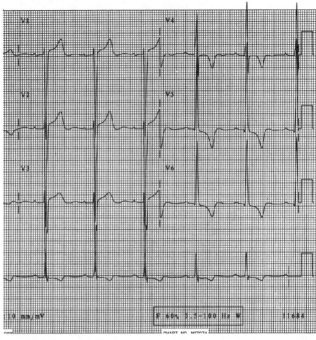

Figure 5–24 □ ECG from a 73-year-old man. S V_1 + R V_6 >35 mm, R aVL + S V_3 >28 mm, and "strain" pattern in V_4 to V_6: left ventricular hypertrophy.

line. ST-T wave changes occur in leads I, aVL, V_5, and V_6. The asymmetric ST-T change should be present in leads V_5 and V_6 and to a lesser degree in lead V_4 (see Figs. 5–25 and 5–26); if these changes are more prominent in leads V_3 and V_4, ischemia should be suspected. The ST-T changes have been termed left ventricular strain, but most cardiologists agree that this change is part of LVH.

Left axis deviation may be present in some cases, but it is not necessary for the diagnosis of LVH. The diagnosis of RVH, however, requires the presence of right axis deviation.

Causes of LVH
1. Hypertension
2. Aortic stenosis and other valvular heart disease
3. Ischemic heart disease
4. Cardiomyopathy
5. Other conditions

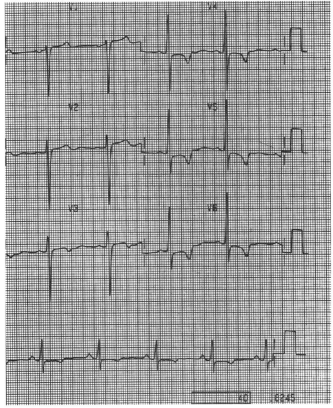

Figure 5-25 □ ECG features typical of left ventricular hypertrophy.

■ RIGHT VENTRICULAR HYPERTROPHY

ECG Criteria for the Diagnosis of RVH. In the absence of RBBB, or absence of anteroseptal and anterolateral MI, the ECG hallmarks of RVH include

1. Right axis deviation of ≥110 degrees; if right axis deviation is absent, consider alternative diagnoses
2. A tall R wave in lead V_1 of ≥7 mm in individuals older than 30 years. The small, normal r wave in lead V_1 usually measures 1 to 4 mm and is caused by vector I. With RVH, vector II is directed to the right and inscribes a tall R wave in lead V_1 and a deep S wave in lead V_6 (Fig. 5-27; see variations of RVH patterns in leads V_1 and V_6).
3. An S wave in lead V_5 or V_6 of ≥7 mm

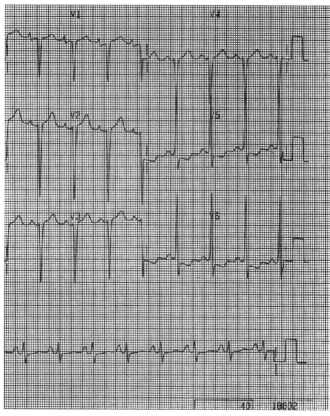

Figure 5–26 □ Left ventricular hypertrophy; left atrial enlargement is frequently present (see Figs. 5–9 and 5–10).

4. An R wave in lead V_1 plus an S wave in lead V_5 or V_6 of >9 mm
5. An R/S ratio in lead V_1 of ≥1 or an R/S ratio in lead V_6 of ≤1 (see Fig. 5–27) (any two of the above criteria indicate RVH; RVH may be well advanced before ECG changes occur)
6. An ST-T strain pattern in leads V_1 to V_3, which may be present and increases the specificity of the ECG criteria
7. Right atrial enlargement, which increases the probability of RVH
8. An S_1, S_2, and S_3 pattern (especially in children)
9. A small q wave in lead V_1. Because the normal location of the septum may be altered by the right ventricular mass, the

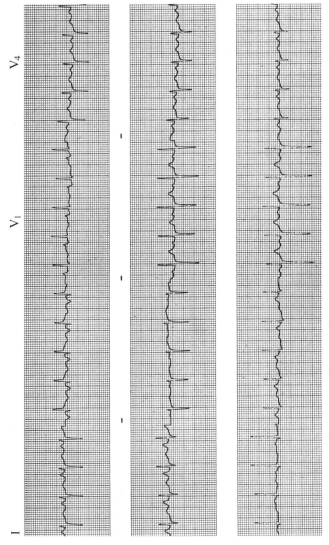

Figure 5-27 □ Right ventricular hypertrophy in a 42-year-old man. Tall R wave in $V_1 \geq 7$ mm; R/S ratio in V_6 ≤ 1; right axis deviation.

initial force that depolarizes the septum (vector I) may be directed from right to left, and thus, a small q wave in lead V_1 may occur, in particular in patients with congenital heart disease and marked RVH

If the QRS duration is ≥0.11 second with a tall R wave in lead V_1, a diagnosis of RBBB or WPW syndrome should be considered. A diagnosis of RVH should not be made in the presence of RBBB or WPW syndrome.

CAUSES OF A TALL R WAVE IN LEAD V_1
1. A normal finding in children
2. RBBB
3. WPW syndrome
4. True posterior infarction
5. Hypertrophic cardiomyopathy
6. Duchenne's muscular dystrophy

Causes of RVH.   These include the following:
1. Congenital heart disease, in particular tetralogy of Fallot and pulmonary stenosis
2. Mitral stenosis
3. Emphysema
4. Recurrent pulmonary embolism
5. Other causes of pulmonary hypertension

■ ACUTE MYOCARDIAL INFARCTION

A rapid, accurate interpretation of the ECG to confirm the clinical suspicion of acute MI is necessary for implementing life-saving therapeutic measures, in particular urgent administration of aspirin and thrombolytic therapy. Despite the advent of expensive and sophisticated cardiologic tests, such as CK-MB, the ECG remains the most reliable and inexpensive tool for the confirmation of acute MI. Thus, it is of paramount importance for trainees to learn to correctly interpret the ECG. Early ECG diagnosis is often made before the development of Q waves or at the stage of evolving Q waves.

Several textbooks on ECG still teach that
- ST segment elevation = current of injury
- Q waves = necrosis = infarction
- ST segment depression = ischemia

These terms are accurate but are inappropriate for early diagnosis of acute infarction. Practices in cardiology have changed drastically, and the following criteria have been accepted internationally.

Diagnosis of Acute MI. In patients presenting with acute onset of chest discomfort, diagnosis of acute MI is based on the following ECG findings:

1. An ST segment elevation of ≥1 mm in two or more contiguous limb leads is diagnostic (Fig. 5–28).
2. An ST segment elevation of ≥1 mm in two or more contiguous precordial leads indicates anterior infarction (Fig. 5–29); abnormal ST elevation in two or more leads has a specificity of 92% for the diagnosis of acute MI; sensitivity increases with the observation of serial ECGs taken every 30 minutes.
3. Abnormal Q waves may not be present on the initial tracing. Patients with diagnostic ST segment elevation are classified as having probable Q wave infarction; Q waves may manifest as early as 2 hours or as late as 12 hours from onset of symptoms and therefore cannot be relied on for early diagnosis.
4. ST elevation and emerging Q waves in two or more leads in patients with acute chest discomfort is diagnostic of acute

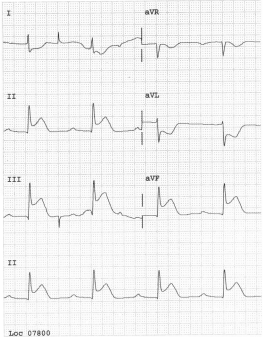

Figure 5–28 □ Acute inferior myocardial infarction: ST elevation in inferior leads; note reciprocal depression in leads I and aVL.

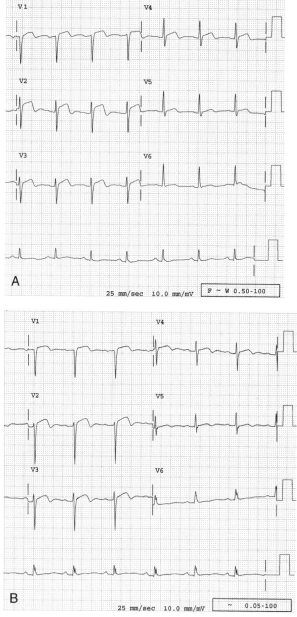

Figure 5–29 □ *A,* Acute anterior myocardial infarction: ST elevation in leads V_1 to V_4. *B,* Acute anterior infarction: same patient as in *A,* 8 hours later.

coronary thrombotic occlusion in >90% of patients; infarction with ST segment elevation and Q waves are shown in Figure 5–30.

5. *Reciprocal depression* in leads opposite to those depicting ST elevation provides important support to confirm the diagnosis (though not in itself diagnostic) (see Fig. 5–28; Fig. 5–31).

6. Evolutionary changes occur over the next 6 to 24 hours; i.e., ST segment elevation recedes, Q waves may become more apparent, and T wave inversion occurs; T wave inversion occurs more rapidly with inferior infarction than with anterior infarction; in some patients, evolutionary changes are delayed over 2 to 3 days.

7. If the initial ECG is nondiagnostic, the ECG should be repeated every 30 minutes for 2 hours to verify changes consistent with the diagnosis of infarction or noninfarction.

8. ST segment depression and positive CK-MB indicate probable MI, now termed non–ST segment elevation MI (the terms "transmural" and "nontransmural" infarction are obsolete) (see page 171).

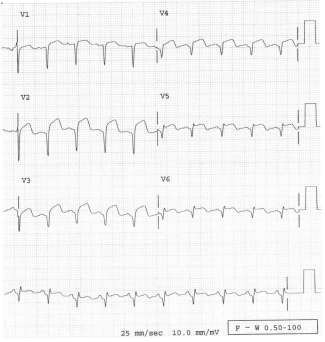

25 mm/sec   10.0 mm/mV   F ~ W 0.50-100

Figure 5–30 □ Acute anterior infarction: marked ST elevation and Q waves in leads V_1 to V_6.

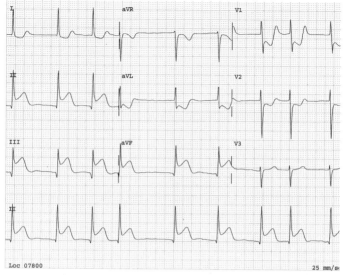

Figure 5–31 □ Acute inferior myocardial infarction: ST elevation in leads II, III, and aVF. Note reciprocal depression in leads V₁, V₂, and aVL.

Because the ECG is the only tool available for rapid diagnosis of acute MI, and because ECG findings are not always diagnostic, it is important to assess the following:

- That the clinical presentation is in keeping with acute MI
- That the several causes of ST elevation that can mimic infarction have been excluded; the presence of reciprocal depression in leads opposite to those depicting ST elevation is not diagnostic but provides important support confirming the diagnosis.

Mimics of Acute Myocardial Infarction

- Acute pericarditis. The ST elevation is not confined to an anatomic coronary blood supply. ST segment elevation occurs in leads I, II, III, and aVF and in the precordial leads. The ST segment elevation is concave, as opposed to convex and upward with infarction (Fig. 5–32).
- So-called early repolarization changes. ST elevation occurs commonly as a normal variant in blacks and some other ethnic groups. The ST segment is commonly elevated in leads V₂, V₃, V₄, and V₅, or in leads II, III, and aVF. ST elevation in the V leads often shows a notched J-point fishhook appearance (see Fig. 5–8; Figs. 5–33 through 5–37). The ST segment

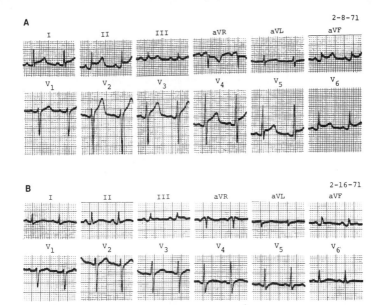

3210   35M

Figure 5–32 □ Serial changes of acute idiopathic pericarditis in a 36-year-old man. *A*, Diffuse ST segment elevation involving all the leads except aVR and aVL. In lead aVR, the ST segment is depressed. The QRS complex is normal. *B*, The ST segment is almost isoelectric, and the T waves are flattened or notched. (From Chou T-C: Electrocardiography in Clinical Practice, 4th ed. Philadelphia, WB Saunders Co., 1996, p 241.)

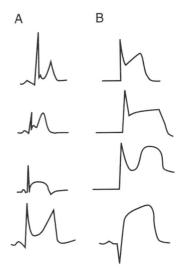

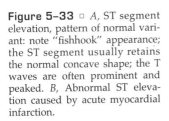

Figure 5–33 □ *A*, ST segment elevation, pattern of normal variant: note "fishhook" appearance; the ST segment usually retains the normal concave shape; the T waves are often prominent and peaked. *B*, Abnormal ST elevation caused by acute myocardial infarction.

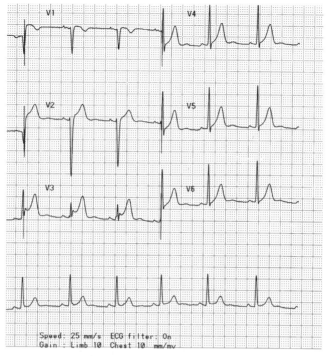

Figure 5–34 □ ECG of a 34-year-old Hispanic man with ST segment elevation with notched J-point "fishhook" in lead V₃.

elevation is usually concave, rather than convex; emergent Q waves and reciprocal depression are absent; the T waves are often peaked and prominent.

- ST elevation caused by left ventricular aneurysm and previous infarction
- LVH, causing poor R wave progression in leads V₁ to V₃ and ST elevation (see Fig. 5–26; Fig. 5–38)
- Acute myocarditis, usually causing nonspecific ST-T wave changes. Cases have been reported, however, with ST segment elevation and Q waves simulating infarction. Chagasic myocarditis should be considered in Hispanic individuals who present with chest pain. In these individuals, ST elevation and Q waves may occur due to **Chagas' disease.** *Reciprocal ST depression* is not a feature, but T wave changes occur and serve to distinguish acute MI.
- Prinzmetal's angina. The ECGs of individuals with coronary artery spasm show ST segment elevation during pain. This situation is rare; pain responds to nitroglycerin, and the ST

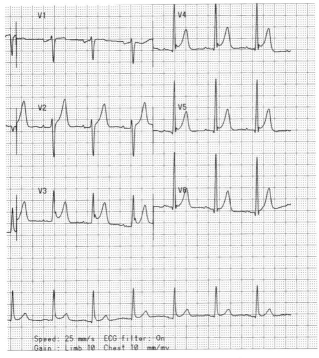

Figure 5–35 □ ECG of a 50-year-old man seen in the emergency room for chest pain. ST elevation in leads V₃ and V₅: note prominent T wave and normal concave ST segment; normal variant.

segment returns to normal. In all patients presenting with atypical features of acute MI, nitroglycerin should be administered before treating with thrombolytic therapy.
- Hyperkalemia or hypothermia, which may cause ST elevation, simulating acute infarction

Infarction Location

- Inferior infarction. Inferior infarction occurs commonly and is identified by ST segment elevation and emerging Q waves in leads II, III, and aVF and reciprocal depression in leads V₁ and V₂ (see Figs. 5–28 and 5–31). Reciprocal depression may not be observed in all cases. Either the right coronary or the circumflex artery is occluded acutely, resulting in a small area of infarction with a good prognosis. Occasionally, inferior infarction occurs in association with infarction of the posterior wall.

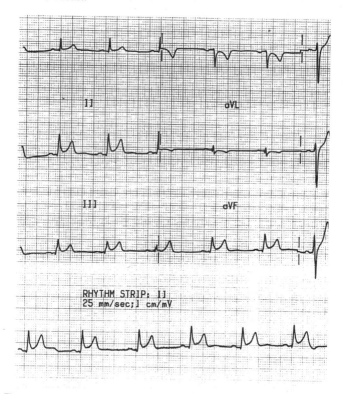

Figure 5–36 □ ECG of a 30-year-old man: concave ST elevation in leads II, III, and aVF; normal variant.

- True posterior infarction. Tall R waves occur in leads V_1 and V_2, because a loss of activation to the posterior wall causes the vector forces to be directed anteriorly (Fig. 5–39). The causes of tall R waves in lead V_1 are given in Table 5–3. The T wave should be upright in leads V_1 and V_2; ST depression occurs in leads V_1 and V_2.
- Anteroseptal infarction. Anteroseptal infarction is indicated by ST segment elevation and Q waves in leads V_1 to V_3 (see Fig. 5–6; Fig. 5–40).
- Anterior MI. Leads V_1 to V_5 (see Figs. 5–29 and 5–30, MI age indeterminate; Fig. 5–41).
- Anterolateral infarction. Leads V_4, V_6, I, and aVL (Fig. 5–42).
- Right ventricular infarction. Right ventricular infarction is indicated by ST segment elevation in leads V_3R and V_4R (Fig. 5–43). This is usually associated with inferior infarction or inferoposterior infarction. The prognosis is worse in patients

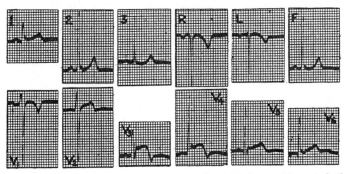

Figure 5–37 □ ECG from a normal 24-year-old black man. Note marked ST elevation and T wave inversion in leads V_3 and V_4. (From Marriott HJL: Practical Electrocardiography, 8th ed. Baltimore, Williams & Wilkins, 1988, p 465.)

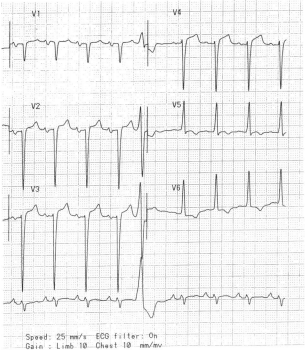

Figure 5–38 □ Poor R wave progression in leads V_1 to V_4 and ST elevation caused by left ventricular hypertrophy; note left atrial enlargement, a common feature of left ventricular hypertrophy.

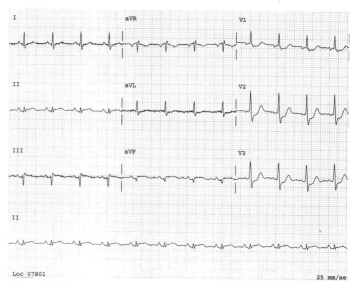

Figure 5–39 □ Inferoposterior infarction. Tall R wave in V_1 and V_2, T wave upright in V_1 and V_2, in association with inferior infarction, and absence of other causes for tall R wave in V_1 and V_2. (From Khan, M Gabriel: Heart Disease Diagnosis and Therapy: A Practical Approach. Baltimore, Williams & Wilkins, 1996, p 11.)

who have inferior infarction complicated with right ventricular infarction. Because therapy is different for patients with inferior as opposed to right ventricular infarction, it is important to include leads V_3R and V_4R in all patients presenting with complicated inferior infarction. The ST elevation in leads V_3R and V_4R may manifest only in the early hours of infarction.

Table 5–3 □ CAUSES OF TALL R WAVES IN LEADS V_1 AND V_2

1. Thin chest wall or normal variant
2. Right bundle branch block
   Note: Slurred S wave in leads I, V_5, and V_6
3. Right ventricular hypertrophy
4. Wolff-Parkinson-White syndrome
5. True posterior infarction
   Note: Associated inferior myocardial infarction and no slurred S wave in leads V_5 and V_6, T wave upright in leads V_1 and V_2
6. Hypertrophic cardiomyopathy
7. Duchenne's muscular dystrophy
8. Low placement of leads V_1 and V_2

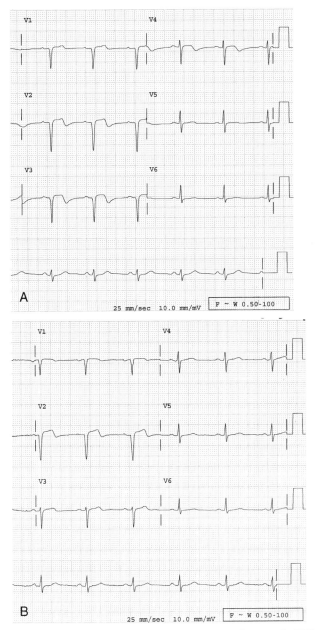

Figure 5–40 □ *A*, Acute anteroseptal myocardial infarction. *B*, ECG of patient shown in *A*, 12 hours later.

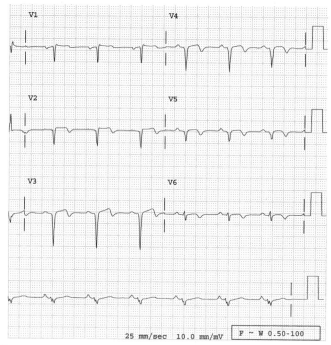

Figure 5–41 □ Q wave in leads V_1 to V_4 with ST abnormalities: correctly reported as anterior infarction, age indeterminate, a term that emphasizes the need for comparison. This ECG is similar to a tracing done 2 years earlier.

- Extensive infarction. Extensive infarction is denoted by ST segment elevation in at least eight leads (Fig. 5–44). A large infarction is reflected by changes in six or seven leads, a moderate-sized infarction by changes in four or five leads, and a small infarction by changes in two or three leads.

■ INFARCTION WITH RBBB

The diagnosis of acute MI in the presence of RBBB can present difficulties. RBBB may produce Q waves in the absence of infarction. The following guidelines should be used:

- RBBB can cause Q waves in leads III and aVF; therefore, the diagnosis of inferior MI should be made only in the presence of significant Q waves in leads II, III, and aVF.
- RBBB may produce Q waves in leads V_1 and V_2; therefore,

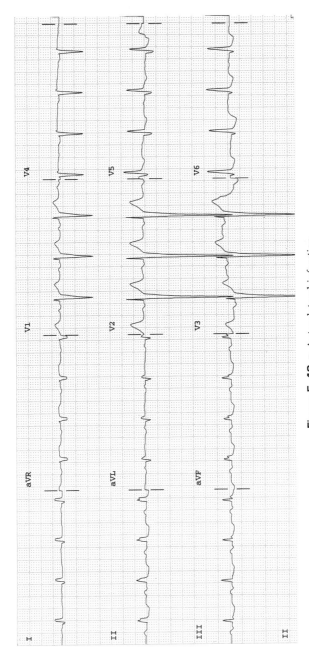

Figure 5-42 □ Anterolateral infarction.

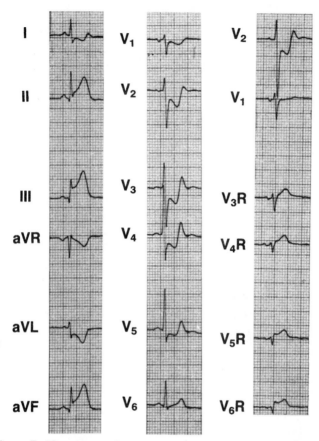

Figure 5–43 □ Acute inferoposterior wall myocardial infarction and right ventricular infarction. Note the elevated ST segment in lead V₄R, indicating an occlusion in the proximal right coronary artery and right ventricular involvement. (From Wellens HJJ, Conover MB: The ECG in Emergency Decision Making. Philadelphia, WB Saunders Co., 1992, p 8.)

the diagnosis of infarction can be made if Q waves are present in precordial leads beyond V_2.

- Uncomplicated RBBB may be associated with ST segment depression and T wave inversion in leads with an RSR′ complex in the absence of ischemia.

■ INFARCTION WITH LBBB

LBBB alters the normal vector forces and causes a marked derangement of the ECG (see Figs. 5–17, 5–18, and 5–19). In most

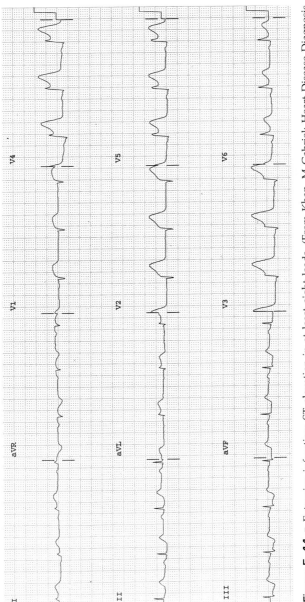

Figure 5–44 □ Extensive infarction: ST elevation in at least eight leads. (From Khan, M Gabriel: Heart Disease Diagnosis and Therapy: A Practical Approach. Baltimore, Williams & Wilkins, 1996, p 9.)

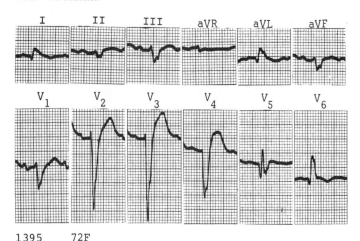

1395   72F

Figure 5–45 □ Complete left bundle branch block with myocardial infarction proved by autopsy. The ECG diagnosis of myocardial infarction is based on the Q waves in leads I, aVL, V_5, and V_6. An autopsy was performed 10 days later and showed severe generalized coronary atherosclerosis with total occlusion of the left circumflex artery. There was an extensive recent lateral wall myocardial infarction in addition to a previous one. Left ventricular hypertrophy also was present. (From Chou T-C: Electrocardiography in Clinical Practice, 4th ed. Philadelphia, WB Saunders Co., 1996, p 181.)

patients a diagnosis of acute or previous infarction cannot be made from the ECG findings. With LBBB, ST segment elevation commonly occurs in leads V_1 to V_4; also, small r waves with poor progression in leads V_1 to V_4 or a QS complex in leads V_1 and V_2 with ST elevation may incorrectly suggest the diagnosis of anteroseptal or anterior infarction. Several cardiology textbooks outline criteria for the diagnosis of acute MI in the presence of LBBB. These guidelines are, unfortunately, misleading and are not supported by the scientific literature. Acute chest pain and the presence of LBBB with Q waves in leads I, aVL, V_5, and V_6 may be caused by anterolateral infarction due to thrombotic occlusion of the left circumflex artery (Figs. 5–45 and 5–46). Norris and Scott studied 85 autopsy-controlled cases; 50 cases had Q waves in leads I, aVL, V_5, and V_6 and showed no infarction at autopsy. When infarction occurred, it usually involved the lateral wall or the septum and lateral wall. In the presence of chest pain, the loss of R waves previously known to be present in leads V_3 and V_4, or the presence of new pathologic Q waves in leads I, V_5, and V_6, is indicative of acute infarction.

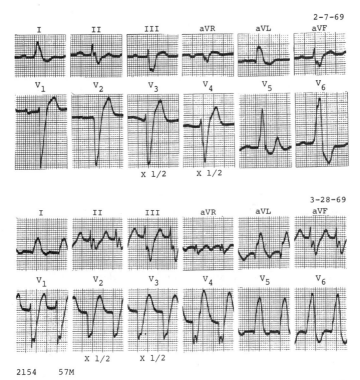

2154   57M

Figure 5–46 □ Left bundle branch block and myocardial infarction. The patient was a 57-year-old man with a history of hypertension and coronary artery disease. The tracing on 2-7-69 was recorded after he developed congestive heart failure and increasing frequency of angina pectoris. It shows first-degree atrioventricular block, complete left bundle branch block with a QRS duration of 0.18 second, and digitalis effect. On 3-28-69, he developed severe substernal chest pain and episodes of ventricular tachycardia. The ECG shows the loss of R waves in leads V_3 and V_4 and the development of a small Q wave in lead V_5. The patient died 5 days later. At autopsy, the heart weighed 1200 g and had marked biventricular hypertrophy. Severe coronary artery disease was present, with a massive acute anterior myocardial infarction. An old myocardial infarction and fatty degeneration and infiltration of the interventricular septum also were observed. (From Chou T-C: Electrocardiography in Clinical Practice, 4th ed. Philadelphia, WB Saunders Co., 1996, p 182.)

■ NON–ST ELEVATION INFARCTION

More than 20% of infarctions occur without the presence of ST segment elevation. In these patients, ST segment depression of >2 mm in two or more leads and associated with an abnormal CK-MB is in keeping with non–Q wave infarction, currently termed non–ST elevation MI (Fig. 5–47). In-hospital prognosis is good, and heart failure or cardiogenic shock is uncommon, except in patients with previous infarction. In patients with non–ST elevation MI, thrombolytic therapy does not provide benefits. The incidence of postinfarction angina is high, however, in these individuals; these patients are at high risk. Note that non–ST elevation MI may occur without much ST depression.

■ OLD MYOCARDIAL INFARCTION

Most infarcts presenting with ST segment elevation develop evolutionary changes with residual Q waves. Q waves may not develop with the rapid administration of thrombolytics. T wave inversion occurs during the second to fourth days, but these T waves often return to near normal configuration. In <10% of patients, T wave inversion persists for many years after infarction. The ST segment is usually normal in most patients within a few days after infarction. In a few patients, some degree of ST elevation persists. Figures 5–5B, 5–41, and 5–48 illustrate the findings in patients with previous infarction.

■ ISCHEMIA

ECG Hallmarks of Myocardial Ischemia

- An ST segment depression of >1 mm after the J-point, persisting in three consecutive complexes; an ST segment depression of ≥2 mm is diagnostic and indicates severe ischemia.
- An ST segment depression that is horizontal, square, or downsloping is considered significant for ischemia (Fig. 5–49); upsloping depression may be misleading and may suggest inaccurate diagnoses.

The ST segment and T wave should normally merge smoothly and imperceptibly. Minor ST segment depression may be associated with T wave inversion and is commonly reported as nonspecific ST-T wave changes.

The ECG is commonly stable in patients with angina. Changes suggestive of ischemia may be present in some patients. Patients with unstable angina may present with the following ECG changes, or changes may occur during pain:

- An ST segment depression of ≥2 mm in several leads
- An ST segment elevation in leads aVR and V_1
- An ST segment isoelectric or slightly elevated (1 mm), con-

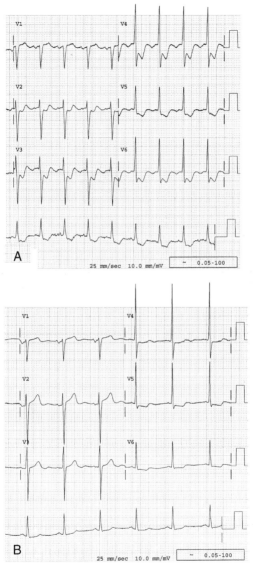

Figure 5–47 □ Non–ST elevation MI (non–Q wave infarction; acute subendocardial infarction). From a patient with a clinical picture of infarction and elevated CK-MB: note widespread ST-T depression in the limb and chest leads but no associated Q waves. *B,* The same patient's ECG tracing 18 hours earlier than depicted in *A.*

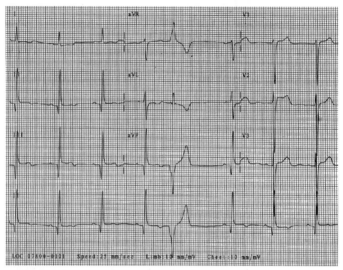

Figure 5–48 □ ECG shows an old inferior myocardial infarction which occurred at age 49 in this 74-year-old woman with severe familial (genetic) hyperlipidemia (total cholesterol >1000 mg in the 1970s).

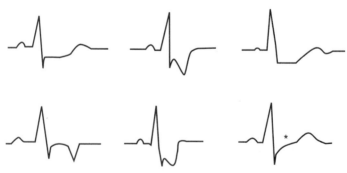

Figure 5–49 □ ECG patterns of myocardial ischemia.

* = upsloping ST depression is nonspecific, commonly seen with tachy-cardia.

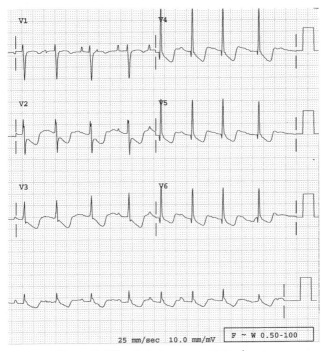

25 mm/sec   10.0 mm/mV   F ~ W 0.50-100

Figure 5–50 □ Anterior myocardial ischemia.

vex, or straight, especially in leads V_2 and V_3 (Fig. 5–50). These changes commonly occur when the patient is pain free and may be present in leads V_1, V_2, and V_3 or in leads V_3 and V_4, and occasionally in leads V_4 and V_5 (Fig. 5–51); these changes are suggestive of proximal, left anterior descending artery stenosis; in patients with left main stem disease, ST segment elevation may be observed in leads V_1 and aVR, and ST segment depression in the remainder of the precordial leads and in leads I, II, and aVL.

■ MISCELLANEOUS CONDITIONS

Pericarditis

Criteria for the Diagnosis of Pericarditis

1. Stage 1, lasting hours to days; i.e., widespread ST segment elevation, 2 to 5 mm concave and upward in leads I, II, III, aVF, and V_2 to V_5 with reciprocal depression in leads aVR and V_1, and slight elevation of the PR segment in lead aVR;

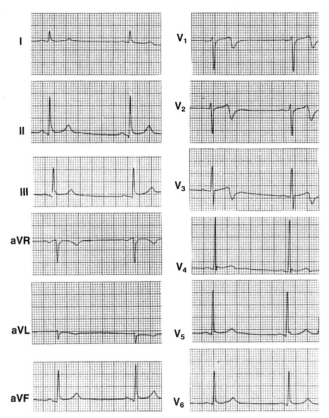

Figure 5–51 □ The ECG pattern in critical proximal left anterior descending stenosis. This pattern is typically present when the patient is pain free. The ST-T segment abnormalities are not limited to leads V_2 and V_3 but are also frequently seen in leads V_3, V_4, and V_5. (From Wellens HJJ, Conover MB: The ECG in Emergency Decision Making. Philadelphia, WB Saunders Co., 1992, p 31.)

the ECG changes do not fit a segmental blood supply (see Fig. 5–32; Fig. 5–52).

2. Stage 2, a few days later; i.e., ST and PR segments become isoelectric, with upright or flattened T waves (see Fig. 5–32).
3. Stage 3; i.e., after normalization of the ST segment, diffuse T wave inversion occurs.
4. Stage 4, lasting from days to weeks; i.e., T waves normalize but rarely remain inverted.

Tachycardia may be the only ECG finding if the ST segment elevation has resolved and the T waves remain normal.

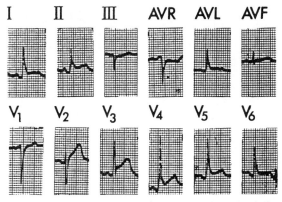

Figure 5–52 □ ECG in a patient with acute purulent pericarditis. Note the ST elevation in all leads except aVR and V_1. (From Gazes PC: Clinical Cardiology, 3rd ed. Philadelphia, Lea & Febiger, 1991, p 368.)

Hypokalemia

ECG Hallmarks of Hypokalemia

1. Progressive ST segment depression, and normally, a small U wave has the same polarity as the T wave; when the serum potassium level falls to <3.5 mEq/L, there is a lowering in the amplitude of the T wave.
2. A marked increase in U wave amplitude; with a serum potassium of <1.5 mEq/L, the T and the U waves may become fused, which is best seen in leads V_2 to V_6 (Fig. 5–53).
3. An increase in the QRS duration
4. Slight prolongation of the PR interval

Hyperkalemia

ECG Hallmarks of Hyperkalemia

1. Mild hyperkalemia at <6 mEq/L, widening of the P wave with a loss in height, prolongation of the PR interval and widening of the QRS complex, and tall, peaked T waves (Figs. 5–54 and 5–55)
2. Severe hyperkalemia at >6 mEq/L and marked widening of the second portion of the QRS complex, which may show notching or slurring; thus, the wide QRS merges with the tall, peaked T waves
3. PR-interval prolongation, high-degree AV block (see Fig. 5–55), and finally, disappearance of the P waves
4. Further widening of the QRS; ventricular fibrillation may occur.

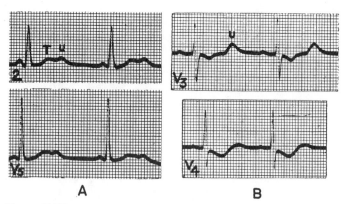

Figure 5–53 □ Hypokalemia. Tracings *A* and *B* are from different patients. *A* shows early changes of hypokalemia with a prominent U wave merging to form a continuous undulating wave with the T wave. *B* shows changes of advanced hypokalemia (1.8 mEq/L) in a patient with cirrhosis; note ST-T depression with very prominent U waves in lead V_3. (From Marriott HJL: Practical Electrocardiography, 8th ed. Baltimore, Williams & Wilkins, 1988, p 523.)

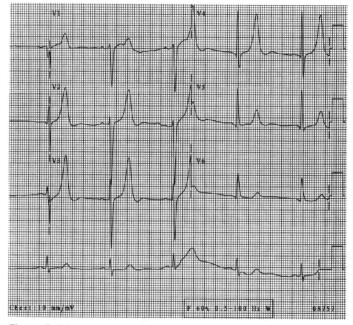

Figure 5–54 □ Hyperkalemia: patient with renal failure and serum potassium of 5.8 mEq/L; tall, peaked T waves.

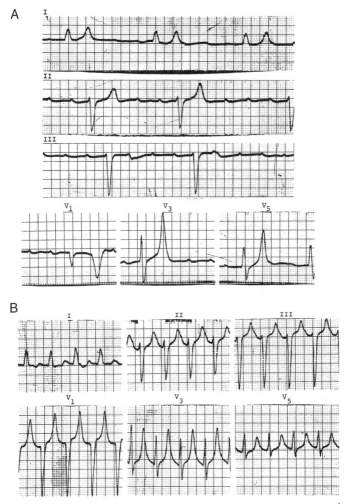

Figure 5–55 □ Hyperkalemia. The patient is a 46-year-old woman with metabolic acidosis. The serum potassium was 8.3 mEq/L; calcium, 5 mEq/L; and blood pH, 7.09. *A,* Tracing showing sinus tachycardia with high-degree atrioventricular block, intraventricular conduction defect, abnormal left axis deviation, and tall, peaked T waves, especially in the precordial leads. *B,* After intravenous administration of sodium bicarbonate and calcium gluconate, the ECG shows first-degree atrioventricular block. The QRS duration decreases to 0.14 second. The T waves remain tall and peaked. (From Chou T-C: Electrocardiography in Clinical Practice, 4th ed. Philadelphia, WB Saunders Co., 1996, p 533.)

Pulmonary Embolism

Nonspecific But Helpful ECG Findings

- Sinus tachycardia, which is common
- Symmetric T wave inversion, strain pattern in leads V_1 to V_3
- ST depression in leads I or II
- S_1, S_2, and S_3 pattern
- RBBB pattern
- Q waves in leads III and aVF
- Qr in lead V_1
- ST segment elevation in leads V_1, aVR, and III
- ST segment depression in leads V_3 to V_6 because of associated myocardial ischemia
- Arrhythmias that include premature beats, atrial flutter, or atrial fibrillation
- Right atrial enlargement

ECG features are shown in Figure 5–56. In the presence of submassive pulmonary embolism, the ECG shows no significant abnormality in <25% of cases. With massive pulmonary embolism causing syncope, cardiogenic shock, or acute right-sided heart failure, one or more of the above-listed ECG changes usually occur.

■ ARRHYTHMIAS

An arrhythmia is defined as
1. Any cardiac rhythm, regular or irregular, that is not driven by the sinus node or
2. Any abnormality of the cardiac rhythm, even if the sinus node is the primary pacemaker

Arrhythmias can be classified as
1. Bradyarrhythmias
2. Tachyarrhythmias

Tachyarrhythmias should be considered under two categories, **narrow QRS tachycardias** and **wide QRS tachycardias.**

Narrow QRS tachycardia
1. Regular
   - Sinus tachycardia
   - AV nodal reentrant tachycardia
   - Atrial tachycardia
   - Atrial flutter with fixed AV conduction
   - WPW syndrome
2. Irregular
   - Atrial fibrillation
   - Atrial flutter when AV conduction is variable
   - Multifocal atrial tachycardia (MAT)

A

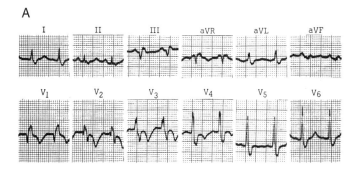

B

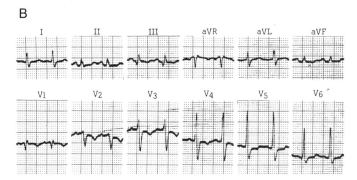

Figure 5–56 □ Massive pulmonary embolism confirmed by autopsy. The patient was a 61-year-old man who had dyspnea and dizziness 3 days before the tracing *(A)* was recorded. The tracing shows sinus tachycardia and complete right bundle branch block. Q waves are present in leads III, aVF, and V_1. There is rather deep T wave inversion in the right and midprecordial leads, suggesting additional primary T wave changes. The ECG recorded on the next day *(B)* shows the $S_1Q_3T_3$ pattern. The complete right bundle branch block is no longer present, but lead V_1 reveals a Qr pattern. There is T wave inversion in leads V_1 through V_5. The patient died the same day. At autopsy, there were large pulmonary emboli that almost totally occluded the lumens of both the left and right pulmonary arteries. No significant coronary artery disease or myocardial infarction was found. (From Chou T-C: Electrocardiography in Clinical Practice, 4th ed. Philadelphia, WB Saunders Co., 1996, p 290.)

Wide QRS tachycardia
1. Regular
   - Ventricular tachycardia
   - Supraventricular tachycardia with bundle branch block or with aberrant conduction
   - Atrial flutter and WPW conduction
   - Preexcited (circus movement) tachycardia (WPW antero-grade conduction)
2. Irregular
   - Atrial fibrillation and WPW anterograde conduction
   - Atrial fibrillation and intraventricular conduction defect

Before discussing narrow and wide QRS complex tachycardias, a discussion of atrial premature beats (APBs), junctional or nodal premature beats, sinus arrhythmia, and ventricular premature beats (VPBs) is relevant.

Atrial Premature Beats

APBs occur commonly at all ages but may be caused by medications and all varieties of heart disease.

ECG Hallmarks of APBs
- A premature P wave, which is different from the sinus P wave. The PR interval may be normal, increased, or decreased.
- Nonconduction of the atrial premature P wave, resulting in a pause. Nonconducted APBs are the most common cause of pauses; if the premature P waves are not identified, the rhythm may be misinterpreted as sinus bradycardia.
- A premature P wave that is usually followed by a QRS complex similar to the normally conducted sinus beat (Fig. 5–57). The QRS may be wide because of aberrant conduction. The premature P wave may be unrecognizable, however, because it may be hidden in the preceding T wave, and hence, the admonition "search the T for the P."
- A cycle after the APB that is less than compensatory; the pause may be compensatory, however, or even longer in some individuals.
- APBs after every sinus beat, causing atrial bigeminy. Early APBs may trigger atrial tachycardia (see Fig. 5–57), atrial flutter, or atrial fibrillation.
- Multiple APBs, which may cause an irregularly irregular (completely irregular) pulse.

Junctional or Nodal Premature Beats

When junctional P waves retrogradely activate the atria, the retrograde P wave may be observed to precede the QRS complex

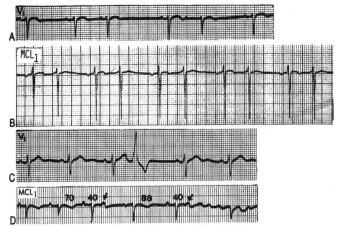

Figure 5–57 □ *A,* The third and fifth beats are atrial premature beats. Note that the shorter RP of the second atrial premature beat is complemented by a much prolonged PR interval. *B,* Atrial bigeminy in which the PR of the atrial premature beats is much prolonged compared with the normal PR of the sinus beats. *C,* The fourth beat is an atrial premature beat with right bundle branch block aberration. Note the deformed T wave and the less than compensatory prostectopic cycle. *D,* When the atrial premature beat is premature enough to make the PR interval (40) less than half the preceding PP interval (88), an atrial tachyarrhythmia is triggered. (From Marriott HJL: Practical Electrocardiography, 8th ed. Baltimore, Williams & Wilkins, 1988, p 151.)

or become lost in the QRS complex and occasionally occur after the QRS complex. The P wave is inverted in leads II, III, aVF, V_1, V_5, and V_6 and upright in leads I, aVR, and aVL. The terms "upper nodal" and "mid" or "lower nodal rhythm" have been replaced by "junctional rhythm."

Sinus Arrhythmia

The ECG shows slight irregularity of RR intervals. The maximum sinus cycle length minus the minimum sinus cycle length should be >120 msec. The P waves are normal and the PP interval varies by >0.16 second (four small squares). This normal irregularity of the heartbeat is physiologic. The minimal change in the heart rhythm may be accentuated during inspiration, and the heart slows slightly during expiration. This normal change is not usually appreciated by individuals, and the ECG depicting such a minimal irregularity gets a cursory look from the interpreting cardiologist. Causes other than respiratory variations may produce sinus arrhythmia and include digitalis, morphine, convalescence from acute illnesses associated with bradycardia, and raised intracranial pressure.

Ventricular Premature Beats

VPBs, termed "extrasystoles" or "ectopic beats," occur commonly in normal and abnormal hearts. The word "beat" denotes an electrical and mechanical event and is preferred to the word "contraction," which implies only a mechanical event. Thus, the text uses the terms VPBs and APBs, not ventricular premature contractions (VPCs) and atrial premature contractions (APCs).

Hallmarks of VPBs
- Wide, bizarre beats (Fig. 5–58)
- Not preceded by premature P waves
- Usually followed by a fully compensatory pause, but this rule is often broken and pauses may be less than compensatory
- >0.11-second duration, but occasionally VPBs can be 0.10 to 0.11 second in duration
- Virtually always different from the adjacent sinus-conducted normal beat
- Typically in lead V_1, left "rabbit ear" is greater than the right one, or a small rS in lead V_6 (see Fig. 5–58)

A run of two VPBs is called a couplet, a run of three consecutive VPBs is called a triplet, and a run of more than three consecutive VPBs is called nonsustained ventricular tachycardia (VT) (Fig. 5–59).

Multifocal VPBs have a varying coupling interval; with unifocal VPBs, the coupling interval is equal. VPBs that are unifocal are of little consequence. VPBs that occur early, close to the T wave or R on T, are multifocal or multiform or may trigger VT (see Fig. 5–59).

VPBs are a common occurrence in individuals with normal hearts, i.e., bigeminy and trigeminy commonly. Increasing the heart rate by walking or stair climbing may suppress some VPBs or mask the symptoms; the patient feels the sensation when the body is at rest.

Causes of VPBs
1. Stimulants, such as caffeine, theophylline, amphetamines, cocaine, and a host of pharmacologic agents, which may stimulate the production of VPBs
2. Acute MI and the chronic phase of myocardial ischemia
3. Valvular heart disease
4. Cardiomyopathy
5. Specific heart muscle disease
6. Cor pulmonale

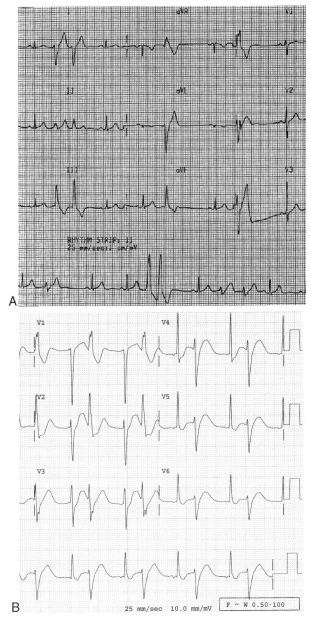

Figure 5–58 □ *A*, Ventricular premature beats, couplets. *B*, Ventricular bigeminy.

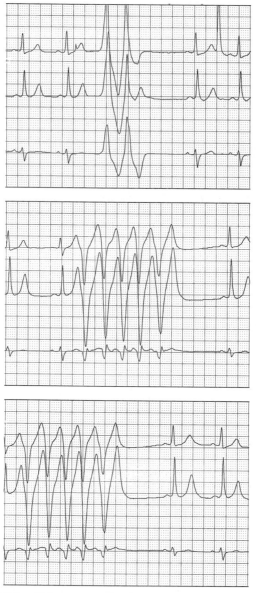

Figure 5–59 □ Holter monitor showing multifocal ventricular premature beats, couplets; salvo: nonsustained ventricular tachycardia.

Narrow QRS Tachycardia

An algorithm for the diagnosis of narrow QRS tachyarrhythmias is given in Figure 5–60. A study of the entire 12-lead ECG during tachycardia and a comparison with the ECG in sinus rhythm are strongly advised. Leads II, III, aVF, V_1, and V_6 deserve careful scrutiny. The lead II rhythm strip is not sufficiently diagnostic.

Sinus Tachycardia

The most common cause of a regular, narrow QRS tachycardia, with a rate of 100 to 140 beats/min, is sinus tachycardia. With rates of <140 beats/min on the ECG at rest, it is advisable to think first of sinus tachycardia (Fig. 5–61*A*), but rates of >160 beats/min at rest may occur in patients with infections and thyrotoxicosis (Fig. 5–61*B*). Occasionally, the sinus P wave is hidden in the T wave and the rhythm mistaken for supraventricular tachycardia or atrial flutter; carotid massage reveals the P wave of sinus tachycardia.

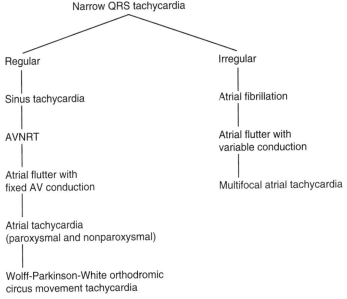

Figure 5–60 □ Algorithm for the diagnosis of narrow QRS tachycardia. AVNRT = atrioventricular nodal reentrant tachycardia. (Redrawn from Khan, M Gabriel: Heart Disease Diagnosis and Therapy: A Practical Approach. Baltimore, Williams & Wilkins, 1996, p 238.)

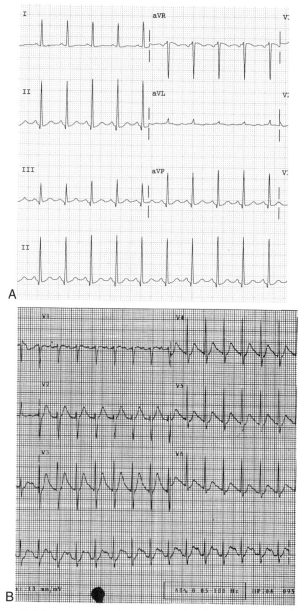

Figure 5–61 □ *A*, Sinus tachycardia, rate 120/min. *B*, Tracing from a 47-year-old woman; sinus tachycardia, 167/min, caused by thyrotoxicosis.

Atrioventricular Nodal Reentrant Tachycardia

Atrioventricular nodal reentrant tachycardia (AVNRT) is the most common cause of a paroxysmal, rapid, narrow, regular QRS tachycardia. The impulse circulates within the AV node; the ventricles are activated from the anterograde path of the circuit with activation of the atrium by the retrograde path (Fig. 5–62).

ECG Hallmarks of AVNRT

- A rapid, regular rhythm, usually 160 to 225 beats/min is present; a rate of >230 beats/min should prompt the search for WPW syndrome
- A QRS complex of <0.12 second

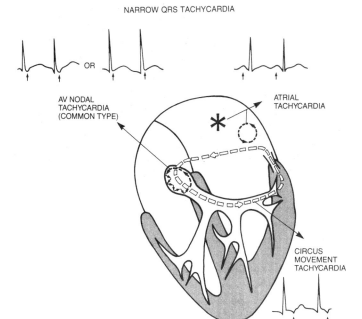

Figure 5–62 □ A representation of the sites of origin and mechanisms of paroxysmal supraventricular tachycardia as determined by the position and polarity of the P waves in relation to the QRS complex. In atrial tachycardia, the P wave precedes the QRS; its polarity in lead III depends on its location. In AV nodal reentry tachycardia, the P wave is buried within the QRS or may distort the end of the QRS; that portion of the QRS is then negative in lead III. In circus movement tachycardia, the P wave follows the QRS. (From Wellens HJJ, Conover MB: The ECG in Emergency Decision Making. Philadelphia, WB Saunders Co., 1992, p 75.)

- In approximately 50% of cases, P waves are hidden within the QRS complex and are not visible; the QRS complex is identical to that of a tracing when in sinus rhythm (see Fig. 5–62; Fig. 5–63).
- In more than 40% of cases, P waves in leads II, III, and aVF occur at the end of the QRS complex and distort the terminal forces of the QRS complex, resulting in pseudo-S waves in leads II, III, and aVF, and a pseudo-r' wave in lead V_1 (see Fig. 5–62; Fig. 5–64).
- In less than 5% of cases P waves are discernible at the beginning of the QRS complex and cause pseudo-q waves in leads II, III, and aVF.
- In a very rare form of AVNRT, P waves are negative in leads II, III, and aVF but follow the QRS complex after a prolonged duration, such that the RP interval is greater than or equal to the PR interval (see Fig. 5–62). It is virtually impossible to distinguish this rare form of AVNRT from the rare-type WPW, circus movement, using the retrograde, slow accessory pathway to activate the atria (see later discussion of WPW; Fig. 5–65).

Atrial Tachycardia

This tachycardia occurs in the following three forms:
- Paroxysmal atrial tachycardia (PAT) with or without AV block
- Persistent ("incessant") atrial tachycardia
- Multifocal atrial tachycardia (MAT)

Paroxysmal Atrial Tachycardia With or Without AV Block

ECG Hallmarks of PAT

- The P wave contour is different from that of the sinus P wave and precedes the QRS. P waves are best identified in lead V_1; they are often small, are not easily identified, and may be hidden in the T wave or QRS; the rhythm may be mistaken for sinus tachycardia or AV junctional tachycardia.
- The atrial rate is commonly 150 to 200 beats/min but may range from 110 to 250 beats/min. If the atrial rate is not rapid and AV conduction is not depressed, each P wave may conduct to the ventricle. Short episodes of nonsustained PAT lasting seconds to a few minutes, with heart rates of 110 to 150 beats/min, are not uncommon findings on routine Holter monitoring. With digitalis excess or other causes, AV conduction may be delayed, resulting in PAT with block.
- Variable AV conduction occurs: A 2:1 conduction (Fig. 5–66) is common; a 3:1 conduction or Wenckebach's phenomenon may occur. At times, the varying AV block results in an irregular ventricular rhythm that may be mistaken for atrial fibrillation.

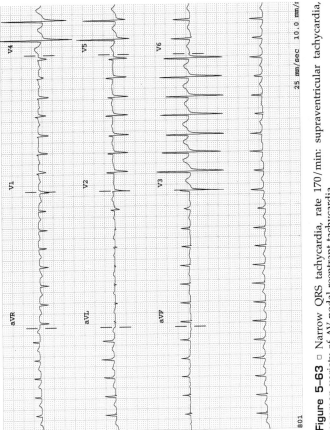

Figure 5–63 □ Narrow QRS tachycardia, rate 170/min: supraventricular tachycardia, common variety of AV nodal reentrant tachycardia.

123

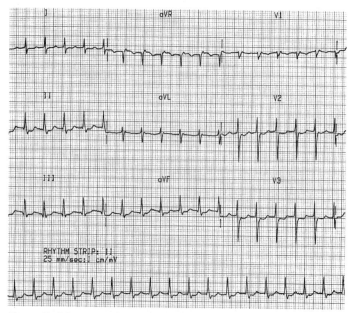

Figure 5–64 □ ECG shows atrioventricular nodal reentrant tachycardia: note the distortion of terminal forces, pseudo-S waves, in leads II, III, and aVF, and a pseudo-r′ wave in lead V_1.

- Isoelectric intervals exist between the P wave and the QRS complex.
- The differentiation of atrial tachycardia and atrial flutter may present difficulties if the atrial rate is rapid, but carotid sinus massage or adenosine would reveal flutter waves in atrial flutter.
- The tachycardia persists despite the development of AV block. This finding excludes the participation of an accessory pathway.

Persistent ("Incessant") Atrial Tachycardia

The incessant nature of this rare tachycardia may cause dilated (congestive) cardiomyopathy. Features include

- Regular rhythm
- P wave preceding the QRS complex, with polarity depending on the site of origin in the atrium
- Variable AV conduction of 1:1, 2:1, including Wenckebach's phenomenon
- Carotid sinus massage or adenosine increasing AV block and facilitating identification

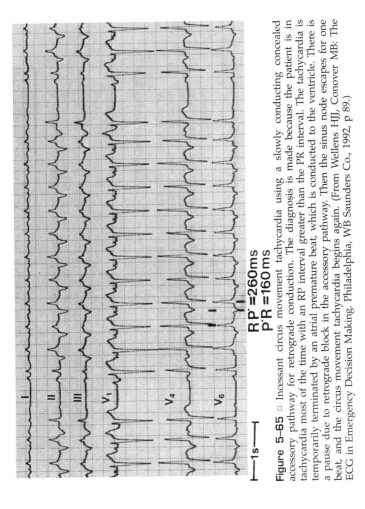

RP'=260ms
P'R=160ms

Figure 5–65 □ Incessant circus movement tachycardia using a slowly conducting concealed accessory pathway for retrograde conduction. The diagnosis is made because the patient is in tachycardia most of the time with an RP interval greater than the PR interval. The tachycardia is temporarily terminated by an atrial premature beat, which is conducted to the ventricle. There is a pause due to retrograde block in the accessory pathway. Then the sinus node escapes for one beat, and the circus movement tachycardia begins again. (From Wellens HJJ, Conover MB: The ECG in Emergency Decision Making, Philadelphia, WB Saunders Co., 1992, p 89.)

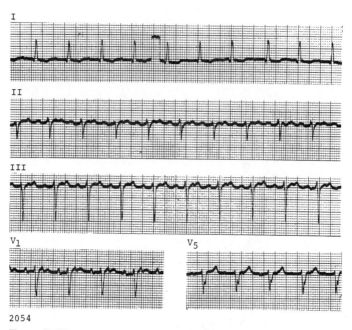

2054

Figure 5–66 □ Paroxysmal atrial tachycardia with block. The atrial rate is 200 beats/min, and there is 2:1 atrioventricular conduction. The P waves are seen best in lead V_1. (From Chou T-C: Electrocardiography in Clinical Practice, 4th ed. Philadelphia, WB Saunders Co., 1996, p 349.)

Multifocal Atrial Tachycardia (Chaotic Atrial Tachycardia)

Hallmarks include
- An atrial rate of 100 to 140 beats/min
- At least three different P wave morphologies with changing PR intervals observed in one lead (Fig. 5–67)
- A completely irregular rhythm
- Usually caused by hypoxemia, chronic obstructive pulmonary disease (COPD), theophylline, (rarely) digitalis; ischemic heart disease

Wolff-Parkinson-White Syndrome

ECG Hallmarks of WPW in Sinus Rhythm
- A QRS complex of >0.12 second (in 20% of individuals, the QRS complex may not be >0.10 second)

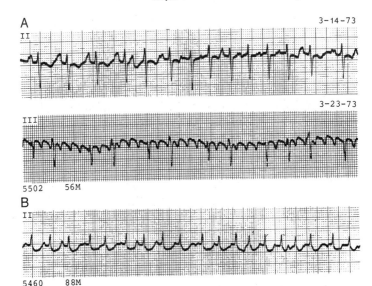

Figure 5–67 □ Multifocal atrial tachycardia. *A,* The patient has chronic obstructive lung disease. The tracing on 3-14-73 shows multifocal atrial tachycardia. The rhythm changes to atrial flutter with varying atrioventricular conduction on 3-23-73. *B,* Tracing obtained from an 88-year-old man with mitral insufficiency. The multifocal atrial tachycardia closely resembles atrial fibrillation with rapid ventricular response. (From Chou T-C: Electrocardiography in Clinical Practice, 4th ed. Philadelphia, WB Saunders Co., 1996, p 353.)

- A PR interval of <0.12 second
- A delta wave present in most (Fig. 5–68) (may be a subtle finding in a few leads)
- A tall R wave in V_1 and V_2 (can mimic RVH or posterior infarction)
- Possible mimicry of inferior MI (Fig. 5–69)

ECG Clues During Tachycardia
- A narrow complex tachycardia, regular rhythm
- Paroxysmal tachycardia
- P waves that are separate from the QRS complex and that, depending on the location of the accessory pathway, may have different shapes; if it is a left lateral accessory pathway, the P wave is negative in lead I; if the location is posteroseptal, the P wave is negative in leads II, III, and aVF and may be positive in leads aVR, aVL, and V_1.
- In the most common type of WPW, orthodromic circus move-

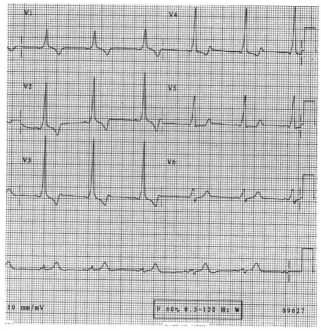

Figure 5–68 □ Wolff-Parkinson-White syndrome has a short PR, a delta wave easily detected in leads V_2 to V_5, and a tall R wave in leads V_1 to V_3.

ment tachycardia, the RP interval is smaller than the PR interval because of retrograde use of the fast accessory pathway to activate the atria (see Fig. 5–62; Figs. 5–70 and 5–71).

- In a very rare form of WPW, orthodromic circus movement with retrograde activation of the atria occurs through a slow conducting accessory pathway retrogradely, causing the late occurrence of the P wave; thus, the RP interval is greater than or equal to the PR interval and the P wave is negative in leads II, III, aVF, and V_3 to V_6. The arrhythmic ECG pattern is similar to the very rare form of AVNRT described earlier (see Fig. 5–65). This rare type of WPW syndrome may manifest as a persistent (incessant) orthodromic circus movement tachycardia and cause a dilated cardiomyopathy with CHF. The condition is resistant to drug therapy but can be cured by ablation.

- Electrical alternans may be present during orthodromic circus movement tachycardia but occurs rarely with other narrow QRS tachycardias.

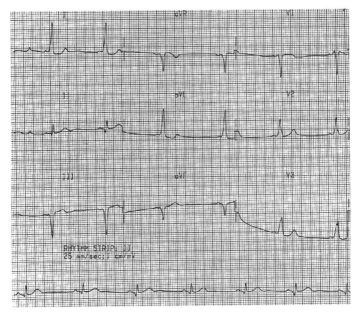

Figure 5–69 □ Wolff-Parkinson-White syndrome may mimic inferior myocardial infarction.

Summary: Diagnosis of Narrow Regular QRS Tachycardia

- If AV block is present or can be produced by carotid sinus massage or adenosine, this rules out WPW syndrome; atrial flutter and atrial tachycardia persist, despite AV block.
- If the P wave is hidden within the QRS or is distorting the terminal QRS complex, causing a pseudo-S wave in leads II, III, and aVF or a pseudo-r' wave in lead V_1, the findings are typical of the common form of AVNRT (see Figs. 5–62, 5–63, and 5–64).
- A negative P wave in lead I suggests WPW or left atrial tachycardia.
- A P wave distant from the QRS complex and RP interval < the PR interval are often seen with the most common type of WPW (see Figs. 5–70 and 5–71).
- An RP interval ≥ the PR interval indicates rare orthodromic-type WPW or the rare type of AVNRT or atrial tachycardia (see Fig. 5–65).
- A positive P wave in leads II, III, and aVF, with atrial tachycardia, rules out AVNRT or WPW tachycardia.

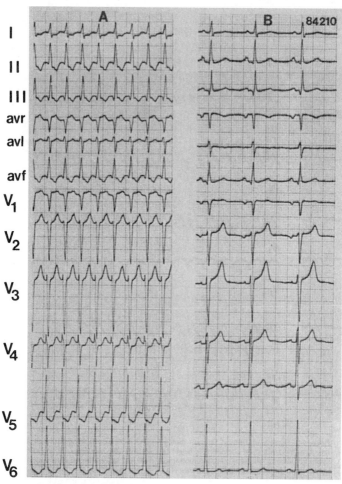

Figure 5–70 □ An example of a circus movement tachycardia using a concealed accessory pathway. The diagnosis is based on the position of the P waves during the tachycardia. *A*, Note that when compared with sinus rhythm *(B)*, negative P waves are clearly visible in leads II, III, and aVF following the QRS complex. The P waves during the tachycardia are positive in leads aVR and aVL, indicating a posteroseptal atrial insertion of the accessory pathway. (From Wellens HJJ, Conover MB: The ECG in Emergency Decision Making. Philadelphia, WB Saunders Co., 1992, p 86.)

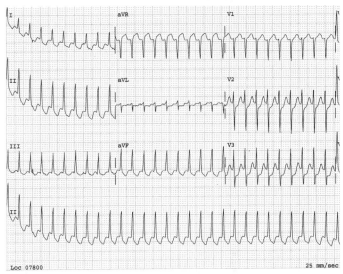

Figure 5–71 □ Narrow QRS regular tachycardia, rate 230/min: orthodromic circus movement tachycardia. Patient with Wolff-Parkinson-White syndrome; resting ECG tracing sinus rhythm shown in Figure 5–68.

- P waves negative in leads II, III, and aVF suggest AVNRT or WPW.
- QRS alternans indicates WPW is likely.
- Ventricular rate >250 beats/min and RR intervals ≤240 msec in duration (six small squares) strongly suggest WPW (see Fig. 5–71).

Summary of the Four Faces of Wolff-Parkinson-White Syndrome

1. Commonly, orthodromic circus movement tachycardia. Activation of the ventricles occurs via the AV node and His bundle; the impulse uses retrogradely the fast accessory tract to activate the atria, and thus, the P wave is close to the preceding QRS complex and the RP interval is < the PR interval.
2. The rare, persistent orthodromic form. Similar activation of the ventricle via the AV node and His bundle but return of the impulse to the atria via the slow accessory tract; therefore, the P wave is distant from the QRS complex and the RP interval is ≥ the PR interval; it requires electrophysiologic studies to distinguish this tachyarrhythmia from the rare form of AVNRT.
3. Rare antidromic tachycardia. Anterograde use of bypass

tract to activate the ventricle, causing tachycardia similar to VT or atrial flutter or fibrillation with a wide QRS. See section on wide QRS tachycardia (page 138).
4. Rare antidromic anterograde conduction using two or more accessory pathways, resulting in a wide QRS tachycardia.

Carotid Sinus Massage or Adenosine IV

Carotid sinus massage or adenosine given intravenously (IV) is an integral part of ECG arrhythmia diagnosis.

- AVNRT reverts to sinus rhythm or no effect.
- Circus movement tachycardia: WPW reverts to sinus rhythm or no effect.
- Persistent atrial tachycardia: increased AV block facilitates recognition of the atrial origin of this arrhythmia, temporary slowing of heart rate with AV block, or no effect.
- Atrial flutter, temporary slowing of the ventricular rate with AV block: reveals flutter waves if not previously visible, or no effect.

Carotid sinus massage or adenosine IV is not required for the verification of atrial fibrillation or sinus tachycardia; both conditions show temporary slowing of the ventricular rate. These arrhythmias, however, are easily recognizable.

Atrial Flutter

Hallmarks

- A sawtooth pattern of flutter (F) waves is present in leads II, III, and aVF (Fig. 5–72). The initial downward deflection of the F waves has a gradual slope followed by an abrupt upward deflection that results in the typical sharp spikes of the sawtooth pattern. There are positive "spiky" P-like waves in lead V_1, negative P-like waves in leads V_5 and V_6, and nearly no atrial activity in lead I; occasionally, leads V_5 and V_6 may show negligible atrial activity (see Fig. 5–72).
- If the ECG reveals a ventricular response of 150 beats/min, the chances of the arrhythmias being atrial flutter are >90%. This situation arises because the atrial rate is often 300 beats/min, and with 2:1 AV conduction, the ventricular response is 150 beats/min. This 2:1 ratio may not be easily apparent, because an F wave may be partially obscured by the QRS complex and the F wave by the T wave; this pattern may be confused with sinus tachycardia or reentrant junctional tachycardia. Carotid sinus massage should reveal sinus P waves or F waves. Conduction ratios of 2:1 and 4:1 occur frequently. The ventricular rate may vary from 100 to 230 beats/min (Fig. 5–73). A ventricular response of >250 beats/min raises suspicion of WPW.
- The rhythm is regular, except when there is variable AV conduction.

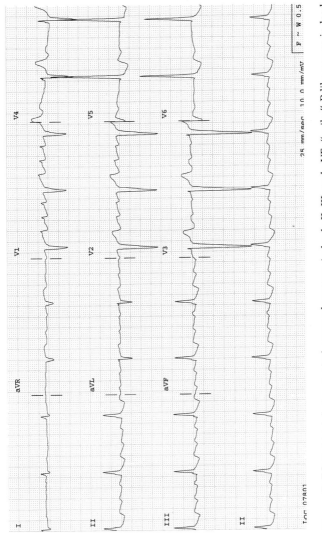

Figure 5–72 □ Atrial flutter: typical sawtooth pattern in leads II, III, and aVF; "spiky" P-like waves in lead V₁; negligible atrial activity in leads I, V₅, and V₆.

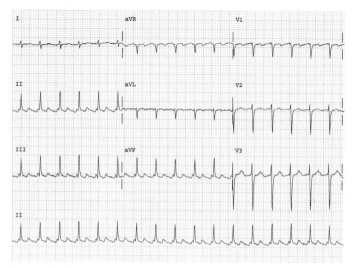

Figure 5–73 □ Atrial flutter with 2:1 atrioventricular conduction, atrial rate 270/min, ventricular response rate 135/min.

- The atrial rate varies from 250 to 400 beats/min but can be <200 beats/min, in particular in patients taking quinidine.
- Flutter waves, if not visible, can be revealed by slowing AV conduction with carotid sinus massage or adenosine IV.
- Digitalis increases the atrial flutter rate and may induce atrial fibrillation before slowing the ventricular response.
- T waves may distort the F wave pattern.
- The incidence of atrial flutter is ½₀th that of atrial fibrillation. Atrial flutter may be caused by ischemic heart disease, valvular heart disease, congenital heart disease, hypoxemia, post–open heart surgery, infections, and any acute illness.

Atrial Fibrillation

Atrial fibrillation is the most common, persistent, significant arrhythmia that is encountered in clinical practice. Causes of atrial fibrillation include diseases that result in left atrial enlargement. Underlying conditions include rheumatic mitral and aortic valve disease, all forms of valvular heart disease including myxomatous MVP, CHF, hypertension, cardiomyopathies, ischemic heart disease, congenital heart disease, constrictive pericarditis, drinking alcohol, specific heart muscle diseases, cor pulmonale, thyrotoxicosis, postthoracotomy, hypoxemia, and ruptured esophagus. Atrial fibrillation may occur in individuals with normal hearts (see Figs. 5–76 and 5–77). Sick sinus syndrome should be considered in patients with syncope, atrial fibrillation, and narrow QRS complexes; if the QRS complex is wide, think of antidromic WPW syndrome.

ECG Hallmarks

- RR intervals that are irregularly irregular (completely irregular) (Figs. 5–74 to 5–77).
- Irregular undulation of the baseline that may be gross and distinct, or barely perceptible, described as coarse (see Fig. 5–77) and fine fibrillation. There may be no recognizable undulations of the baseline, in particular in lead V_1, where it is best seen; in this situation, careful measurement of the RR intervals is necessary to detect slight irregularities. Coarse fibrillation is frequently seen with rheumatic valvular heart disease and significant atrial enlargement.
- Occasionally, small P-like waves or atrial premature beats
- The atrial rate ranges from 350 to 500 beats/min, and thus,

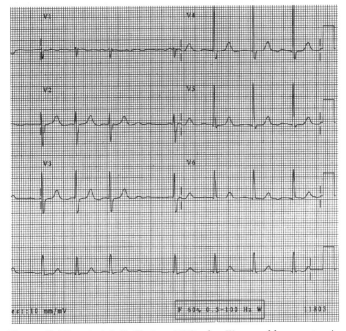

Figure 5–74 □ Atrial fibrillation: ECG of a 71-year-old normotensive woman with a 5-year history of stable angina and no valvular or other heart disease. RR intervals are irregularly irregular; no P waves; controlled ventricular rate.

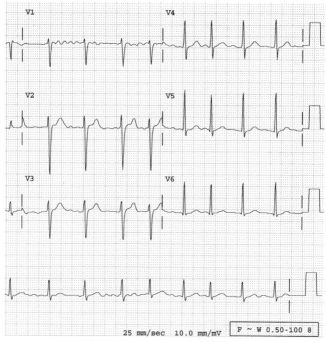

Figure 5–75 □ Atrial fibrillation in a 29-year-old man with a normal heart. Coarse undulations in V_1; RR intervals completely irregular; ventricular response 102/min.

there is variable AV conduction, resulting in a chaotic ventricular response.
- QRS complexes often varying in amplitude
- The heart rate is commonly 100 to 180 beats/min but possibly accelerates to >200 beats/min. Rates of >200 beats/min should suggest WPW. With WPW antidromic tachycardia, wide QRS tachycardia with rates of 250 to 320 beats/min may occur.

Differential Diagnosis in Patients With an Irregularly Irregular (Completely Irregular) Rhythm
- Atrial fibrillation
- MAT; the varying morphology of P waves preceding most QRS complexes and the changing PR, RR, and PP intervals should confirm MAT; at least three different morphologic P waves should be observed in the same lead.
- PAT with variable AV block (see earlier discussion)
- Atrial flutter with variable AV conduction; the sawtooth pat-

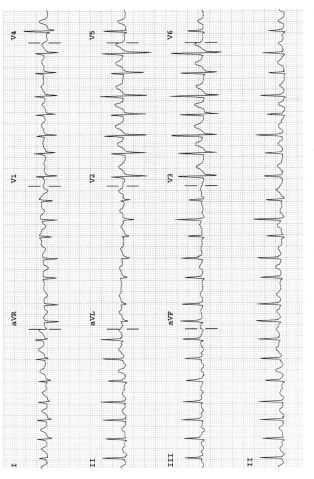

Figure 5-76 □ Atrial fibrillation in a 38-year-old man with a "normal heart"; uncontrolled ventricular response 166/min.

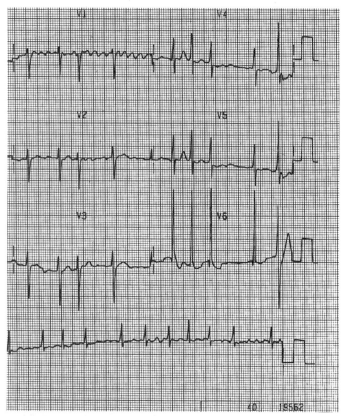

Figure 5–77 □ Atrial fibrillation in a 68-year-old man with significant mitral regurgitation: completely irregular RR interval; coarse oscillations (fibrillatory waves) in lead V₁.

tern in leads II, III, and aVF, and little or no atrial activity in leads I, V₅, and V₆, are clues to flutter.
- Artifacts caused by somatic tremors that may occur mainly in the limb leads, in particular in patients with Parkinson's syndrome: P waves should be visible in lead V₁ or the precordial leads.

Wide QRS Tachycardia

The differential diagnosis of wide QRS tachycardias is shown in Figure 5–78. The differential diagnosis of a wide QRS complex tachycardia includes

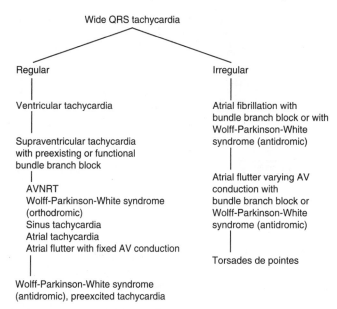

Figure 5–78 □ The differential diagnosis of wide QRS tachycardia. AVNRT = atrioventricular nodal reentrant tachycardia. (Redrawn from Khan, M Gabriel: Heart Disease Diagnosis and Therapy: A Practical Approach. Baltimore, Williams & Wilkins, 1996, p 273.)

- Ventricular tachycardia (coronary and noncoronary)
- All types of supraventricular tachycardia with preexisting or functional bundle branch block (aberration)
- Preexcited tachycardia, WPW with anterograde conduction over an accessory pathway (antidromic) (see Fig. 5–78).

Ventricular Tachycardia

All wide QRS regular tachycardias should be treated as VT until proved otherwise. An algorithm for the differential diagnosis of wide QRS complex tachycardia, as it should be used in clinical practice, is given in Figure 5–79.

You need to assess a complete 12-lead ECG, and in particular leads V_1 to V_6, to observe the hallmarks of VT.

Hallmarks of VT

- Predominantly negative QRS complexes in precordial leads V_4 to V_6 (Fig. 5–80)
- The presence of a QR complex in one or more of the precordial leads V_2 to V_6 (see Figs. 5–79 and 5–80). Negative precordial concordance is diagnostic of VT (Fig. 5–81), but pos-

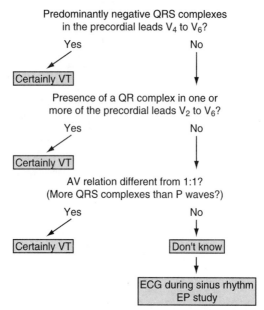

Predominantly negative QRS complexes
in the precordial leads V₄ to V₆?

Yes ———— No

Certainly VT

Presence of a QR complex in one or
more of the precordial leads V₂ to V₆?

Yes ———— No

Certainly VT

AV relation different from 1:1?
(More QRS complexes than P waves?)

Yes ———— No

Certainly VT | Don't know

ECG during sinus rhythm
EP study

Figure 5–79 □ Algorithm for the differential diagnosis of wide QRS complex tachycardia as it should be used in clinical practice. EP = Electrophysiologic; VT = ventricular tachycardia. (Redrawn from Steurer G, Gursoy S, Frey B, et al: The Differential Diagnosis on the Electrocardiogram Between Ventricular Tachycardia and Preexcited Tachycardia. Clin Cardiol 1994;17:306. Reprinted with permission from Clinical Cardiology Publishing Company, Inc.)

itive concordance (all complexes positive in leads V_1 to V_6) can be VT or circus movement antidromic WPW tachycardia.

- An RS interval of >0.10 second in any precordial lead
- AV dissociation; more QRS complexes than P waves. P wave identification may be difficult, however. T waves or the terminal or initial parts of the QRS complex may resemble P waves, causing an incorrect diagnosis of supraventricular tachycardia. Thus, AV dissociation is not a reliable diagnostic point.

Other suggestive features include
- Positive concordance
- A QS or rS in lead V_6 or net negative QRS complex in lead V_6; a small r wave with a deep S in lead V_6 is typical of VT
- Left rabbit ear taller than the right rabbit ear in lead V_1 (see Fig. 5–80). The rabbit ear may be very subtle; a slurred or notched S downstroke in lead V_1 or V_2 is suggestive of VT.
- Axis commonly −90 to ±180 degrees. The axis may, how-

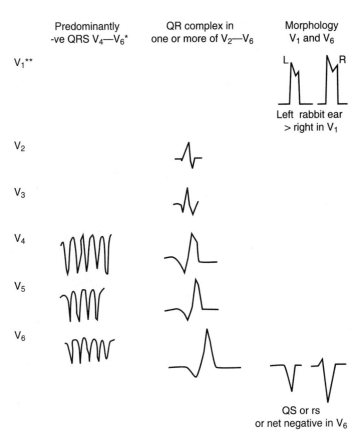

Figure 5–80 □ Electrocardiographic hallmarks of ventricular tachycardia.

* = or concordant negativity in leads V_1 to V_6 (see Fig. 5–81); positive concordance in leads V_1 to V_6 can be caused by VT or Wolff-Parkinson-White antidromic (preexcited) tachycardia (see Fig. 5–83*B*).

** = it is necessary to study the entire 12-lead tracing with particular emphasis on leads V_1 to V_6; lead II may be useful for assessment of P waves and AV dissociation.

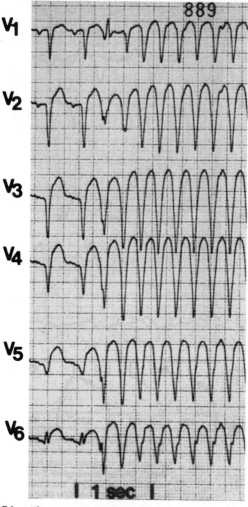

Figure 5–81 □ The onset of a tachycardia with negative precordial concordance. Negative precordial concordance indicates ventricular tachycardia, because such a pattern does not occur during anterograde conduction over an accessory pathway. (From Wellens HJJ, Conover MB: The ECG in Emergency Decision Making. Philadelphia, WB Saunders Co., 1992, p 60.)

ever, be normal in patients with idiopathic VT and some other varieties.

- Negative precordial concordance; an important feature of VT, because this pattern does not occur during antidromic WPW using anterograde conduction over the bypass tract; in this situation, positive concordance occurs.

The diagnosis of VT can be confidently made, therefore, by a careful study of the morphologic pattern of the QRS complex in leads V_1 to V_6 (see Figs. 5–79, 5–80, and 5–81).

Torsades de Pointes

Torsades de pointes is a polymorphic VT that usually occurs in the presence of a prolonged QT interval. The RR interval is irregular; the QRS complexes show a typical twisting of the points. The amplitudes of complexes vary and appear alternately above and below the baseline (Fig. 5–82). The ventricular rate varies from 200 to 300 beats/min but can reach 400 beats/min and is usually nonsustained, lasting 0.5 to 1 minute. Longer episodes degenerate into VT.

Drugs and conditions that increase the QT interval may precipitate torsades de pointes and include quinidine, procainamide, amiodarone, disopyramide, sotalol, tricyclic antidepressants, phenothiazines, histamine H_1 antagonists such as terfenadine, antiviral and antifungal agents, hypokalemia, hypomagnesemia, insecticide poisoning, bradyarrhythmias, congenital long QT syndrome, cirrhosis, and subarachnoid hemorrhage.

Supraventricular Tachycardias With Wide QRS

A wide QRS tachycardia and a diagnosis of aberration should be made only in special circumstances in which patients were known to have bundle branch block earlier and supraventricular tachycardia has ensued. Supraventricular tachycardia with a wide QRS complex is the likely diagnosis when atrial flutter or fibrillation occurs in a patient with WPW syndrome. An example of this form of preexcited tachycardia is shown in Figure 5–83A. Antidromic circus movement tachycardia (anterograde conduction over an accessory pathway) may cause a wide QRS tachycardia with positive concordance in leads V_1 to V_6 that resembles VT (see Figs. 5–79 and 5–83B).

In patients with irregular wide QRS tachycardias, the differential diagnosis includes atrial fibrillation with aberrant conduction or WPW syndrome with conduction over an accessory pathway (see Fig. 5–83A). In patients with very fast ventricular rates, in particular RR intervals ≤240 msec (fewer than six small spaces), WPW should be strongly considered.

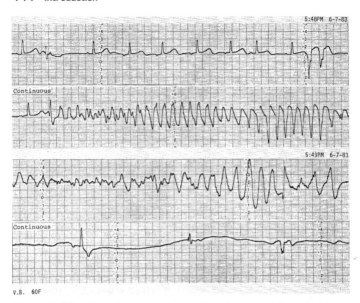

Figure 5–82 □ Torsades de pointes resulting from quinidine administration. The patient was a 60-year-old woman who had a previous myocardial infarction and was receiving digoxin and quinidine for the control of supraventricular and ventricular tachyarrhythmias. Because of recurrent dizziness, an ambulatory ECG was obtained. During the recording, she had a syncope episode. The tracing at the time of syncope (5:48 P.M.) shows torsades de pointes followed by ventricular fibrillation, and sinus arrest with ventricular space beats. Sinus rhythm returns in about 1 minute. Note the prolongation of the QT interval (0.48 second) in the top strip during sinus and ectopic atrial rhythm. There is a ventricular couplet followed by a pause and a supraventricular beat that falls on the terminal part of the T wave and initiates a 45-second episode of torsades de pointes. Thus, a long–short cycle initiating sequence is present. The quinidine and digoxin levels were within the therapeutic range. The patient did not have recurrence of syncope after quinidine administration was discontinued. (From Chou T-C: Electrocardiography in Clinical Practice, 4th ed. Philadelphia, WB Saunders Co., 1996, p 431.)

Bradyarrhythmias

Sinus Bradycardia

Sinus rhythm with rates of 45 to 60 beats/min is commonly observed in healthy individuals, and rates as low as 36 to 42 beats/min occur in most athletes. Causes of sinus bradycardia include physiologic causes, ischemic heart disease, sick sinus syndrome, hypothyroidism, and cardioactive drugs, in particular beta blockers, digoxin, and verapamil.

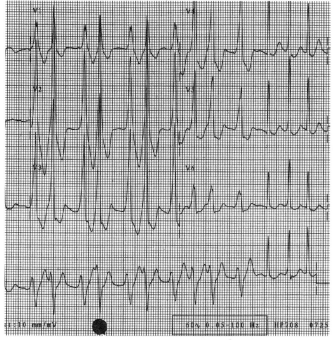

A

Figure 5–83 □ *A*, ECG from a 46-year-old man with a few short bouts of nonbothersome palpitations over 3 years. Onset of rapid tachycardia with presyncope resulted in an emergency room assessment. ECG reveals atrial fibrillation, rapid ventricular response, and wide QRS indicating conduction down the accessory pathway (antidromic, preexcited circus movement). Intravenous procainamide caused reversion; the ECG in sinus rhythm showed Wolff-Parkinson-White syndrome. The patient had electrophysiologic studies and successful ablation.

Illustration continued on following page

First-Degree AV Block

The normal PR interval ranges from 0.12 to 0.20 second (see Fig. 5–5*B*). Some normal individuals have intervals of 0.22 second.

Second-Degree AV Block

Patients with second-degree AV block should be categorized as having Mobitz type I (Wenckebach) or Mobitz type II. Two types of second-degree AV block were originally described by Wenckebach and Hay from their analysis of the A, C, and V waves in the jugular venous pulse; with the introduction of the ECG, Mobitz classified these blocks as type I and type II.

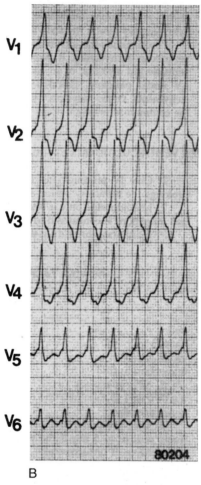

B

Figure 5–83 □ *Continued (B)* Broad QRS tachycardia with positive precordial concordance. The mechanism is atrial flutter with 2:1 conduction over a left-sided accessory pathway. (From Wellens HJJ, Conover MB: The ECG in Emergency Decision Making. Philadelphia, WB Saunders Co., 1992, p 61.)

Mobitz Type I AV Block

Mobitz type I (Wenckebach) is shown in Figure 5–84.

Hallmarks of Wenckebach

- The PR interval may begin within normal limits or may be slightly prolonged, and then with each beat, the PR interval gradually lengthens. Finally, the impulse fails to reach the ventricles and the QRS complex is dropped.
- Following the dropped beat, the PR interval reverts to near normal.
- The beats are grouped in pairs or trios (bigeminy, trigeminy).
- The long cycle containing the dropped beat (pause) is shorter than two of the shorter cycles because it contains the shortest PR interval.
- This type of benign block is observed with acute inferior MI, rheumatic fever, acute myocarditis, PAT, old age, digitalis toxicity, and administration of verapamil and diltiazem.
- Block is at the level of the AV node and rarely progresses to Mobitz type II or complete AV block.

Mobitz Type II AV Block

Diagnostic Features

- At least two regular and consecutive atrial impulses are conducted with the same PR interval before the dropped beat (Fig. 5–85).
- With high-grade block (2:1, 3:1), two or more consecutive atrial impulses fail to be conducted, in particular when the atrial rate is slow, at <135 beats/min, and in the absence of interference by an escaping subsidiary pacemaker.
- The QRS complex may be narrow if the conduction problem is in the His bundle and >0.12 second if the lesion is situated below the His bundle. Thus, the condition may precipitate third-degree AV block.

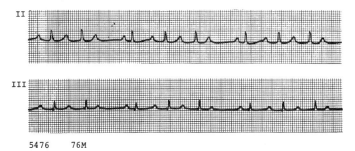

5476   76M

Figure 5–84 □ Type I second-degree atrioventricular block with typical Wenckebach's phenomenon. (From Chou T-C: Electrocardiography in Clinical Practice, 4th ed. Philadelphia, WB Saunders Co., 1996, p 451.)

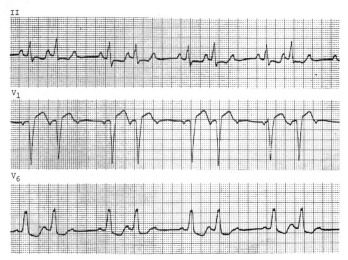

Figure 5–85 □ Mobitz type II second-degree atrioventricular block. There is a 3:2 conduction. The QRS complex has a left bundle branch block morphology. (From Chou T-C: Electrocardiography in Clinical Practice, 4th ed. Philadelphia, WB Saunders Co., 1996, p 453.)

- The PR interval is normal or slightly prolonged but remains constant, as opposed to Mobitz type I, in which the PR interval gradually becomes prolonged before the dropped beat.
- Ventricular rhythm is irregular because of nonconducted beats.

Mobitz type II block is usually caused by fibrotic disease of the conduction system or anteroseptal MI and may cause syncope or complete AV block. The condition is made worse by atropine, exercise, or catecholamines, whereas Mobitz type I block improves with atropine or exercise.

Third-Degree AV Block

Complete AV block is a serious condition and requires prompt diagnosis and treatment.

ECG Hallmarks

- P waves are sinus waves and plentiful with very few QRS complexes.
- AV dissociation; no relationship between P waves and QRS complexes; complete absence of AV conduction (Fig. 5–86A)
- The RR intervals are regular. The QRS complex is narrow if the site of block is in the AV node with an escape rhythm originating in the AV junction. The QRS complex is wide if

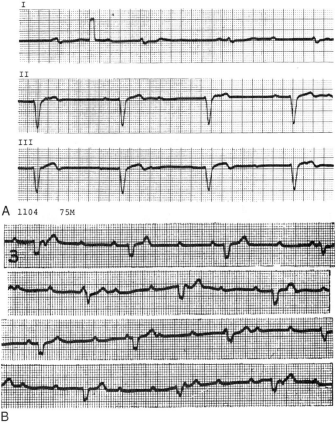

Figure 5–86 □ *A,* Complete atrioventricular block with idioventricular rhythm. The QRS complexes are abnormally wide and are different from those seen during sinus rhythm. The ventricular rate is 36 beats/min. (From Chou T-C: Electrocardiography in Clinical Practice, 4th ed. Philadelphia, WB Saunders Co., 1996, p 457.) *B,* Complete atrioventricular block with idioventricular rate of 36 and atrial rate of 104/min. The four strips are continuous. Atrial and ventricular activities are independent except for the first and last ventricular beats; each of these is conducted retrogradely to the atria (note that inverted P waves deformed the ST segments of these beats). (From Marriott HJL: Practical Electrocardiography, 8th ed. Baltimore, Williams & Wilkins, 1988, p 372.)

the escape rhythm originates from the ventricle or in the AV junction in the presence of bundle branch block.

- The ventricular rate is very slow, usually <45 beats/min, but with congenital AV block, rates may be 40 to 60 beats/min.
- With complete AV block, anterograde conduction never occurs, but in <20% of complete AV blocks, retrograde conduction to the atria occurs (Fig. 5–86B).

Note that AV dissociation may occur without the presence of third-degree AV block.

PATIENT-RELATED PROBLEMS: THE COMMON CALLS

6 | Chest Pain

Chest pain is one of the most important and common symptoms of heart disease and must be quickly assigned a cause. The resolution of the symptom is sometimes easy, but on many occasions it presents considerable difficulty for the physician. A systematic approach is necessary; taking an accurate and relevant history is crucial to the diagnosis.

■ PHONE CALL

Questions

1. Is the patient in the emergency room, the coronary care unit (CCU), or the ward?
2. What are the vital signs?
3. Is the patient stable or unstable?
4. Is the pain in the central, the left, or the right lateral chest?
5. Is there associated shortness of breath, and is it mild, moderate, or severe?
6. What is the age of the patient?

Orders

1. Give an IV of 5% dextrose in water, to keep veins open.
2. If the patient is unstable, instruct the RN to call the medical resident if this has not been done.
3. Order an electrocardiogram (ECG) immediately.
4. Give nitroglycerin 0.3 or 0.4 mg sublingually twice as needed (PRN).
5. Give oxygen by nasal prongs; start at 2 L/min.

Inform RN

"Will arrive at the bedside in . . . minutes."

■ ELEVATOR THOUGHTS

What are the common causes of chest pain? (Table 6–1)
1. **Cardiac causes.** Cardiac pain can be life threatening and

Table 6–1 □ CAUSES OF CHEST PAIN

Cardiac	Gastrointestinal
Myocardial infarction	Reflux esophagitis
Stable angina	Esophageal spasm
Unstable angina	Hiatal hernia
Pericarditis	Peptic ulcer
Aortic dissection	Chest wall pain
Pulmonary hypertension	Costochondritis
Pulmonary	Muscular
Pulmonary embolism	Rib fracture
Pleurisy	Nerve route pain
Pneumothorax	Cervical disk disease
Pneumonia	Cervical osteoarthritis
Mediastinal emphysema	Intercostal neuritis
Lung tumor	Herpes zoster (shingles)
Pleurodynia	Psychogenic

should be assessed rapidly. The following are the three sources of cardiac pain:

- The myocardium: acute myocardial infarction (MI) and unstable angina. The pattern of pain in stable angina is discussed in Chapter 8.
- The pericardium: pericarditis
- The great vessels: aortic dissection, pulmonary embolism, and pulmonary arterial hypertension

2. **Pulmonary causes**

- **Pleurisy:** The pain becomes worse on deep breathing and coughing and is unrelated to change in posture. There may be associated cough and pyrexia due to underlying chest infection.

- **Pulmonary embolism:** The pain may be severe, central, or pleuritic and is often associated with acute shortness of breath; the patient is often apprehensive and may be sweaty. Pulmonary embolism should be suspected when chest pain occurs in a setting that predisposes to thromboembolism, e.g., after surgery or with sudden immobilization for >2 days. Request arterial blood gas (ABG) study and ventilation-perfusion lung scan (see Chapter 16).

- **Pneumothorax:** Chest pain is usually associated with acute shortness of breath. Chest pain is often located in the lateral chest. Underlying causes include asthma, pneumocystis pneumonia, emphysema, tuberculosis, cystic fibrosis, interstitial pulmonary fibrosis, sarcoidosis, eosinophilic granuloma, blunt or penetrating trauma, and positive pressure ventilation.

- **Pneumonia:** Shortness of breath, fever, and chills, associated with pleuritic or nonpleuritic pain and cough, with or without sputum production

3. **Chest wall pain.** A common cause of chest wall pain is costochondritis. Pain is usually mild to moderate; it is usually localized to a fingertip area and is often present over the second or third costochondral junction. Chest wall pain from other causes may last from seconds to several hours. Pain is unrelated to exertion or activites and may appear to respond to nitroglycerin in some patients; unfortunately, it accompanies most types of heart disease, particularly ischemic heart disease and mitral valve prolapse syndrome.

4. **Pain of gastrointestinal (GI) origin:** Reflux esophagitis may mimic cardiac pain and may radiate from the upper epigastrium to the substernal area, the upper chest, the throat, and the arms. Pain does not radiate to the lower jaw, a feature of anginal pain. Pain lasting minutes to several hours may be mild to moderate but can be severe. Pain is not usually associated with profuse sweating or shortness of breath. The discomfort is worse on lying flat or on stooping but may start in the upright position. Pain is unrelated to exertional activities.

■ MAJOR THREAT TO LIFE

- Acute MI (see Chapter 7)
- Aortic dissection (see Chapter 11)
- Pulmonary embolism (see Chapter 16)
- Tension pneumothorax

The patient in cardiogenic shock is usually sweaty, pale, and apprehensive; there may be associated clouding of consciousness.

■ BEDSIDE

Quick Look Test

Does the patient look well (comfortable), sick (uncomfortable or distressed), or critical (about to die)?

If the patient is critically ill or is unstable, i.e., systolic blood pressure (BP) is <100 mm Hg; pulse rate is < 40 beats/min or >150 beats/min with a cardiac arrhythmia; or there is clouding of consciousness, call your resident immediately.

Airway and Vital Signs

What is the blood pressure?

Although the BP may be normal in patients with unstable angina and acute MI, many patients with MI, pulmonary embolism, or cardiac tamponade have systolic BPs of <100 mm Hg and require aggressive management.

What is the heart rate?
1. Does the patient have tachycardia?
   If so, is this related to chest pain, shortness of breath, or clouding of consciousness? Request a rhythm strip, and hook up the patient to a cardiac monitor (see Chapters 5 and 19).
2. Does the patient have bradycardia?
   This may be caused by treatment with beta blockers, diltiazem, or a combination of these two agents. Also, inferior MI commonly causes sinus bradycardia. Bradycardia usually requires no treatment unless it is symptomatic (see Chapter 19).

What is the breathing pattern?
   Tachypnea may occur with pulmonary embolism and status asthmaticus. Orthopnea may be present in patients with acute MI. Painful breathing on inspiration suggests a pleuritic or pleuropericardial origin.

Selective History and Chart Review

It is necessary to become familiar with the description of cardiac pain so that the diagnosis of stable angina, unstable angina, or MI can be made clinically within a few minutes. Because urgent administration of thrombolytic therapy is crucial to reducing morbidity and mortality, it is vital to make the diagnosis of acute MI within a few minutes of the patient's arrival in the emergency room or the physician's office.

Salient features of cardiac pain are as follows:

- The pain of acute MI is usually described as crushing, vise-like, or a tightness or a heaviness (see Chapter 7).
- The location of pain in acute MI is usually substernal across the chest, often accompanied by diaphoresis and sometimes shortness of breath.
- Figure 6–1 gives the location and the radiation of cardiac pain. The pain is unlikely due to MI if it can be located with one fingertip or if it is made worse by deep breathing or coughing.

If the patient is stable and the diagnosis is not yet clarified, obtain relevant information from all sources, i.e., the patient, the spouse, a relative, a chart review, and the nursing staff.

- The pain of MI usually lasts from minutes to several hours.
- The pain of angina is typically a retrosternal discomfort, precipitated by a particular activity, especially walking quickly up an incline or against a wind. Pain or discomfort disappears within seconds to minutes of stopping the precipitating activity, in keeping with the concept of oxygen supply

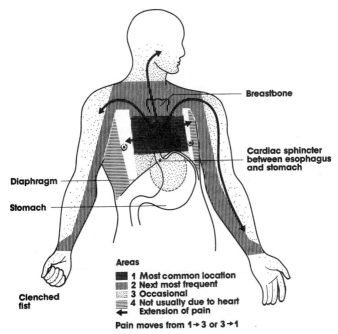

Breastbone

Cardiac sphincter between esophagus and stomach

Diaphragm

Stomach

Areas

▓ 1 Most common location
▥ 2 Next most frequent
▦ 3 Occasional
▤ 4 Not usually due to heart
← Extension of pain

Pain moves from 1→3 or 3→1

Clenched fist

Figure 6–1 □ Common locations of cardiac pain. (From Khan, M Gabriel: Heart Disease Diagnosis and Therapy: A Practical Approach. Baltimore, Williams & Wilkins, 1996, p 143.)

insufficient to meet myocardial demand. The discomfort is usually located in the lower, middle, or upper substernal area, the arm, or the lower jaw. The discomfort is usually described as tightness, squeezing, heaviness, pressure, constriction, strangulation, burning, nausea, or an indigestion-like feeling of gradual onset that disappears at rest, except with unstable anginal syndromes (see Chapter 8).

- The area of pain in MI is usually at least the size of a clenched fist and often occupies most of the central chest area. The patient uses more than two fingers, the fist, or the entire palm of the hand to indicate the site. Patients with unstable angina have pain that has changed in pattern and frequency.
- Pericardial pain is usually sharp or stabbing, is relieved by sitting and leaning forward or standing, is made worse on lying down or on deep inspiration, and does not usually radiate to the neck or arms (see Chapter 9).
- Pain of dissecting aneurysm is sudden like a gunshot; the pain is excruciating and persists with the same intensity for hours; pain may radiate to the back.

Warning: Myocardial ischemia or infarction may cause only minimal chest discomfort for a few minutes; pain may range from minor distress to being severe and unbearable.

What does the electrocardiogram (ECG) show?

Is the ECG in keeping with acute MI? Acute MI poses a threat to life; the diagnosis must be made rapidly. Thrombolytic therapy has proved effective in saving life if given within 6 hours of the onset of chest pain. It is important, however, that triage through the emergency room be efficient; patients presenting with chest pain caused by acute MI should receive thrombolytic therapy within 15 minutes of presentation to the emergency room (see Chapter 7).

Selective Physical Examination

1. Assess the BP and heart rate.
2. Assess the cardiovascular system.

Is the patient orthopneic? Apprehensive or sweaty? Assess for elevated jugular venous pressure or abnormal venous waves. With the bell of the stethoscope placed gently on the chest wall, listen for gallop sounds. Listen with the diaphragm of the stethoscope for murmurs and, with the patient leaning forward with the breath held in deep expiration, for an aortic diastolic murmur and pericardial friction rubs (see Chapters 4 and 9).

3. Assess the respiratory system.

Assess for crackles over the lower lung fields that may indicate left ventricular failure; unilaterally decreased air entry and hyperresonance suggest a pneumothorax.

■ MANAGEMENT

- Acute MI (see Chapter 7)
- Unstable angina (see Chapter 8)
- Pericarditis (see Chapter 9)
- Aortic dissection (see Chapter 11)
- Pulmonary embolism (see Chapter 16)

Pneumothorax.   Intervention is necessary for symptomatic primary pneumothoraces or if the pneumothorax is >40%. Tension pneumothorax causes severe respiratory distress and is a medical emergency that requires urgent relief of the pressure by using a 16-gauge IV catheter. Call your senior resident for assistance. After rapid radiologic confirmation, insert a 16-gauge IV catheter as follows:

1. Put on sterile gloves; clean the area of the second intercostal space in the midclavicular line on the affected side of the chest.

2. Infiltrate the area with lidocaine, and insert a 16-gauge IV catheter above the rib into the site until air is aspirated. Remove the inner needle and attach the catheter to a three-way stopcock and a 60-ml syringe to allow repeated aspirations. Aspiration is discontinued when no more air can be withdrawn, or when about 2.5 L has been removed. Occlude the catheter for about 6 hours, and if the chest radiograph shows no recurrence, remove the catheter.

The insertion of a chest tube (tube thoracostomy) is required in patients with underlying lung disease, with respiratory compromise, or for failure of simple aspiration. A small, asymptomatic pneumothorax usually resolves spontaneously over a few days.

Esophagitis and Reflux Syndrome

1. Elevate the head of the patient's bed.
2. Give **Maalox or a similar antacid 30 ml at 1 hour and 3 hours after meals plus at bedtime.**
3. Give **omeprazole 20 mg daily** or similar agent.
4. If candidiasis is suspected in an immunocompromised patient, request a GI consultation for endoscopic confirmation, then order **ketoconazole 200 to 400 mg daily.**

Calls concerning acute myocardial infarction (MI) and its complications are frequent. In >95% of cases, an acute MI is caused by occlusion of a coronary artery by a thrombus overlying a ruptured atheromatous plaque. The ruptured plaque, by direct release of tissue factor and exposure of the subintima, is highly thrombogenic. The diagnosis must be made rapidly to allow the timely initiation of therapy that improves survival, prevents long-term complications of MI, and results in a better quality of life. Such therapy consists of **aspirin, a beta-blocking drug, a thrombolytic agent, an angiotensin-converting enzyme (ACE) inhibitor, and a statin.**

■ PHONE CALL

Questions

1. Is the chest pain relieved by 2 nitroglycerin tablets or nitrolingual spray? If not, is the pain mild, moderate, or severe?
2. Is the electrocardiogram (ECG) now available?
3. Is the patient stable or unstable?
4. Is the patient acutely short of breath?

Orders

If the patient's chest pain is persistent after nitroglycerin, give **morphine 4 mg intravenously (IV) immediately and aspirin 160 or 325 mg chewed and swallowed.** Contraindications to the use of morphine include status asthmaticus, severe chronic obstructive pulmonary disease (COPD), and severe, untreated hypothyroidism. Further small incremental doses of 2 to 4 mg intravenously (IV) should be given only after assessment of the patient.

Inform RN

"Will arrive at the bedside in <2 minutes."

Patients with chest pain and suspected acute MI or proven infarction must be assessed immediately to obtain a brief and relevant history and interpretation of the ECG to document acute infarction.

■ ELEVATOR THOUGHTS

1. Prepare to assess the chest pain, and ensure that it is consi̇tent with acute MI (see Chapter 6, Table 6–1, Fig. 6–1, and page 178).
2. Be prepared to give IV streptokinase, tissue plasminogen activator (tPA), or other thrombolytic, depending on your emergency room (ER) policy, as soon as the ECG confirms the diagnosis.
3. Ask about a history of asthma, because the use of a beta blocker is contraindicated in patients with asthma.

■ MAJOR THREAT TO LIFE

- Extensive infarction
- Moderate to severe acute pulmonary edema
- Moderate to severe heart failure, in particular in patients with a second infarct and in elderly patients
- Cardiogenic shock
- Mycardial rupture

■ BEDSIDE

Quick Look Test

Does the patient look relatively well (comfortable), sick (uncomfortable or distressed), or critical (about to die)?
Is the patient orthopneic and in respiratory distress, and is there clouding of consciousness?

Airway and Vital Signs

What is the BP?
Most patients with acute MI have a fall in blood pressure (BP). If severe hypotension is present, if systolic pressure is <100 mm Hg, call your resident for assistance.

What is the heart rate?
1. Does the patient have tachycardia?
   A sinus tachycardia of 100 to 125 beats/min is not uncommon in patients with anterior MI in the absence of heart failure. These patients respond well to a small dose of a beta-blocking drug. If an arrhythmia is present, request assistance from the resident.
2. Does the patient have bradycardia?
   A heart rate <60 beats/min is commonly seen in patients with acute inferior MI, which initiates vagal overactivity. Severe bradycardia <50 beats/min may predispose to ventricular fibrillation (VF), especially if hypotension is present.

Symptomatic bradycardia <50 beats/min with hypotension or associated with ventricular premature beats (VPBs) should be managed with administration of **atropine 0.5 or 0.6 mg IV given slowly** to increase the heart rate to about 60 beats/min. Asymptomatic bradycardia should not be treated with atropine.

What is the breathing pattern?

Orthopnea with tachypnea occurs in >20% of patients, and careful clinical assessment to determine the degree of heart failure is necessary. The majority of patients with mild heart failure do not exhibit significant orthopnea.

Selective History

Reassess the chest pain for location, radiation, intensity, and what makes it better or worse.

Selective Physical Examination

1. Assess the jugular venous pressure (JVP); elevation to >2 cm above the sternal angle indicates heart failure.
2. Auscultate the heart.
   - Gallop rhythm; an S_4 is commonly present; an S_3 is heard if there is congestive heart failure (CHF), a previous large infarct, or a left ventricular aneurysm.
   - New systolic murmurs may be caused by mitral regurgitation, secondary to infarction and ischemia of the papillary muscle that produces papillary muscle dysfunction. The murmur may be early systolic, midsystolic, late systolic, or holosystolic in timing. Mitral regurgitation secondary to papillary muscle rupture is rare and causes hemodynamic compromise and pulmonary edema. The murmur caused by a ventricular septal defect secondary to rupture of the septum usually occurs 2 to 5 days after infarction. Pericardial friction rubs may occur occasionally within hours of acute infarction, but most are heard during the second to fifth days after infarction. A rub is best heard with the patient upright and leaning forward with the breath held at the end of complete exhalation, and auscultating with the diaphragm firmly pressed.
3. Listen over the lung fields for crepitations (crackles); these may be more prominent over the lower two-thirds of the lung fields in patients with left ventricular failure.

■ DIAGNOSTIC TESTING

Electrocardiographic Diagnosis

The ECG is the single most valuable test for documenting the diagnosis of acute MI at the earliest stage. **Because creatine** kinase (CK) and cardiac troponin T (cardiac TnT) elevation occur only from 6 to 12 hours after the onset of symptoms, their measurements are not relevant to the early management of ST-elevation MI with thrombolytic agents. Therefore, it is important for all students, house staff, and ER physicians to learn how to accurately interpret the ECG (see Chapter 5).

Electrocardiographic Hallmarks of Acute Myocardial Infarction

- ST segment elevation of ≥1 mm in two or more contiguous limb leads (see Fig. 5–28) or ST elevation ≥1 mm in two or more contiguous precordial leads (see Fig. 5–29A).
- Several conditions may cause ST elevation and thus mimic acute MI (see discussion in Chapter 5).
- Small Q waves may be visible from 2 hours after the onset of chest pain but are not essential for the early diagnosis. Q waves may develop early or from 4 to 12 hours after the onset of symptoms. Patients with chest pain and ST segment elevation who are unresponsive to nitroglycerin usually develop a Q wave infarct.
- **In patients with ST segment elevation, the presence of reciprocal ST segment depression is an important confirming sign** (see Fig. 5–31).
- Chest pain and ST segment depression and CK MB band (CK-MB) elevation without ST segment elevation is categorized as **non–ST elevation MI** (non–Q wave infarction) (see Fig. 5–47).
- The terms "transmural" and "nontransmural" infarction are no longer used.
- ST-T wave abnormalities, termed "evolutionary changes," occur during the next 12 to 36 hours (see Chapter 5).

Location of Infarction

The location of the infarct site depends on the coronary artery involved and is usually categorized as

- Anteroseptal, with ST elevation in leads V_1 to V_3 (see Fig. 5–40A).
- Anterior, with ST elevation in leads V_3 to V_5.
- Anterolateral, with ST elevation in leads V_4 to V_6, 1, and aVL.
- Inferior, with ST elevation in leads, II, III, and aVF, and reciprocal depression in leads V_1, V_2, and V_3 (see Fig. 5–31).
- Inferoposterior, with ST elevation in leads II, III, and aVF and a tall R wave in leads V_1 and V_2 (see Fig. 5–43).
- Right ventricular, with ST elevation in leads V_3R and V_4R.

Size of Infarction

- Involvement of two to three leads indicates a small infarct.
- Involvement of four to five leads indicates a moderate infarct.
- Involvement of six to seven leads indicates a large infarct.

- Involvement of eight or more leads indicates an extensive infarct (see Fig. 5–44).

■ MANAGEMENT

Aspirin

Aspirin should be given within minutes of the patient's arrival in the ER; **160 to 325 mg chewed and swallowed, then enteric-coated aspirin 160 to 325 mg swallowed once daily.** Aspirin enhances the efficacy of thrombolytic agents.

Pain Relief

It is necessary to relieve pain promptly, because pain precipitates autonomic disturbances that may trigger malignant arrhythmias and hypotension and may increase infarct size.

Morphine. Morphine **4 mg IV at a rate of 1 mg/min** should be given and **repeated if necessary at a dose of 2 to 4 mg at intervals of 5 to 15 minutes** until pain is completely relieved. Morphine may cause hypotension and respiratory depression. Assess the BP and respiratory rate before each dose. Morphine allays anxiety and causes venodilation, thus reducing preload; also, the drug increases VF threshold. Respiratory depression related to morphine peaks about 7 minutes after IV dosing. Respiratory depression can be reversed with the narcotic antagonist **naloxone (Narcan) 0.4 to 0.8 mg every 15 minutes, to a maximum of 1.2 mg. Metoclopramide 5 to 10 mg IV** may be given if the first or second dose of morphine causes vomiting or severe nausea. In the United Kingdom, diamorphine is preferred, i.e., 2 to 5 mg IV every 4 hours. **Meperidine (pethidine) 25 to 50 mg IV by slow injection** may be used if pain relief is required in patients with inferior MI and bradycardia; morphine may cause bradycardia.

Beta Blockers. If morphine fails to completely relieve pain, a beta-blocking drug should be given intravenously if there is no contraindication (Table 7–1). If beta blockers are contraindicated, nitroglycerin IV should be administered for the relief of pain.

Treatment of ST Elevation Myocardial Infarction

Thrombolytic Therapy

Both tPA (alteplase) and streptokinase (SK) have proved effective in saving lives when given to patients within 6 hours of onset of symptoms. Some clinical trials have provided (weak) evidence that a few lives can be saved when thrombolytic therapy is administered between the 6th and 12th hours. In large random-

Table 7–1 □ **DOSAGE OF BETA BLOCKERS IN ACUTE MYOCARDIAL INFARCTION***

IV†	Oral Dosage First 7 Days	1 Week to 2 Years
Atenolol (IV 5 mg over 5 min, 10 min later 5 mg over 5 min)	10 min after last IV dose give 50 mg oral daily	50 mg daily
Metoprolol (IV 5 mg at a rate of 1 mg/min, 5 min later 2nd 5-mg bolus, 5 min later 3rd 5-mg bolus)	8 hr after IV 25–50 mg twice daily	50–100 mg twice daily
Propranolol (IV not approved for MI in USA)	20 mg 3 times daily	80 mg long acting, increasing to 160 mg once daily; maximum 240 mg daily
Timolol	5 mg twice daily	5–10 mg twice daily

Modified from Khan, M Gabriel: Heart Disease Diagnosis and Therapy: A Practical Approach. Baltimore, Williams & Wilkins, 1996, p 35.

*Contraindications: bronchial asthma, severe heart failure, systolic BP <100 mm Hg, second- or third-degree AV block.

†Halt IV if the following events develop: heart rate <50 beats/min, second- or third-degree AV block, PR >0.24, systolic BP <95 mm Hg, marked shortness of breath, wheezes, or crackles in more than one-third of the lung fields, or pulmonary capillary wedge pressure >22 mm Hg, if this parameter is being monitored.

IV = intravenous; MI = myocardial infarction; BP = blood pressure; AV = atrioventricular.

ized trials in which thrombolytic therapy was given 1, 3, 4 to 6, and 7 to 12 hours from the onset of symptoms, the numbers of lives saved were 65, 27, 25, and 8, respectively, per 1000-treated patients. It is therefore imperative that the thrombolytic agent be given within 30 minutes of the patient's arrival in the ER (Fig. 7–1).

Choice of Thrombolytic Agent

None of the large randomized trials that have compared SK with tPA in some 80,000 patients (without restricting data only to GUSTO-I) found any significant difference in outcome. **Experts in the United Kingdom strongly advise that the choice of SK versus accelerated tPA is of little consequence to public health measures provided that either agent is used within 2 hours of onset of symptoms. Rapidity of administration is the key to improved survival and quality of life.** In the GUSTO trial, accelerated tPA caused a modest 14% reduction in mortality over SK IV, and this beneficial effect at 30 days was sustained at 1 year.

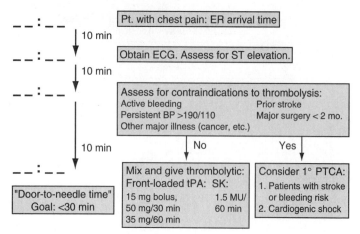

Figure 7–1 □ Algorithm for rapid triage of patients in the emergency room (ER) to provide thrombolysis with the shortest possible "door-to-needle" time. tPA = tissue plasminogen activator; SK = streptokinase; PTCA = percutaneous transluminal coronary angioplasty. (Courtesy of Dr. Chris Cannon, Brigham and Women's Hospital, Boston, MA. Redrawn from Julian D, Braunwald E, eds: Management of Acute Myocardial Infarction. London, WB Saunders Co., 1994, p 48.)

However, tPA is much more expensive than SK, requires several days of heparin IV to ensure vessel patency, and causes a slightly higher rate of intracranial hemorrhage (ICH), particularly in patients older than 75 years. The rate of ICH for alteplase was approximately 0.7%, but **in recent studies it is 0.8% to 0.9%. The rate for SK is 0.44%.** In patients over age 75 the incidence of stroke is >4% for tPA versus <2.8% for SK. The choice of tPA or SK depends on the preference of the hospital.

The following guidelines have been suggested for patients in the United States:

- Do a composite assessment of risk based on age of the patient, location and size of the infarct, presence of a previous infarction, and degree of heart failure (Table 7–2).
- Patients at high risk are given accelerated tPA and heparin (see heparin infusion pump chart [Table A–3]).
- For low-risk patients—e.g., those with inferior MI, absence of CHF, and no prior infarction—SK plus aspirin (no heparin) is used in some hospitals.
- SK is advisable in patients older than age 75 because of a higher risk of bleeding with the combination of tPA and heparin than with SK. SK is routinely used in the United Kingdom for most patients. Many hospitals in the United States are wisely switching from tPA to SK because the cum-

Table 7–2 □ TISSUE PLASMINOGEN ACTIVATOR PREFERRED THERAPY

1. Patient with extensive infarction: (ST segment ↑ in ≥8 leads)
2. Patient younger than 75 years with anterior infarction. In patient older than 75 years, streptokinase carries less risk of cerebral bleeding than accelerated tPA.
3. Patient with second infarction, in particular if it is complicated by pulmonary edema, indicating very high risk
4. Patient allergic to streptokinase or if streptokinase was used in prior 12 months.

tPA = tissue plasminogen activator.

bersome use of heparin is not required, the ICH rate is significantly less, and the cost per dose is $294 for SK and $2196 for tPA (Tables 7–3 and 7–4). Nonetheless, tPA is used in this setting in most hospitals in the United States.

Streptokinase.   SK forms an activator complex with plasminogen and converts circulating plasminogen to plasmin, which causes lysis of fibrin. Dosage: **1.5 million U in 100 mg 0.9% saline over 30 to 60 minutes.**

Alteplase tPA (Activase).   tPA binds specifically to fibrin and its substrate plasminogen, resulting in activation of plasminogen to plasmin, which causes lysis of fibrin. Dosage: **15-mg bolus, then 0.75 mg/kg over 30 minutes, not to exceed 50 mg; then 0.5 mg/kg over 30 minutes, not to exceed 35 mg.** tPA has a very short half-life.

tPA interacts with diltiazem, which may cause an increase in the incidence of cerebral hemorrhage; nitroglycerin IV impairs the thrombolytic effects of tPA.

Reteplase (Retavase).   Reteplase is administered in a 10 U plus 10 U double-bolus dose, each over 2 minutes, given 30 minutes apart. The patency rate is similar to tPA, but without the need for an infusion pump, administration is easy.

Tenecteplase (TNKase).   A single-bolus injection of tenecteplase **is a major advance that is clinically meaningful** and should gain widespread acceptance. **(Consult the product monograph and your hospital's MI thrombolytic protocols and Table C–2.)**

Adverse Effects of Thrombolytic Agents

1. Bleeding, particularly in patients with invasive procedures. Intracranial bleeding in 0.3 to 1% of patients; the incidence of intracranial bleeding is higher in patients older than 75 years
2. Rarely, myocardial or splenic rupture
3. Allergic reactions to streptokinase in 5 to 10% of patients

Table 7–3 □ INTRACRANIAL HEMORRHAGE IN RECENT THROMBOLYTIC TRIALS

Patient Characteristics	GUSTO-I (497)	GUSTO-II (805)	COBALT (832)	GUSTO-III (802,833)	ASSENT-2*	In Time-II*
Number	41,021	3473	7169	15,059	16,950	15,078
Average age (y)	62	62.5	62.4	63	—	—
>75 y [%]	10.5	11.8	13.0	13.6	—	—
Female [%]	25.2	22.4	23.4	27.4	—	—
Intracranial Hemorrhage Rates						
SK	0.51	0.37	—	—	—	—
tPA	0.70	0.72	Double bolus 1.12 Accl infusion 0.81	0.87	0.93	0.62
nPA	—	—	—	0.91	—	—
TNK-tPA	0.7	0.72	—	—	0.94	—
nPA	—	—	—	—	—	1.13

From Ryan TJ, Antman EM, Brooks NH, et al: ACC/AHA guidelines for the management of patients with acute myocardial infarction. J Am Coll Cardiol 1999;34:890–911. © 1999 by the American College of Cardiology and American Heart Association, Inc. Reproduced with permission.
*Data based on preliminary results.
accl = accelerated; nPA = lanetoplase; nPA = reteplase; TNK-tPA = a genetically engineered variant of tPA; tPA = tissue plasminogen activator; SK = streptokinase.

Table 7-4 □ COMPARISON OF APPROVED THROMBOLYTIC AGENTS

	Streptokinase	Anistreplase	Alteplase	Reteplase
Dose	1.5 MU in 30–60 min	30 mg in 5 min	100 mg in 90 min	10 U × 2 over 30 min
Bolus administration	No	Yes	No	Yes
Antigenic	Yes	Yes	No	No
Allergic reactions [hypotension most common]	Yes	Yes	No	No
Systemic fibrinogen depletion	Marked	Marked	Mild	Moderate
90-min patency rates [%]	≈50	≈65	≈75	≈75
TIMI grade 3 flow [%]	32	43	54	60
Mortality rate in most recent comparative trials [%]	7.3	10.5	7.2	7.5
Cost per dose [US]	$294	$2116	$2196	$2196

From Ryan TJ, Antman EM, Brooks NH, et al: ACC/AHA guidelines for the management of patients with acute myocardial infarction. J Am Coll Cardiol 1999;34:890–911. © 1999 by the American College of Cardiology and American Heart Association, Inc. Reproduced with p⟶ :⟶n.
TIMI = Thrombolysis in Myocardial Infarction.

ı hemorrhage occurs, discontinue streptokinase and administer ıood products.

Contraindications to Use of Thrombolytic Agents

1. Recent hemorrhage within prior weeks
2. Previous cerebral hemorrhage
3. Nonhemorrhagic stroke within 6 months
4. Major surgery or major trauma within 2 months
5. Severe hypertension, i.e., systolic BP >200 mm Hg, diastolic BP >110 mm Hg
6. Diabetic proliferative retinopathy
7. Suspected aortic dissection
8. Underlying malignancy
9. Significant dementia
10. Neurologic operation in prior 6 months

Use of Beta Blockers

Therapy is indicated in all patients but, in particular, in those with acute anterior infarction.

Contraindications include
1. Asthma
2. Severe CHF
3. Hypotension, i.e., systolic BP <100 mm Hg
4. Heart rate <60 beats/min

IV and oral dosages are given in Table 7–1. Beta blockers decrease the incidence of cardiac rupture, decrease the infarct size, and improve survival if administered within 4 hours of onset of symptoms. Most clinical trials administered beta blockers after the fourth hour of onset of symptoms. **The American College of Cardiology–American Heart Association (ACC-AHA) task force committee strongly recommends the use of a beta-blocking drug unless there are contraindications** (see study section at end of chapter).

Use of ACE Inhibitors

The ACC-AHA recommends ACE inhibitors within the first 24 hours of a suspected anterior MI with ST segment elevation in >2 anterior precordial leads or with CHF in the absence of hypotension (systolic BP <100 mm Hg) or known contraindication. They should be initiated at low doses, e.g., captopril in a 6-mg test dose, then 12.5 mg 3 times per day, or enalapril 2.5 mg twice daily. The dose should be increased cautiously over a few days, but hypotension must be avoided.

Use of Nitrates

The GISSI-3 and the ISIS-4 trials yielded an insignificant mortality reduction among patients randomized to 24 hours of IV nitroglycerin. The ACC-AHA task force committee recommends IV nitroglycerin for 24 to 48 hours in patients with CHF, persistent ischemia, hypertension, and extensive transmural anterior MI. Nitroglycerin IV and other preload-reducing agents are contraindicated in patients with right ventricular infarction (RVI), hypotension, and aortic stenosis. The combination of nitroglycerin IV and a beta blocker is complementary and is advisable in patients with recurrence of ischemic pain.

Nonspecific Therapy

- Order bedrest with bedside commode for 24 hours.
- Give oxygen by nasal prongs, 2 to 4 L/min for 12 hours, then continue only if there is evidence of pulmonary edema or proven hypoxemia. Use a Venturi or similar low-flow oxygen delivery system if COPD is present.
- Give a stool softener, e.g., **docusate 100 mg 2 or 3 times daily.**
- Order sedation, **oxazepam 15 mg or lorazepam 1 mg once daily and at bedtime** for a few days.

Arrhythmia Management

VPBs that are asymptomatic require no medication. Prophylactic lidocaine is used only where facilities for monitoring cardiac rhythm are poor; in areas where a cardiac monitor and a defibrillator are available, lidocaine is unnecessary, is potentially toxic, and adds to expense. Lidocaine is used in the following subsets of patients:

1. Those having VPBs causing hemodynamic disturbance
2. Those having multiform VPBs, triplets, or nonsustained ventricular tachycardia, or R on T phenomenon, if observed
3. Those having had an episode of VF
4. Those having had an episode of VT that occurred within 24 hours of infarction

Dosage: **Lidocaine IV, initial bolus of 1 to 1.5 mg/kg (75–100 mg).** After 5 to 10 minutes, **give a second bolus of 1 mg/kg.** The second or subsequent doses should be reduced in the presence of liver disease or CHF and in patients older than 70 years. Start an infusion at the same time the bolus is given, and continue the **intravenous infusion at 2 mg/min,** or a maximum of 3 mg/min.

Treatment of Non–ST Elevation Myocardial Infarction

Patients with chest pain and no ST elevation but CK-MB elevation were categorized as having non–Q wave infarction. The terminology "non–Q wave MI" has become redundant but is still used in current cardiology journals. The mortality for these patients is low within the first 2 weeks of infarction; thereafter, the incidence of angina and mortality increases.

Thrombolytic therapy does not improve survival and is not recommended. Therapy includes aspirin, beta blockers, and statins. If beta blockers are contraindicated, diltiazem may be given if the EF is >40%, until catheterization is evaluated with regard to possible angioplasty or bypass surgery.

Cardiac Enzymes

Creatine Kinase. A total CK >220 U/L with a CK-MB mass >10 μg/L and a relative index >3.9 is consistent with myocardial damage. A CK-MB mass <5 μg/L and a relative index <2.0 is negative. Other combinations of results are equivocal. The CK-MB is not specific and may be elevated in patients with rhabdomyolysis, head injuries, bowel infarction, and end-stage renal failure. The relative index is low in these situations. CK-MB isoforms are useful serum cardiac markers; they exist in only one form in the myocardium—CK-MB2—but occur in different isoforms in plasma. **An absolute level of CK-MB2 >1 U/L or a ratio of CK-MB2 to CK-MB1 of 1.5** has improved sensitivity and specificity for the diagnosis of MI within the first 6 hours compared with CK-MB assays.

Troponin. Troponin levels are not required in patients with ST segment elevation MI, but they are more useful than CK-MB in the risk stratification of patients with non–ST segment elevation MI (non–Q wave MI) and those with unstable angina, and they are efficient for the late diagnosis of MI.

Cardiac-specific troponins (TnI and TnT) may not be detectable for up to 6 hours after onset of chest pain, but their elevation in these patients and even in the presence of normal CK-MB indicates an increased risk of death or reinfarction (see Chapter 8). TnT levels may be elevated (>0.1 μg/L) in patients with end-stage renal failure or severe CHF. In end-stage renal disease (due to diabetes, glomerulonephritis, hypertension, and other causes), these increases are stable over short periods, and measuring TnT in a subsequent sample will clarify the situation. The CK-MB elevation in MI may occur 1 to 2 hours earlier than troponin and is not elevated in CHF. Measurement of troponin levels is of greatest value in patients with unstable angina and normal CK-MB.

Treatment of Complications of Infarction

Congestive Heart Failure. Mild CHF occurs commonly and responds to small doses of **furosemide 20 to 40 mg daily for 2 to 3 days.** Invasive hemodynamic monitoring is not required if the systolic BP is >100 mm Hg and there is no evidence of hypoperfusion or oliguria.

SEVERE CHF. Dyspnea, accompanied by crepitations over more than one-third of the lower lung fields and increased JVP, requires aggressive management with furosemide and nitroglycerin IV; dobutamine IV may be required if hypotension is present. Insert a balloon flotation (Swan-Ganz) catheter. Pharmacologic therapy should be guided by hemodynamic parameters. Patients with a pulmonary capillary wedge pressure (PCWP) >22 mm Hg and a cardiac index <2.2 L/min/m² have a poor prognosis.

Management is as follows:

- Have the patient propped up and the trunk and the head maintained at a >45-degree angle.
- Give oxygen by nasal prongs at 2 to 4 L/min.
- Give **furosemide 40 to 80 mg IV** but ensure that the serum potassium is >4 mEq/L (mmol/L).
- Start **dobutamine IV** if the systolic BP is 70 to 100 mm Hg. Start at **2.5 μg/kg/min, and titrate the dose to the range of 3 to 10 μg/kg/min.**
- Administer **nitroglycerin IV** if the PCWP is >24 mm Hg and the systolic BP is >95 mm Hg. Start with **5 μg/min** and **increase by 5 μg/min every 5 minutes to the range of 20 to 40 μg/min.** Decrease the rate if the systolic BP is <95 mm Hg.
- Use a combination of dobutamine and nitroglycerin, depending on hemodynamic parameters.
- Add **digoxin 0.5 mg immediately, then 0.125 to 0.25 mg daily,** when the patient has stabilized and it is appropriate to wean off dobutamine over 2 to 4 days.
- Start **captopril, at a test dose of 3 mg,** when the BP is >100 mm Hg and stable for >24 hours; then **increase the dose over days to 12.5 mg two times per day, then to 25 mg 2 or 3 times per day** at the time of discharge. Captopril is easier to use than enalapril, because the 3- or 6-mg test dose causes less hypotension, and an observation of 2 hours is required, versus 4 hours with enalapril dosing. If needed, on discharge, the patient can be switched to **enalapril 2.5 to 5 mg twice daily** and, on follow-up, **5 to 10 mg once or twice daily,** depending on the level of the systolic BP and the patient's tolerance of the drug.

Right Ventricular Infarction. RVI is strongly suspected when a patient presents with an inferior infarct with complications. An RVI diagnosis is made when an ECG shows signs of an inferior infarct plus ST elevation in lead V_4R or V_3R (see Fig. 5–43). The JVP may be elevated but with clear lung fields. A normal PCWP and a right atrial pressure of >10 mm Hg strengthens the diagnosis; Kussmaul's sign may be present.

Management is as follows:
- Avoid preload reducing agents, such as diuretics, ACE inhibitors, and nitroglycerin.
- Start plasma volume expansion combined with dobutamine.
- If hemodynamic deterioration occurs, arrange for coronary angiography for a possible angioplasty. Coronary balloon angioplasty has been shown to produce beneficial effects in patients with RVI.

Postinfarction Angina. Chest pain should not recur after infarction because necrotic myocardium does not cause pain. Thus, if pain occurs after day 1, search for pericarditis or recurrent ischemia. Patients with a stuttering pattern of pain due to ischemia should be started on a beta-blocking drug and nitroglycerin IV. Assess further for coronary angiography for a possible angioplasty or coronary artery bypass surgery.

Cardiogenic Shock. See Chapter 12.

Mechanical Complications. If called to see a patient after infarction who was stable for at least 24 hours and then developed sudden hemodynamic deterioration, strongly suspect a mechanical complication. These are
- **Severe acute mitral regurgitation.** Transient mitral regurgitation with a soft murmur is often present with acute MI caused by papillary muscle dysfunction. Severe mitral regurgitation is rare and occurs in <5% of patients with acute MI. This catastrophic event is usually caused by papillary muscle rupture or rupture of chordae tendineae. These patients usually manifest pulmonary edema. Management includes the use of dobutamine and nitroglycerin IV, depending on BP response, and the use of an intra-aortic balloon pump for support in preparation for interventional therapy.
- **Ventricular septal rupture.** Ventricular septal rupture usually occurs from 3 to 5 days after infarction.
- **Pericarditis.** Pericarditis most often occurs during the second to fifth days after infarction. Pain is worse when lying down and is relieved on leaning forward. A pericardial friction rub is best heard with the diaphragm, with the patient leaning forward and the breath held at the end of complete exhalation (see Fig. 9–1). Management includes discontinuing heparin if pericarditis is proved, and **aspirin** given in full doses of **650 mg twice daily;** but other nonsteroidal anti-inflammatory drugs should be avoided (e.g., **indomethacin, which may cause increased incidence of myocardial rupture**).

Discharge Medications

1. Aspirin. **Enteric-coated aspirin 81 to 325 mg once daily** is given to all patients.

2. Nitroglycerin. **Nitroglycerin 0.3 or 0.4 mg tablets or nitolingual spray** to be used when needed.
3. Beta blockers. **Metoprolol 50 mg twice daily or timolol 5 mg twice daily** is given for at least the next 2 years to prevent recurrence of fatal events or reinfarction. These agents have been proven to decrease the incidence of sudden death and the early morning incidence of MI and death.
4. ACE inhibitors. These agents improve survival and decrease the incidence of CHF in patients with anterior infarcts and prior infarction and in those with CHF or EF of <35%. **Captopril 25 mg 3 times per day, or enalapril 10 mg once daily,** is given if the systolic BP is >110 mm Hg after a test dose and an initial phase of a low dosage. ACE inhibitors are continued for at least 1 year in patients with CHF or EF of <35%.
5. Agents to lower low-density lipoprotein (LDL) cholesterol. Statins have proved effective in improving survival and decreasing the incidence of reinfarction in patients after MI. **Simvastatin (Zocor) 10 to 20 mg after the evening meal or pravastatin (Pravachol) 20 mg at bedtime or atorvastatin (Lipitor) 10 to 20 mg** to maintain the LDL cholesterol at <100 mg/dl (2.5 mmol/L), is advisable.

Study Section: Acute Myocardial Infarction

■ PATHOPHYSIOLOGY

Acute MI is nearly always caused by occlusion of a coronary artery by thrombus overlying a fissured or ruptured atheromatous plaque. Owing to direct release of tissue factor and exposure of the subintima, the ruptured plaque is highly thrombogenic. Exposed collagen provokes platelet aggregation. Coronary angiography performed during the early hours of infarction has confirmed the presence of total occlusion of the infarct-related artery in over 90% of patients. It is not surprising that aspirin, through inhibition of platelet aggregation, reduces the incidence of coronary thrombosis and is especially useful in preventing progression of unstable angina to thrombosis and MI. Aspirin is particularly useful when given at the onset of chest pain produced by infarction. Aspirin, however, does not block all pathways that relate to platelet aggregation. In addition, aspirin does not decrease the incidence of sudden death in patients with acute MI. Aspirin reduces the incidence of MI in patients after an infarction and in those with unstable and stable angina. Thus, aspirin administration plays a key role in the prevention and management of acute MI.

The increased morning incidence of acute MI documented in several studies of the diurnal variation of infarction is related to the early-morning catecholamine surges, which induce platelet aggregation, and to an increase in blood pressure and hydraulic stress, which may lead to plaque rupture. **Beta-adrenergic blockers have been shown to decrease the early-morning peak incidence of acute infarction and sudden death.**

Unfortunately, when an atheromatous plaque ruptures, the thrombogenic effect of plaque contents cannot be completely nullified by the inhibition of all aspects of platelet aggregation, and chemical agents that can arrest the effects of these thrombogenic substances deserve intensive study. Agents such as hirudin, bivalirudin (Hirulog), and agatroban, which are direct antagonists of thrombin, have been shown to be superior to heparin in preventing coronary thrombosis in experimental models. Preliminary studies in patients suggest that direct thrombin inhibitors administered with aspirin are effective in the prevention of coronary thrombosis. These studies may pave the way for further research that may uncover newer types of antithrombotic agents, more specific than and superior to the coumarins, in preventing coronary thrombosis. The combination of a thrombin inhibitor, therefore, with aspirin may cause a significant increase in survival of patients with ischemic heart disease, and large-scale clinical trials are in progress.

Coronary artery spasm appears to play a lesser role in the pathogenesis of coronary occlusion leading to infarction. Evidence of coronary vasoconstriction was found when angioscopy was performed shortly after infarction, and intermittent occlusion, presumably on a vasomotor basis, has been apparent in some cases. Vasoconstriction appears to be a secondary factor, however, and because sudden plaque rupture is now proved to be the initiating event in coronary thrombosis, the mechanisms underlying plaque rupture and its prevention deserve intensive study to no lesser degree than does prevention of atheroma formation.

Use of a beta-blocking agent may inhibit plaque rupture, perhaps by its ability to decrease cardiac ejection velocity. This action reduces hydraulic stress on the arterial wall, stress that might be critical at the arterial site where the atheromatous plaque is predisposed to rupture (Fig. 7–2). **Recent data suggest that statins have the capacity to decrease plaque growth and perhaps decrease rupture.**

Occlusion of a coronary artery leads, in about 20 minutes, to death of cells in areas of severely ischemic tissue, which usually become necrotic over 4 to 6 hours. Because early and late mortality are directly related to the size of the infarct, limitation of infarct size (or even prevention of necrosis) by means of thrombo-

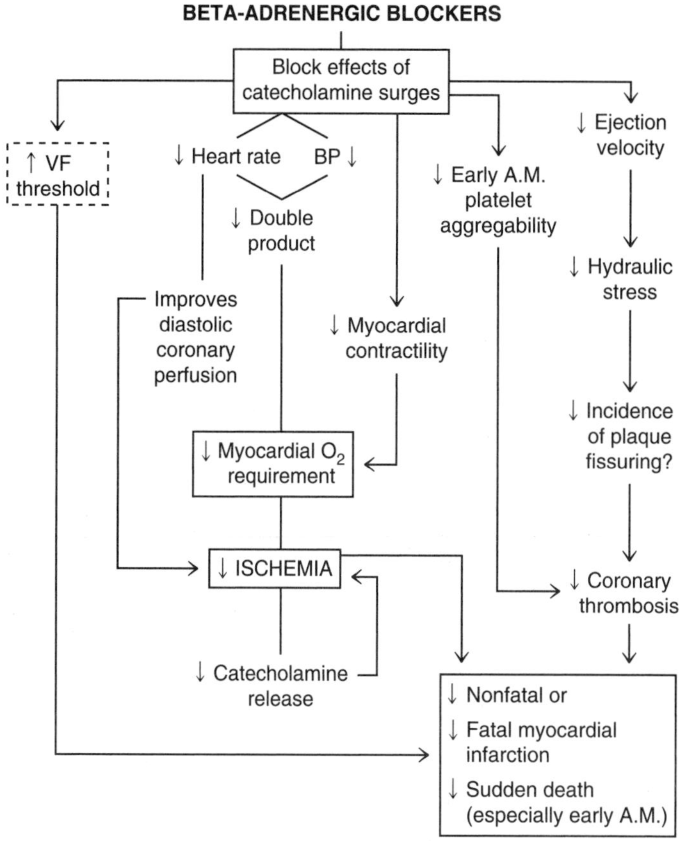

BETA-ADRENERGIC BLOCKERS

Figure 7–2 □ Salutary effects of beta-adrenergic blockade. ↑ = increase; ↓ = decrease. (Redrawn from Khan, M Gabriel: Heart Disease Diagnosis and Therapy: A Practical Approach. Baltimore, Williams & Wilkins, 1996, p 2.)

lytic therapy initiated at the earliest possible moment is of the utmost importance.

The ischemic zone surrounding the necrotic tissue provides electrophysiologic inhomogeneity that predisposes to the occurrence of lethal arrhythmias. These arrhythmias are most common during the early hours after onset and contribute to one of the major mechanisms of sudden death.

Extensive myocardial necrosis is the major determinant of heart failure; papillary, septal, and free-wall rupture; and cardiogenic shock, in which more than 35% of the myocardium is usually infarcted. The most effective means of reducing the extent of myocardial necrosis is the administration of thrombolytic therapy, aspirin, and a beta-blocking agent as soon as possible after the onset of symptoms of coronary thrombosis.

■ DIAGNOSTIC POINTS

Chest Pain

- Usually lasts more than 20 minutes and often persists for several hours. However, the pain of infarction can last for only 15 minutes, and occasionally, fatal infarction occurs after only a few minutes of severe pain or even unheralded cardiac arrest. Infarction may be silent, particularly in diabetic patients and in the elderly.
- Typically retrosternal and across the chest
- Variations of a crushing, vise-like, heavy weight on the chest; pressure; tightness; strangling; aching
- At times, only a discomfort with an oppression and burning or indigestion-like feeling
- May radiate to the throat, jaws, neck, shoulders, arms, scapulae, or epigastrium. At times, pain is centered at any one of these areas, e.g., the left wrist or shoulder, without radiation
- Usually builds up over minutes or hours, as opposed to aortic dissection, in which pain has an abrupt onset like a gunshot

Associated Symptoms and Factors

- Diaphoresis; cold, clammy skin; apprehension
- Shortness of breath, nausea, vomiting, dizziness
- Presyncope and, rarely, syncope may occur owing to bradyarrhythmias, especially in inferior MI.
- Occasionally, no pain. A marked decrease in blood pressure with associated symptoms, along with ECG findings, should suffice in making the diagnosis.
- Painless infarcts (in about 10% of patients), especially in diabetics or the elderly. In these patients, associated symptoms are often prominent and serve as clues to diagnosis.
- Over 50% of patients have a history of angina or prior infarction.
- Approximately 33% of patients with acute infarction have no major risk factors: death of a parent or sibling <age 55, hypercholesterolemia, cigarette smoking, hypertension, or diabetes. Absence of these factors should not influence the diagnosis.

Physical Signs

- The patient appears apprehensive, anxious, cold, and clammy.
- The area of chest pain may be indicated with a clenched fist.
- Tachycardia of 100 to 120 beats/min. An increase in blood pressure due to increased sympathetic tone is observed in approximately 50% of patients with anterior infarction.
- Bradycardia <60 beats/min and a decrease in blood pressure in about ⅔ of inferior infarcts; many of these patients become hypotensive, sometimes profoundly.
- S_4 gallop is common; S_3 and S_4 heart sounds are heard if the patient is in heart failure or cardiogenic shock.
- Murmur of mitral regurgitation due to papillary muscle dysfunction
- Crepitations, more prominent over the lower third of the lung fields, may be present.
- Elevated jugular venous pressure due to left- and right-sided heart failure or a very high venous pressure in the presence of right ventricular infarction or cardiac tamponade
- Frequently, there are no abnormal physical signs; this situation in a patient with suggestive symptoms should not decrease the level of suspicion that the patient may have an MI.

Although sophisticated tests evolved in the 1980s to improve diagnostic accuracy, they are of limited value in the era of thrombolysis. Thus, **a relevant history and correct interpretation of the ECG are of paramount importance in the implementation of early thrombolytic therapy,** which is of greatest benefit if given very early after symptom onset (<60 minutes).

Electrocardiogram

Despite the advent of new and expensive diagnostic technologies, the ECG has retained its prominent and vital role as an irreplaceable noninvasive and inexpensive test for the diagnosis of acute MI.

Diagnostic Features of ST Elevation Acute MI

- ST segment elevation >1 mm in ≥2 limb leads (see Figs. 5–28 to 5–31)
- At least 2-mm ST elevation in two or more precordial leads. When symptoms are not typical, the response to nitroglycerin is ascertained. Also, minimal ST segment elevation in black patients must be reassessed to exclude the occasional normal variant. There is clear recognition that Q waves may evolve early or late and cannot be relied on for early diagnosis. Thus, the terms "transmural" and "nontransmural" have

been abandoned, and Q wave or non–Q wave infarction cannot be categorized in the early phase. The best differentiating feature is ST segment elevation, which is present in >90% of patients with acute coronary thrombotic occlusion. **Thus, the new terminology, ST elevation MI and non–ST elevation MI, replaces the term non–Q wave MI,** but non–Q wave MI is still commonly used in many countries and in journal articles.

In addition, later ECG signs of infarction include

- Diminution of R waves (poor R wave progression)
- Evolving Q waves
- The simultaneous presence of reciprocal ST segment depression is not diagnostic of MI, but it provides major support to confirm the electrocardiographic diagnosis (see Figs. 5–28 and 5–31).
- Patients who are developing non–ST elevation MI (non–Q wave infarction) often manifest ST depression or T wave change (Fig. 5–47); see later discussion of non–Q wave infarction.

In patients with ischemic-type chest discomfort, ST segment elevation in two leads reportedly has a specificity of 91% and sensitivity of 46% for diagnosing acute MI. The sensitivity increases with serial ECG done every 30 minutes for 2 or more hours in patients in whom the initial ECG reveals no ST segment elevation. See discussion of ST depression and non–Q wave infarction later in Study Section.

Because the ECG is a vital yet nonspecific tool, it is necessary to correlate the ECG findings with the clinical presentation. In this regard, it is wise to recall Marriott's "warnings":

- An "abnormal-looking" ECG does not necessarily mean an abnormal heart.
- Exclude normal variants; see discussion of mimics later in Study Section.
- Consider causes of heart disease other than coronary.

If the first ECG is not diagnostic of acute injury or infarction, but the patient is strongly suspected of having an acute coronary syndrome, the ECG is repeated every 30 minutes until diagnostic changes are observed or until the CK-MB fraction or troponin results are reported. If the ECG is equivocal and there is a strong clinical impression that acute MI is present, valuable confirmatory information may be obtained from an echocardiogram.

Because the initial abnormality may not be fully diagnostic in up to 40% of cases, it is imperative to correlate the findings with accurate historical details. In patients with chest pain, new or presumably new Q waves in two leads with ST elevation are diagnostic of acute MI in over 90% of cases.

ECG signs in these patients:

- Q waves are fully developed in 4 to 12 hours and may

manifest as early as 2 hours from onset of chest discomfort or associated symptoms.

- Evolutionary ST-T changes occur during 12 to 24 hours but may be delayed up to 30 hours.
- Inferior MI ST elevation in leads II, III, and aVF with evolving Q waves and reciprocal depression in V_1 to V_3. The latter depression may be due to reciprocal changes, but there is evidence to suggest that in some patients it is due to left anterior descending artery disease. The evolutionary changes in repolarization that occur with inferior infarction evolve more rapidly than with anterior infarcts.
- Tachycardia may increase ischemic injury, causing elevation of the ST segment that must be differentiated from extension of infarction or pericarditis. Reciprocal depression does not occur in pericarditis, however.

Nondiagnostic Electrocardiogram

Acute MI may be present with ECG changes that are nonspecific in 10 to 20% of cases and may result from

- Slow evolution of ECG changes; the tracing may remain normal for several hours
- Old infarct masking the ECG effect of a new infarct
- Inferior MI associated with left anterior hemiblock in which R waves are expected to be small in leads III and aVF
- LBBB
- Apical infarction
- Posterior infarction not associated with ST elevation or Q waves but manifested by ST depression in leads V_1 and V_2 and often inferior or inferolateral infarct signs
- Right ventricular infarction: ST segment elevation in leads V_3R and V_4R, associated with inferior infarction

■ MIMICS OF ACUTE MYOCARDIAL INFARCTION

Types of ST segment elevation caused by acute MI are illustrated in Figure 5–33. ST elevation of infarction must be distinguished from the following:

- Acute pericarditis, in which the ST segment elevation is not confined to leads referable to an anatomic segmental blood supply. Thus, elevation in lead I is accompanied by elevation in leads II, III, and aVF; the ST elevation is concave, as opposed to convex upward with an injury current of infarction; and reciprocal depression is absent except in aVR (see Fig. 5–32).
- Early repolarization changes may mimic infarction but are often observed in leads V_2–V_3 and V_5–V_6 with a subtle "fish-

hook" configuration. This feature is common in black people (see Fig. 5–37).

- Myocardial infarction age indeterminate with mild ST elevation in the absence of true aneurysm is not uncommon; previous ECG may be required for comparison to exclude acute MI (see Fig. 5–41).
- Left ventricular aneurysm, in which there may be permanent ST elevation
- Left bundle branch block (LBBB). The V leads commonly show small r waves in V_1 or V_2 or QS complexes with ST elevation that can be misinterpreted as an anteroseptal infarct if the physician fails to note a QRS duration >0.11 second (see Fig. 5–19).
- Left ventricular hypertrophy (LVH) is a common cause of poor R wave progression in leads V_1 to V_3, and occasionally ST segment elevation occurs (see Fig. 5–38).
- Hypothermia with rectal temperatures below 93°F (34°C) may cause distortion of the earliest stage of repolarization; the ST segment appears elevated in a curious "hitched-up" pattern.
- Primary or secondary tumors may cause ST elevation and Q waves.
- Acute myocarditis may present with ST elevation with or without Q waves. Chagasic myocarditis can cause ST and Q wave changes.
- Subarachnoid hemorrhage or intracranial hemorrhage may cause ST segment shifts, or alteration of the QT interval. Torsades de pointes and transient left ventricular dysfunction have been associated with both entities.
- Hypertrophic cardiomyopathy (HCM) usually causes Q waves, but it can present with Q waves and ST elevation.
- Acute cor pulmonale, especially caused by pulmonary embolism, may cause ST elevation and Q waves, simulating acute MI.
- Severe trauma may cause myocardial injury and thus ST segment elevation with or without Q waves.
- Electrocution may cause ST segment elevation and occasionally Q waves and recurrent ventricular fibrillation (VF).
- Scorpion sting may cause ST segment elevation, with or without Q waves, right bundle branch block (RBBB), and other conduction defects.

■ MIMICS OF OLD MYOCARDIAL INFARCTION

It is necessary to make the ECG diagnosis of old MI because patients with acute MI and previous infarction are at high risk for complications, including decreased long-term survival. Mimics of old MI include the following:

- Incorrect chest lead placement may simulate old infarction. A QS pattern in leads V_1 and V_2 or a small r wave in lead V_2 may be observed in some women, even with correct lead placement.
- LVH commonly causes poor R wave progression in leads V_1 to V_3 and can thus mimic anteroseptal infarction. Other mimics include incomplete LBBB, cardiomyopathy, and myocardial replacement, e.g., tumor or fibrosis. In an autopsied series of 63 patients a QS in leads V_1, V_2, V_1–V_3, or V_1–V_4 indicated anteroseptal infarction in 20%, 66%, and 100%, respectively.
- Severe right ventricular hypertrophy may produce small q waves in leads V_1 to V_3, simulating anteroseptal infarction.
- Cor pulmonale caused by chronic bronchitis and emphysema is a common cause of poor R wave progression or QS patterns in the precordial leads. The finding of right atrial enlargement and an S wave in leads V_4 or V_5 equal to, or greater than, the R wave in leads V_4 or V_5 favors the diagnosis of cor pulmonale.
- Wolff-Parkinson-White (WPW) syndrome may simulate inferior or anterior infarction. Pseudo-Q waves are commonly seen in leads III and aVF but can occur in leads II, III, and aVF; the diagnosis of inferior MI is a common error (see Fig. 5–69). The P wave is usually stuck into the commencement of the Q wave. If the ECG suggests inferior MI but looks somewhat atypical, the suspicion of WPW should be entertained; the delta wave and short PR become obvious to the eye at this point. WPW may also mask the ECG findings of acute MI.
- The ECG hallmarks of HCM include narrow Q waves in leads II, III, aVF, or I, aVL, V_5 and V_6, or V_1 and V_2.
- Dilated cardiomyopathy. Involvement by neoplasms or amyloid is a well-known cause of Q waves in the absence of coronary artery disease.
- Chagas' disease. The presence of Q waves, T wave inversion, and conduction defects in an individual who has previously lived in an endemic area should suggest chagasic heart muscle disease.
- Myotonic dystrophy and other neuromuscular disorders commonly cause Q waves and conduction defects.
- Rare causes include hemochromatosis, scleroderma, sarcoidosis, and echinococcal cyst. These diseases and other conditions that cause myocardial fibrosis and thinning of the left ventricular wall can produce Q waves, and some may produce bulging with aneurysm-like formation, thus resulting in some degree of ST elevation.

■ THERAPY

Thrombolytic Therapy

Guidelines for the administration of thrombolytic therapy include the following patient subsets:

- Patients irrespective of age who are seen within 12 hours of onset of symptoms with clinical and ECG diagnoses consistent with acute ST elevation MI.
- Most importantly, patients older than age 75 in good general health should *not* be excluded if seen within 6 hours of pain onset when the impending infarction is large or extensive and there is no contraindication to thrombolytic therapy. ISIS-3 indicated that patients older than age 75 showed the greatest absolute benefit.
- Patients with new LBBB seen within 6 hours of onset of chest pain. This subset represents a high-risk group and was shown to benefit in the ISIS-3 study.
- Patients with new RBBB and proven acute infarction, associated with heart failure.
- Patients seen within 12 hours from onset of symptoms with evidence of ongoing ischemia. Pain is still present or stuttering episodes occur in the presence of continuing elevation of ST segments and CK and CK-MB elevation. Caution is required in patients seen after 12 hours because late reperfusion appears to increase the risk of myocardial rupture, and it is necessary to weigh the risks involved.

Rapid door to needle time (<15 minutes) is more important than the choice of thrombolytic agent. In patients older than age 75 mortality is high, but inferior MI carries a low risk and can be treated with streptokinase because of the high risk of intracranial bleeding with tPA and similar agents. See Table 7–3 for further details. For cost comparisons of approved thrombolytic agents, see Table 7–4.

Beta-Blocker Therapy

The ACC-AHA task force recommends that beta-blocker IV therapy be given at the same time as aspirin, as soon as the diagnosis of acute MI is considered. This is especially important in patients with anteroseptal and anterior MI with a heart rate >100 and/or systolic blood pressure >110 mm Hg, in which no contraindication to beta blockade exists. In this subset, beta blockers should be given in the emergency room at the same time as aspirin and sublingual nitroglycerin. No harm can ensue if the patient is not later selected for thrombolytic therapy. Beta-blocker therapy from day 7 for 2 years is expected to save 3 lives annually per 100 treated.

Early IV followed by oral beta-blocker therapy should be

strongly considered for all patients presenting with definite or probable acute infarction in whom contraindications do not exist. These agents are particularly strongly indicated in the following situations:

- Sinus tachycardia unassociated with hypotension or clinically apparent heart failure
- Rapid ventricular response to atrial fibrillation or atrial flutter
- Administration of thrombolytic agents to prevent arrhythmias and/or ischemia and improve survival

Calcium Antagonists

Verapamil should not be used in patients with acute MI because of its negative inotropic effect and strong propensity to precipitate heart failure, sinus arrest, or asystole. The drug is advisable in selected patients with SVT or AF with an uncontrolled ventricular response after a trial of beta blockers or digoxin in the absence of heart failure. Other calcium antagonists are contraindicated. Diltiazem is not indicated in acute ST elevation MI because it increases mortality in patients who manifest left ventricular dysfunction or in those with an ejection fraction (EF) <40%.

Magnesium

IV magnesium was associated with small but significant increases in heart failure, hypotension, bradycardia, and deaths attributed to cardiogenic shock. Thus, magnesium is not recommended in the management of acute ST elevation MI.

Interventional Therapy

If excellent cardiac expertise is readily available, PTCA with stent is considered first-line therapy for high-risk patients or if thrombolytics are contraindicated in patients with ST elevation MI.

■ NON–ST ELEVATION MI (NON–Q WAVE MI)

The term "non–Q wave infarction" was often used to embrace nontransmural infarction and the term "Q wave infarction" to denote transmural infarction. Because of anatomic inconsistencies, however, the use of the terms "transmural" and "nontransmural" is no longer recommended. It is established that patients with non–ST elevation MI, so-called non–Q wave infarction, represent a group at high risk for the occurrence of reinfarction within 3 months of hospital discharge.

Timolol has been shown to decrease mortality in patients with non–Q wave infarction. All patients with non–Q wave infarction should be treated with aspirin and a beta blocker if no contraindication exists to beta blockade. Patients who have good left ventricular function with an EF >40% and in whom beta blockers are contraindicated should receive diltiazem in addition to aspirin. Patients with non–Q wave infarction and postinfarction angina or those who continue to have transient ischemic ECG changes from day 2 onward, congestive heart failure (CHF), or elevated troponin levels require urgent coronary angiography prior to discharge (2–5 days), with a view to PTCA or CABG. A platelet IIb/IIIa receptor blocker significantly reduces adverse outcomes and is administered judiciously.

Patients with uncomplicated non–Q wave infarction are discharged on aspirin, a beta blocker, and/or diltiazem and with coronary angiography done within 2 weeks or earlier, depending on departmental preferences and results of exercise testing and nuclear imaging.

Beta blockers play an important role along with aspirin, IV nitroglycerin, low-molecular-weight heparin, and a statin in the management of non–ST elevation MI and unstable angina up to the moment of interventional therapy. A statin should be administered from day 1 because total cholesterol and LDL cholesterol levels are usually not available until after day 2, and >70% of patients are expected to exceed the LDL cholesterol goal of <2.6 mmol/L. Statins and aspirin play an important role in plaque stabilization.

■ IMPORTANT UPDATE FROM THE ACC, MARCH 2001

1. Committee guidelines recommend the assessment of cardiac troponin levels for the diagnosis and management of suspected non–ST elevation acute coronary syndromes [non–ST elevation MI and unstable angina]. In this large subset of patients CK-MB determination is not required. The committee's recommendations specify a diagnostic limit for MI using troponins based on the 99th percentile levels among healthy controls rather than comparison to CK-MB.

2. The CAPRICORN study has shown conclusive evidence that carvedilol administered to patients with acute MI and LV dysfunction from day 3 and followed for 1.3 years caused significant reduction in mortality and cardiac hospitalization to the same degree as obtained with ACE inhibitors, but this salutary beta-blocker effect is additive.

8 | Unstable Angina

Angina pectoris is a common manifestation of coronary artery disease. Chest pain occurs usually when at least one coronary artery is >70% obstructed by an atheromatous plaque. Pain occurs on exertion and is relieved within 1 to 5 minutes of cessation of the precipitating activity. Angina is said to be stable when there has been no change in pain frequency, duration, and precipitating causes in the past 60 days.

Braunwald's classification of patients with unstable angina is given in Table 8–1. Basically, there is a change in the pattern of pain, an increase in the frequency, severity, or duration of pain, and a lesser degree of known precipitating factors. Pain may occur on exertion only, or on exertion and at rest. New-onset angina, <60 days' duration, occurring on exertion or at rest is classified as unstable angina.

In patients with unstable angina, atheromatous plaques are eccentric with irregular borders; plaques may become fissured and covered with platelet thrombi. **Plaques with a rich lipid core, an abundance of inflammatory cells, and a thin protective fibrous cap are prone to rupture** (see Atherosclerotic Plaque in the Study Section at the end of this chapter).

■ PHONE CALL

Questions

1. Is the patient in the emergency room, coronary care unit (CCU), or ward?
2. Is the chest pain relieved by nitroglycerin?
3. Has the pain recurred within hours of taking nitroglycerin?
4. What are the patient's vital signs?

Orders

1. Order an electrocardiogram (ECG) immediately and repeat during the next episode of pain.
2. Give nitroglycerin sublingually as the occasion arises, provided systolic blood pressure (BP) is >90 mm Hg.
3. Give aspirin (plain) 160 to 325 mg to be chewed and swallowed immediately if no aspirin has been administered in the past 12 hours.

Table 8-1 □ CLASSIFICATION OF UNSTABLE ANGINA

Severity	Clinical Circumstances		
	A—Develops in Presence of Extracardiac Condition That Intensifies Myocardial Ischemia (Secondary UA)	B—Develops in Absence of Extracardiac Condition (Primary UA)	C—Develops Within 2 Wk of AMI (Postinfarction UA)
I—New onset of severe angina or accelerated angina; no rest pain	IA	IB	IC
II—Angina at rest within past month but not within preceding 48 hr [angina at rest, subacute]	IIA	IIB	IIC
III—Angina at rest within 48 hr [angina at rest, acute]	IIIA	$IIIB-T_{neg}$ $IIIB-T_{pos}$	IIIC

From Hamm CW, Braunwald E: A classification of unstable angina revisited. Circulation 2000:102:118–122.
UA = unstable angina; AMI = acute myocardial infarction.

Inform RN

"Will arrive at the bedside in . . . minutes."
The patient with recurrent chest pain or unstable angina must be assessed immediately.

■ ELEVATOR THOUGHTS

What is the classification of unstable angina?
Review the classification of unstable angina and be ready to categorize the patient as low or high risk (see Table 8–1). This will assist treatment strategy.

■ MAJOR THREAT TO LIFE

Patients with unstable angina may develop acute myocardial infarction (MI) within minutes to hours.

■ BEDSIDE

Quick Look Test

Does the patient look relatively well (comfortable), sick (uncomfortable or distressed), or critical (about to die)?

Selective History and Chart Review

1. How does the patient describe the pain?
2. Is the pain similar to that of angina but now more severe and more frequent?
   - Does the pain occur only on exertion?
   - Does the pain occur on exertion and at rest?
   - Does the pain occur at rest only?
   - Did the pain occur only in the past 48 hours?
   - Is there a relation to meals and posture to suggest a gastrointestinal (GI) cause, esophageal spasm, or reflux or gallbladder disease?

Pain lasting longer than 30 minutes suggests MI and not unstable angina.

Selective Physical Examination

1. Assess the BP and heart rate.
2. Physical examination may be normal.

3. An S_4 heart sound is commonly heard during pain.
4. Assess for signs of congestive heart failure (CHF).

■ DIAGNOSTIC TESTING

What does the ECG show?
- The ECG may be normal.
- ECG abnormalities during pain: mild ST segment elevation with positive T waves or horizontal or downsloping ST depression with positive or negative T waves (Fig. 8–1).
- During pain-free periods, some patients develop ST segment abnormalities and progressive symmetric T wave inversion (Fig. 8–2). Abnormal ST-T changes may be seen mainly in leads V_2, V_3, or V_4 and sometimes in leads V_5 and V_6 (see Fig. 5–51).

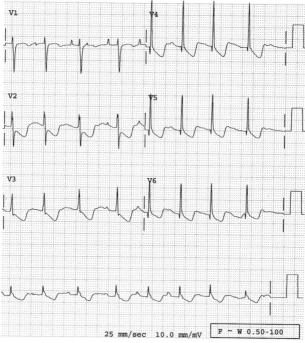

25 mm/sec   10.0 mm/mV   F ~ W 0.50-100

Figure 8–1 □ Anterior myocardial ischemia: ST segment depression in leads V_2 to V_6.

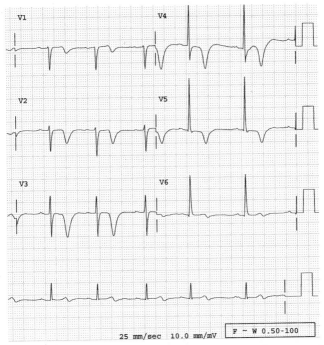

Figure 8–2 □ Anterior ischemia: abnormal ST segment; deep symmetric T wave inversion in leads V_2 to V_6.

- ECG changes may occur over 24 hours but may be delayed up to 4 days.

Cardiac Troponins

In patients with acute coronary syndromes *not associated with ST segment elevation* the following statements are clinically relevant:

1. Cardiac troponins (cTnT, cTnI) have replaced creatine kinase (CK) and the MB band of CK (CK-MB) as the cardiac enzyme marker of choice for diagnosis and risk stratification. They are useful predictors of short- and long-term cardiac mortality and morbidity. The CK-MB is also assessed; if it is abnormal, consider MI.
2. The relative risk (RR) for evolving MI and/or mortality in a cTnT-positive group ranges from 2.5 to 5.6.
3. Elevation of troponins, particularly TnT (TnI has been less studied), is correlated with angiographic findings of more complex coronary lesions, more thrombus, and less TIMI flow.

4. Elevated TnT identifies patients who would benefit the most from expensive but salutary therapy with platelet IIb/IIIa receptor blockers and **expedited invasive therapy** (Fig. 8–3).
5. TnT may be elevated >0.1 μg/L after cardiac surgery, in patients with renal failure, in those with CHF, and in patients with positive rheumatoid factor. A recent TnT isoform assay claims not to cause false-positive results with renal failure.

■ MANAGEMENT

A treatment strategy for patients who present with unstable angina is given in Figure 8–3.

1. High-risk patients and those requiring intravenous (IV) nitroglycerin should be admitted to the CCU.
2. Low-risk patients can be admitted to the ward provided that there are adequate facilities for monitoring BP and heart rate half-hourly for a few hours, then hourly for 12 hours with repeat ECG every 12 hours or during pain.
3. **Aspirin 160 mg (chewable aspirin) or 325 mg (plain aspirin),** chewed and swallowed for rapid effect, then **325 mg enteric-coated aspirin daily.**
4. **Heparin 5000 units IV immediately, then continuous infusion** (see Table A–3). Low-molecular-weight heparin (LMWH) administered subcutaneously is as good as IV heparin and is often used routinely in combination with aspirin.
5. Monitor the cardiac rhythm for 36 to 48 hours, although arrhythmias are uncommon in patients with unstable angina. If there is no recurrence of pain within 48 hours, the patient can be discharged to the ward. A stress test is not required for high-risk cases. These patients should undergo coronary angiography to determine the extent of coronary stenosis and the number of vessels involved. All low-risk

---

Figure 8–3 □ Algorithm for the management of unstable angina (see classification given in Table 8–1). CABG = coronary artery bypass graft; EF = ejection fraction; IV = intravenous; MI = myocardial infarction.

   * = **risk categories subject to modification by departmental cardiologist**

  ** = risk of death and MI: 24 hours <1%; 30 days <2%; 6 months <5%

 *** = prisk of death and MI: 24 hours 5%; 30 days 15–20%; 6 months 25%

**** = keep for 4 months even if LDL cholesterol <100 mg/dl (2.6 mmol/ L), then alter dose to goal LDL

   † = Left main, CABG; 3-vessel, 2-vessel with proximal left anterior descending artery and EF <40% or diabetes, recommend CABG; but EF >40% and no diabetes, CABG or angioplasty/stent

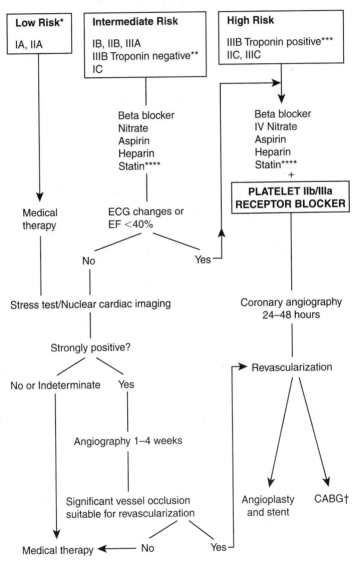

Figure 8-3 □ *See legend on opposite page*

patients should have an exercise stress test. In some units, a nuclear scan or dobutamine echocardiography is used for further assessment.

6. Evaluate the BP every 30 minutes for 4 hours, then every 2 hours as needed.

7. **IV nitroglycerin: Start with 5 to 10 μg/min; increase 5 to 10 μg/min every 5 or 10 minutes, if needed, to 100 to 200 μg/min.** Do not lower the systolic BP to <100 mm Hg.

8. **Beta blockers:** If there is no history of asthma or CHF, give **metoprolol 50 mg every 8 hours, then 100 mg every 12 hours,** or the equivalent of another beta blocker depending on the preference of your staff physician. The combination of a beta blocker and IV nitroglycerin should suffice to relieve pain within the next 24 to 48 hours.

9. **Calcium antagonists:** There is no evidence to suggest that beneficial effects can be obtained by the addition of a calcium antagonist to the combination of IV nitroglycerin and a beta blocker. Nifedipine used without a beta blocker increases mortality. **Diltiazem 60 mg 4 times daily or Cardizem CD 180 to 240 mg once daily added to IV nitroglycerin** may be used if a beta blocker is contraindicated. The combination of nitroglycerin, beta blocker, diltiazem, and aspirin/heparin constitutes optimal medical therapy. The combination of beta blocker and diltiazem should be avoided if bradycardia occurs, if the ejection fraction is <35%, or if there is documented CHF in the past. Verapamil is contraindicated because this agent may cause CHF, and if acute MI supervenes, mortality increases.

10. **Platelet IIb/IIIa receptor blockers** should be administered early to high-risk patients with a positive TnT test or those in whom implantation of coronary stents is anticipated (see Fig. 8–3).

    Interventional therapy: All high-risk patients, most intermediate-risk patients, and all those with positive troponin tests should have coronary angiograms done within 1 to 3 days of admission with the hope of early percutaneous transluminal coronary angioplasty (PTCA) and stenting; some will require coronary artery bypass surgery. Many cardiologists do not endorse the strategy for all intermediate-risk patients as outlined in Figure 8–3 and proceed to angiography without resorting to perfusion scintigraphy. It is important to recognize that studies comparing **aggressive** medical therapy and the impressive results of stents are not available. Comparison of medical therapy with PTCA is available, but stents confer significantly greater relief.

11. **Statins** should be administered to all patients as soon as the diagnosis of unstable angina is made regardless of cholesterol level results, which take more than 24 hours to

be obtained. These agents favorably influence the endothelial dysfunction that promotes the unstable state. The MIRACL study demonstrated that 80 mg atorvastatin in this setting for 16 weeks reduced the risk of cardiac events. The majority of patients admitted with unstable angina or non–ST-elevation MI have low-density lipoprotein (LDL) levels >2.5 mmol/L. It is necessary to ensure aggressive lipid lowering immediately after PTCA and stenting.

12. Although bacteria appear to play a small role, currently antibiotics have not proved to be successful. The role of antibiotics will emerge from the results of current randomized trials. The levels of **C-reactive protein** should be assessed in all patients because it is an independent marker for prognosis beyond troponins and ECG changes; levels appear to relate to the intense nonspecific inflammatory reaction observed in vulnerable plaques. The inflammatory change may be subdued by the combination of powerful statins and aspirin and perhaps by experimental agents such as newer nonsteroidal anti-inflammatory drugs (e.g., rofecoxib [Vioxx]) or colchicine-like agents that inhibit the pseudopodia of white cells.

Study Section: Stable Angina

■ ATHEROSCLEROTIC PLAQUE

An understanding of the pathogenesis of atherosclerotic plaque is essential because atheroma is the underlying lesion in most patients with coronary ischemic syndromes, i.e., stable angina, unstable angina, acute myocardial infarction, and sudden cardiac death. These clinical manifestations occur because plaques partially or almost totally occlude the lumen of the affected artery or because plaque ruptures, and the intensely thrombogenic material triggers thrombosis (Fig. 8–4).

The atherosclerotic plaque consists of a soft central core that has a variable lipid-laden content, covered by a fibrous cap that varies in thickness, smoothness, and fragility. The surface of some plaques is smooth, or it may be rough and bumpy. Plaques project into the lumen of the artery, causing variable obstruction, and over time the surface of plaques may ulcerate or become fissured. Plaques tend to occur at bending points, i.e., bifurcations of arteries, or in regions of oscillating shear stress, which results in endothelial injury or dysfunction.

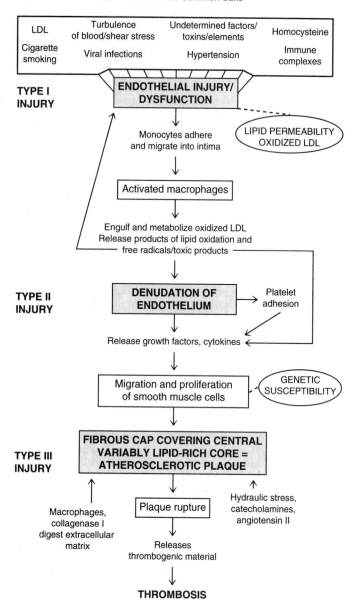

Figure 8–4 □ Pathogenesis of the atherosclerotic plaque. LDL = low-density lipoproteins. (From Khan, M Gabriel: Heart Disease Diagnosis and Therapy. Baltimore, Williams & Wilkins, 1996, p 135.)

Response to Injury Hypothesis

The initiating event in the development of the atherosclerotic plaque is believed to be injury to the endothelium of the artery. Endothelial dysfunction or injury incites a host of intricate biologic reactions that eventually lead, over several years, to the development of plaque. These reactions appear to occur as a healing response to the injury, but the response becomes counterproductive.

The principal cells and elements involved in atheroma formation include

- Endothelium. The injured endothelium appears to secrete chemotatic factors that attract leukocytes, monocytes, and smooth muscle cells to protect the endothelial monolayer.
- In leukocytes, several beta-integrins, which bind to extracellular matrix proteins, are expressed in T and B lymphocytes.
- Platelets
- T and B lymphocytes in cells. These lymphocytes are transformed to proliferative smooth muscle cells by cytokine and growth factors. Beta-integrins are implicated in smooth muscle cell migration.
- Smooth muscle cells
- Oxidized LDL cholesterol
- Free radicals, products of lipid oxidation
- Cytokines
- Mitogenic factors, such as platelet-derived growth factor (PDGF), released from injured endothelial cells, platelets, and macrophages
- Angiotensin II

The endothelium forms a protective monolayer lining the arterial tree and produces vasoactive substances:

- Prostacyclin (PGI$_2$), a potent vasodilator
- Endothelium-derived relaxing factor (EDRF), a form of nitric oxide, causes vasodilation
- Surface molecules, e.g., heparan sulfate, PGI$_2$, and plasminogen, which lyse fibrin clot to ensure a nonthrombogenic surface
- Procoagulant materials, e.g., von Willebrand's factor

The endothelium grows only in an obligate monolayer, and endothelial sheets cannot crawl over one another. Thus, at sites of endothelial injury, monocytes, platelets, and smooth muscle cells play a crucial role in the repair reaction.

Type I Injury. Turbulence of blood, i.e., oscillatory shear stress at arterial bifurcations and/or bending points, results in endothelial injury or dysfunction, which appears to be provoked by atherogenic factors: LDL cholesterol, diabetes, hypertension, cigarette smoking, viral infection, *Helicobacter pylori* and *Chlamydia pneumoniae* infections, immune complexes, and undefined toxins and elements (see Fig. 8–4). Endothelial injury provokes the surface expression of adhesive molecules with monocyte and platelet–vessel wall interaction. Monocytes migrate between endothelial cells into the subendothelial space. They convert to macrophages that engulf and become laden with oxidized LDL.

Type II Injury.   Activated macrophages metabolize oxidized LDLs and release products of lipid oxidation and free radicals. These toxic products may cause denudation of the endothelium and platelet adhesion. Macrophages, platelets, and endothelial cells release growth factors and cytokines that cause the proliferation of smooth muscle cells and their migration from the media to the intima. Smooth muscle cells have the capacity to contract and have receptors for several substances including LDLs, angiotensin II, and chemotatic and mitogenic factors. Smooth muscle cells can produce their own mitogenic factors. By proliferation they form elastin and collagen, which play a major role in producing a fibrous cap that covers the core of the lipid-laden atherosclerotic plaque. Fuster and colleagues have observed that plaques, which cause less than 50% of coronary stenosis but are lipid rich, especially with relatively increased ratios of monounsaturated to polyunsaturated fatty acids, are prone to rupture.

Type III Injury.   Plaque rupture or fissuring, ulceration, and thrombosis occur. The mechanisms underlying plaque rupture are not clearly understood. It appears that in soft-centered lesions, macrophages release collagenase I, which digests extracellular matrix predisposing to rupture.

Other Factors.   It is not clearly understood how the other risk factors (hypertension, diabetes, smoking, and genetics) relate to the aforementioned cells and elements to produce the atherosclerotic lesion. There is little doubt that there is a genetic predisposition to the development of plaques, especially those that are prone to rupture. It is not surprising that patients who do not have angina or silent ischemia but who have plaques that cause <60% stenosis die from heart attack or fatal infarction. Lesions prone to rupture often cause <60% stenosis and have a high-lipid core filled with inflammatory foam cells with a thin protective fibrous cap.

■ PATIENT HISTORY

A relevant history is essential for the diagnosis of angina. Myocardial ischemia signals impulses via afferent sympathetic nerves, the cervical and upper thoracic sympathetic ganglia, spinal cord, and dorsal roots of thoracic segments, T1–T5. Discomfort or pain is thus typically located in the retrosternal area (T1–T6), left arm (T1), hypothenar eminence (C8), and fourth and fifth fingers (C7, C8) and may radiate widely or poorly. Because the nerve pathways are finally referred to somatic nerves, pain may be referred to the lower jaw, to the neck, to both arms, across the shoulders, or to interscapular areas that extend from C2 to T10 (see Fig. 6–1). Pain may occur in a small segment (1–2 square inches) of the C2–T10 zone, e.g., only in the jaw, a small area of the arm, the wrist, or the throat, and not involve the chest. Discomfort localized to any of these areas outside the chest, occurring during exertion and rapidly relieved on discontinuation of the activity, is a hallmark of angina.

The discomfort or pain of angina is typically a squeezing, pressure-like sensation under the breastbone, precipitated by a particular activity, such as walking quickly up an incline. The discomfort is usually described as an unpleasant sensation: "strangling in the chest," "choking," or "burning."

When requested to point to the area of pain, the patient usually uses two or more fingers, the entire palm of the hand, or a clenched fist to indicate the pain site. A fingertip area of pain is rarely caused by myocardial ischemia. In an individual with *stable angina*, relief of the discomfort always occurs within 1 to 7 minutes of cessation of the precipitating exertional or emotional activity. Sublingual nitroglycerin causes relief within 1 to 2 minutes but is not diagnostic of angina because similar relief of pain may be observed in some patients with esophageal spasm and sphincter of Oddi spasm.

In patients with *unstable angina*, chest pain may occur on exertion and/or at rest; there is a change in the pattern of pain: it may increase in severity, frequency, and duration; and the pain is actuated by a lesser degree of known precipitating factors.

Patients do not always experience chest discomfort during episodes of myocardial ischemia; this condition is termed *silent ischemia*. Patients with unstable angina may have daily episodes of silent ischemia.

■ DIFFERENTIAL DIAGNOSIS

Except when symptoms are typical, as described previously, the following conditions should be considered.

Chest Wall Pain. Costochondritis is an extremely common occurrence. Patients usually localize the pain with one fingertip directed to the second, third, or fourth left costal cartilage; pain occurs less often on the right side. Sharp, dull, or aching pain may last for seconds or minutes, to several days. The costochondral junctional area is usually tender to palpation. Caution is necessary because angina and costochondritis may coexist, and a relevant history is crucial. Other causes of chest wall pain and gastro-esophageal reflux may require consideration.

Signs. The physical examination is not helpful in establishing a diagnosis of angina. Assess for abnormal cardiac pulsations, S_4 gallop, aortic stenosis, absent peripheral pulses, and signs of anemia.

■ INVESTIGATIONS

Investigations relate to the important observation that patients with similar clinical symptoms may have different prognoses depending on coronary anatomy (e.g., one-, two-, three-vessel or left main coronary artery disease) and on left ventricular (LV) function. It is necessary to stratify the risk so that patients at higher risk can progress to angiography early. Exercise stress testing and, in some patients, thallium or sestamibi scintigraphy and echocardiography are required to stratify the risk (see Fig. 8–3).

Blood Work

Lipid Levels. It is rational to request the total cholesterol and the high-density lipoprotein (HDL) cholesterol levels with the patient in a nonfasting state at the same time as the outpatient visit, because the levels are not affected by daily food intake and this routine saves the patient's time. If the total cholesterol exceeds 190 mg/dl (4.9 mmol/L), then prior to the next visit, request tests for total cholesterol, HDL, LDL, triglycerides, and glucose with the patient fasting 14 hours before testing.

Hemoglobin. This estimation is necessary to exclude the rare occurrence of angina precipitated by anemia in patients with atheromatous coronary stenosis.

Electrocardiogram

The ECG is normal in >50% of patients with stable angina. The ECG may reveal evidence of previous infarction, left ventricular hypertrophy, or nondiagnostic ST-T wave changes. Most important, a normal record makes a valuable baseline with which to compare future tracings. If the ECG is recorded during an episode of chest pain, ischemia is denoted by downsloping or horizontal ST segment depression ≥1 mm (see Fig. 5–49).

Exercise Electrocardiography

Unlike the resting ECG, which is not useful in confirming a diagnosis of angina and cannot be used for defining outcomes, the ECG exercise test is useful in assessing coronary reserve and in formulating therapeutic strategies. The test is *contraindicated* in patients with aortic stenosis and obstructive cardiomyopathy.

The **Bruce protocol** is commonly used; patients are exercised on the treadmill until one of the following occurs:

- Angina
- ST segment depression that signifies ischemia
- A fall in blood pressure
- Greater than 90% of maximal heart rate is achieved
- Intolerable fatigue or shortness of breath

Patients who can tolerate >9 minutes of a Bruce protocol without the occurrence of angina or ischemia have a good prognosis. A positive test is indicated by flat or downsloping ST segment depression >1 mm. The precipitation of angina and a ≥2-mm ST depression is virtually diagnostic of ischemic heart disease. Patients who develop chest pain within 4 minutes of exercise and/or ST segment depression of ≥2 mm, persisting for more than 4 minutes on cessation of exercise associated with a systolic pressure <130 mm Hg, or a fall in blood pressure, have a poor prognosis.

Stress Echocardiography

Echocardiography using exercise, arbutamine, or dobutamine may reveal new or worsening regional wall motion abnormality and can be useful in the assessment of patients, particularly in females.

Nuclear Imaging

Thallium is a potassium analogue. Thallium-201 is taken up by normal myocardial cells. Ischemic or infarcted areas cannot take up thallium, resulting in a "cold spot" on imaging. Thallium-201 is injected into a peripheral vein at maximal exercise. If a cold spot is observed, a repeat image is done 3 hours later. A cold spot that fills in indicates transient ischemia on exercise. A permanent cold spot is usually caused by prior infarction. The test is approximately 87% sensitive and 77% specific. It is advisable to consider the following:

- Methodology and interpretation must be sound.
- Image artifacts are common.
- Apical thinning may cause lack of thallium uptake and incorrectly suggest ischemia.
- Overlying breast shadows may cause false-positive results.
- **Negative scans may manifest in patients with lesions in the circumflex and diagonal arteries.**
- A negative result may be reported in patients with global reduction in thallium uptake caused by widespread disease.

Technetium-99m sestamibi (Cardiolite) or tetrofosmin (Myoview) nuclear perfusion imaging is used in preference to thallium-201 in many hospitals.

Dipyridamole, Dobutamine, or Adenosine-Thallium Imaging. If a decision is reached that therapeutic strategies can be altered by performing this test, then testing is justifiable. Patients with class 2 angina, with the absence of pain at rest, who are unable to exercise because of arthritis or peripheral vascular disease may benefit. Patients with class 3 angina require coronary angiographic assessment; thus this test is not warranted. Dipyridamole-thallium scintigraphy is contraindicated in patients with unstable angina, postinfarction angina, and non–Q wave infarction within 1 month of infarction; these patients require coronary angiography. Also dipyridamole-thallium or adenosine-thallium scintigraphy is contraindicated in patients with asthma and chronic obstructive pulmonary disease (COPD).

Thallium imaging, using single photon emission computed tomography (SPECT), gives superior images with a three-dimensional view. Both sensitivity and specificity of SPECT are approximately 92%.

Echocardiography

Echocardiography is not routinely required in patients with angina. Patients with previous heart failure, suspected LV dysfunction, or concomitant valvular lesions benefit from echocardiographic assessment. Assessment of LV systolic function and ejection fraction (EF) are useful parameters in patient selection for angioplasty vs. coronary artery bypass surgery (CABS). Individuals with EF ≤35% usually are not suitable candidates for angioplasty or treatment with diltiazem or verapamil. Patients with poor LV function and EF <25% have a poor prognosis with CABS.

■ THERAPY

The first step is to control the risk factors that contribute to the development of obstructive atherosclerotic plaques.

- **Serum cholesterol** must be maintained at <190 mg/dl (4.9 mmol/L), and LDL cholesterol at <100 mg/dl (2.6 mmol/L). Lipid-lowering strategies must be more aggressive if the HDL cholesterol is <35 mg/dl (0.9 mmol/L). There is sufficient evidence to indicate that regression of plaques can occur and progression of the disease can be ameliorated. The evidence of plaque rupture may decrease on long-term therapy with statins.
- **Hypertension.** Strict control of hypertension with agents that

decrease cardiac work, oxygen requirement, and the deleterious effects of catecholamines causes improvement in angina and outcome. A beta-blocking agent and/or angiotensin-converting enzyme (ACE) inhibitor is a rational choice.

- **Cigarette smoking.** Cessation of smoking is vital. The patient should be informed that smoking increases the size of obstructing plaques and increases the incidence of sudden cardiac death. Cigarette smoking also decreases the effectiveness of most antianginal drugs. These statements should provide the powerful motivation that is necessary to assist the patient to stop smoking.
- **Weight reduction.** The patient should be informed that weight reduction exceeding 20 lb often results in about a 25% decrease in anginal symptoms and, in conjunction with cessation of smoking, may prevent resorting to very expensive drug and/or interventional therapy. The appropriate bedside approach of a caring physician is important in discussing these issues; words must be carefully chosen to accomplish the difficult task of motivating the patient to decrease weight and to stop smoking.
- **Stress.** Removal or avoidance of stressful situations is important.

Drug Therapy

Most patients with class 1 and 2 stable angina are adequately managed with nitroglycerin and one-a-day beta blocker. The rationale for a beta-blocking drug as a first-choice oral antianginal agent is discussed shortly.

Many patients cope with mild angina that quickly disappears on cessation of the precipitating activity. However, failure to achieve about a 50% symptomatic relief with an adequate dose of a beta blocker should result in the addition of a second agent. Either a calcium antagonist or an oral nitrate is considered second choice. If a beta blocker is being used, then **nifedipine extended release 30 to 60 mg daily** or **amlodipine 5 mg** is advisable. If beta-blocking agents are contraindicated, but verapamil is not, then verapamil should be used as the drug of first choice, because it is the most effective antianginal calcium antagonist. A sustained-release nitrate is given once daily or, at most, twice daily, with the last dose prior to 3 P.M. to avoid nitrate tolerance. Triple therapy with a beta-blocking agent, nitrate, and calcium antagonist is warranted if angina remains bothersome; however, this step should prompt consideration for coronary angiography and interventional therapy.

Beta Blockers. Release of catecholamines plays a major role in the initiation and perpetuation of myocardial ischemia in patients with angina. Beta blockers can inhibit the initiation of ischemia and the effects of catecholamines, interrupt the dynamic process, and provide rational and effective therapy, as well as prolong life. Calcium antagonists and/or nitrates do not prolong life, do not ameliorate the effects of catecholamines, and are thus less effective antianginal agents.

Beta-adrenergic blockers are competitive inhibitors of catecholamines, and their action depends on the ratio of drug to catecholamine concentration at beta-adrenoceptor sites. Beta receptors are situated in the cell membrane and are part of the adenyl cyclase system. The ventricle contains mainly beta$_1$- and some beta$_2$-adrenergic receptors; beta$_2$ receptors predominate in the lung. Adenyl cyclase converts adenosine triphosphate to cyclic adenosine monophosphate (cyclic AMP), the intracellular messenger of beta stimulation.

Beta-adrenergic blockade causes

- A decrease in heart rate; the increased diastolic interval results in improved diastolic coronary perfusion, especially during exercise (see Fig. 7–2).
- A decrease in the velocity of myocardial contraction; this further reduces myocardial oxygen demand, which is particularly important during exertional activities.
- A fall in systolic blood pressure and a decrease in the heart rate–pressure product and, thus, a reduction in myocardial oxygen requirement.
- A decrease in shearing forces imposed on the arterial wall; this may reduce the incidence of plaque rupture and the incidence of fatal or nonfatal infarction.
- An increase in ventricular fibrillation (VF) threshhold; this causes a decrease in the incidence of VF and sudden death in postinfarction patients.
- A decrease in catecholamine surges; this has been shown to eliminate and decrease the incidence of early-morning mortality from myocardial infarction (see Fig. 7–2).

Dosages of available beta blockers are given in Table C–4. Cardioprotection occurs with timolol in smokers and in nonsmokers; metoprolol and propranolol protect only nonsmokers. Beta blockers are *contraindicated* in patients with asthma, severe COPD, bradycardia, and heart block.

Nitrates. Isosorbide dinitrate undergoes hepatic metabolism. Mononitrates are unaffected by the liver and, on entering the walls of veins and arteries, combine with sulfhydryl (SH) groups to form nitric oxide, which activates guanylate cyclase to produce cyclic guanosine monophosphate. This action causes relaxation of vascular smooth muscle with dilatation of veins and minimal dilatation of arteries. Continued exposure to nitrates causes a depletion of SH groups. **Round-the-clock administration of oral**

or transdermal preparations results in nitrate tolerance after a few days, and an ineffectiveness of the drug. A daily 10-hour nitrate-free interval is essential for the regeneration of SH and the effectiveness of nitrates. Nitrates are mainly venodilators. They reduce preload ventricular volume and myocardial wall stress. A small reduction in afterload occurs, with an increase in heart rate. Because nitrates decrease preload, they are *contraindicated* in hypertrophic cardiomyopathy, constrictive pericarditis, cardiac tamponade, right ventricular infarction, and hypovolemia.

Nitrate preparations and their dosages are given in Table C–4.

Calcium Antagonists.   Verapamil is a more powerful antianginal agent than diltiazem and nifedipine because of a more prominent negative inotropic effect. Dihydropyridines, such as nifedipine and amlodipine, have no electrophysiologic effects and minimal negative inotropic effects. Dihydropyridines are a rational choice for use in conjunction with beta blockers. Verapamil should not be combined with a beta blocker because severe bradyarrhythmias and/or CHF may occur; the combination of diltiazem and a beta blocker may cause similar adverse effects, but the interaction is not as intense.

Preparations and dosages of calcium antagonists are given in Table C–4. Calcium antagonists are *contraindicated* in patients with aortic stenosis, sick sinus syndrome, CHF or suspected LV dysfunction, and myocardial infarction.

Interventional Therapy

Patients with an EF >35%, and lesions that are angiographically acceptable for angioplasty, are preferably managed with angioplasty, and often with a stent. Bypass is reserved for later use. When surgery is indicated for left anterior descending (LAD) artery obstruction, left internal mammary artery anastomosis is used in patients less than age 65, and vein bypass grafting is used in older patients. The 10-year occlusion rate is 5% for internal mammary artery anastomosis, as opposed to 10% for internal mammary artery bypass grafting, and 50% for vein grafting.

■ PRINZMETAL'S (VARIANT) ANGINA

Variant angina is a rare form of angina and is caused by coronary artery spasm, often without identifiable stimuli. The resulting myocardial ischemia in this condition also stimulates catecholamine release. During the pain, the ECG shows ST segment elevation, which resolves when pain subsides. Rarely, exposure to cold, smoking, emotional stress, aspirin ingestion, or cocaine may trigger coronary spasm. Pain relief is obtained with the administration of nitrates and/or calcium antagonists. Beta-blocking agents may allow alpha activity with resulting vasoconstriction and can increase pain.

Pericarditis is caused by many conditions. Pericarditis may be fibrinous, serofibrinous, hemorrhagic, or purulent. Chest pain caused by pericarditis may mimic acute myocardial infarction (MI) with radiation to the neck, jaw, arm, trapezius muscle, interscapular region, or upper abdomen. Pain is not always pleuritic. **Pain may be absent, because the visceral pericardium has no pain fibers, and only the lower part of the parietal pericardium is innervated by the phrenic nerve.**

■ PHONE CALL

Questions

1. What are the vital signs?
2. Is the patient in distress and does the patient have severe shortness of breath, suggesting tamponade?
3. Is the pain made worse by deep breathing and lying down?
4. Is the pain relieved when the patient sits upright?

Orders

If the patient is distressed by shortness of breath or is hypotensive or has had presyncope, start an IV of 5% dextrose in water (D5W) to keep the vein open.

■ ELEVATOR THOUGHTS

What are the causes of pericarditis?
The common causes of pericarditis are given in Table 9–1.

■ MAJOR THREAT TO LIFE

- Cardiac tamponade

■ BEDSIDE

Quick Look Test

Does the patient look sick (uncomfortable or distressed) or critical (about to die)?

Table 9–1 □ CAUSES OF PERICARDITIS

Obvious Underlying Diseases	Drugs	Other
Post MI	Anticoagulants	Idiopathic
Early	Cromolyn	(probable viral)
Late (Dressler's)	Daunorubicin	Viruses
Renal failure	Dantrolene	Coxsackie B5,
Neoplastic tuberculosis	Hydralazine	B6
Septicemia (purulent)	Isoniazid	Echovirus
Endocarditis	Methysergide	HIV, Epstein-
Collagen disease	Minoxidil	Barr
Rheumatic fever	Procainamide	Influenza,
Rheumatoid arthritis	Phenytoin	mumps,
Lupus		varicella,
Scleroderma		rubella
Myxedema		Tuberculosis
Trauma		Other bacteria
Surgery		Mycoplasma
Catheter		
Pacemaker		
Radiation		

HIV = human immunodeficiency virus; MI = myocardial infarction.

Selective History and Chart Review

1. How does the patient describe the pain?
2. Is the chest pain made worse with deep breathing or with postural change?

    The pain of pericarditis usually gets worse when lying down and is relieved by sitting upright or standing, **but pain is not always typical**.
3. Is the pain worse on swallowing, suggesting pericarditis or an esophageal problem?
4. Is the pain oppressive or is it a vague ache?
5. Is there genuine shortness of breath, or is the patient splinting because of pain on inspiration?
6. Is there actual lightheadedness, presyncope, nausea, or vomiting?
7. Is there an underlying disease that can cause pericarditis (see Table 9–1)?
8. Is there fever or are there chills?
9. Are palpitations or is tachycardia a feature?

Selective Physical Examination

1. Assess the jugular venous pressure (JVP): This should be normal (<2 cm); if >4 cm and the patient is short of breath or distressed, consider cardiac tamponade.

2. Check for pulsus paradoxus (see Chapter 10).
3. Listen for a pericardial friction rub: The rub is best heard at the cardiac apex and left sternal border. Listen with the diaphragm pressed firmly against the chest wall with the patient sitting and leaning forward with the breath held in deep expiration. Another technique is shown in Figure 9–1. The rub may increase in intensity on inspiration if the pleura is involved; pleuropericarditis may be present.
4. The rub is usually triphasic, consisting of a systolic component during ventricular systole, an early diastolic sound during the early phase of ventricular filling, and a presystolic component during atrial systole. Occasionally, the rub is biphasic, consisting of a systolic component and a diastolic component; a monophasic systolic rub is uncommon.
5. The rub may be transient. If a rub is not heard initially, listen at different intervals during the course of the examination and after completing the orders and at different times of the day.
6. A rub may occur even in the presence of a large pericardial effusion.

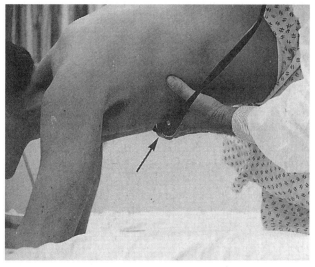

Figure 9–1 □ A technique for eliciting a pericardial rub. The diaphragm of the stethoscope is firmly applied to the precordium *(arrow)* while the patient rests on elbows and knees. (From Braunwald E: Heart Disease, 5th ed. Philadelphia, WB Saunders Co., 1997, p 49.)

■ DIAGNOSTIC TESTING

1. Electrocardiogram
   - During stage 1, that is, in the early phase of pericarditis, hours to days, there is widespread ST segment elevation 2 to 5 mm concave upward in at least 8 of the 12 precordial leads and often mild depression in aVR and sometimes in V_1 (see Fig. 5–32).
   - A few days later: ST and PR segments become isoelectric, with upright or flattened T waves.
   - After normalization of the ST segment, diffuse T wave inversion occurs. This is unlike acute MI, in which T wave inversion occurs often before the ST segment has returned to normal.
   - Stage 4: Days to weeks later, the T waves normalize, but rarely they may remain inverted.
   - Sinus tachycardia is a common finding during the early phase of acute pericarditis and may be the only electrocardiographic (ECG) finding.
   - Q waves do not occur except when there is prominent myocarditis occurring with pericarditis. Note that the ST segment elevation of inferior infarction occurs in leads II, III, and aVF and does not involve leads I and aVL, whereas in pericarditis, leads I, II, III, and aVL are elevated (see Chapter 5).
2. Chest x-ray
   A chest x-ray is not diagnostic but may reveal pulmonary or mediastinal abnormalities, in particular neoplastic or infectious processes that may be the underlying cause of pericarditis.
3. Echocardiography
   This is necessary to detect the presence of pericardial effusion and in assessing tamponade.

■ MANAGEMENT

1. Pain is usually relieved by aspirin or nonsteroidal anti-inflammatory drugs (NSAIDs): **ibuprofen 400 mg every 8 hours or indomethacin 25 to 50 mg every 8 hours, naproxen 250 mg 3 times daily.**
2. Modified bedrest for a few days. The patient should ambulate in the room to prevent deep venous thrombosis.
3. **Dexamethasone 4 mg IV** may be required if pain is recurrent and uncontrolled with NSAIDs; 4 mg IV given as a bolus may relieve pain in 4 to 6 hours.
4. Corticosteroids are not used routinely; they may be tried for relapsing pericarditis not controlled with NSAIDs.

5. Colchicine may be tried for relapsing pericarditis.
6. Determine and treat the underlying cause.
   - Purulent pericarditis may occur during septicemia caused by pneumococcus, *Haemophilus*, gonococcus, and other organisms. If purulent pericarditis is suspected, arrange for pericardiocentesis to obtain fluid and to determine culture and sensitivities. The thoracic surgery service should be consulted to accomplish adequate drainage.
   - Uremic pericarditis usually improves with increased frequency of dialysis. Pericardiocentesis is not required except if purulent infection is suspected.
   - Postinfarction pericarditis (see Chapter 7).
   - Drug-induced: Discontinue the offending agent (see Table 9–1).
   - Connective tissue diseases including lupus and rheumatoid arthritis may cause pericarditis and require control.
   - Neoplastic involvement by carcinoma of the lung or breast, melanoma, lymphomas, leukemia, or mesothelioma should be considered. Radiation or chemotherapy may cause significant resolution and decrease the size of effusion over a period of months. Pericardiocentesis is not required for moderate or large effusions except if tamponade is documented.

Study Section: Constrictive Pericarditis

The proper management of constrictive pericarditis begins with correct diagnosis. Common causes include neoplastic disease—especially carcinoma of the lung or breast, asbestosis, and lymphoma; mediastinal irradiation; nonviral pericardial infections; viral pericarditis; tuberculosis; post–cardiac surgery; chest trauma; connective tissue diseases; and chronic renal failure and dialysis.

■ DIAGNOSTIC HALLMARKS

- If the jugular venous pressure is both markedly and chronically elevated and the history and physical examination fail to suggest an apparent cardiac cause in the presence of a small quiet heart, then a restrictive syndrome must be considered, the most common cause being constrictive pericarditis.
- Neck vein examination should reveal Kussmaul's sign, which may be difficult to elicit when the venous pressure is severely elevated.
- The venous pulse usually has a prominent Y descent, coinci-

dent with the early rapid diastolic filling of the ventricle. A prominent X descent, coincident with filling of the atrium, is often observed in patients with sinus rhythm. The exaggerated X and Y descents give the venous pressure a characteristic M- or W-shaped pattern.

- Auscultation should reveal the presence of an early high-frequency third heart sound (S_3) caused by abrupt cessation of early diastolic filling. This sound, referred to as a pericardial knock, occurs earlier than the conventional third heart sound of heart failure and has a sharp, high-pitched quality that is easily heard with the diaphragm and may mimic an opening snap or early filling sound heard in endomyocardial fibrosis (see Fig. 4–1).

- Atrial fibrillation occurs in approximately 33% of cases of constrictive pericarditis.

- The presence of **marked ascites, occurring days to weeks before the presence of significant edema, points strongly to constrictive pericarditis** and serves to distinguish the condition from heart failure, in which prominent edema occurs and is followed weeks later by mild ascites. In a few patients with long-standing constriction and congestion, protein-losing gastroenteropathy may ensue.

■ DIFFERENTIAL DIAGNOSIS

Patients who present with noncalcific constrictive pericarditis pose a diagnostic problem.

- **Heart failure** not caused by constrictive pericarditis can be difficult to differentiate. The presence of a pericardial knock and marked ascites developing prior to leg edema favor the diagnosis of constrictive pericarditis. Also, severe heart failure causing chronically elevated JVP is invariably associated with tricuspid regurgitation and prominent V waves. The heart size is usually normal with constrictive pericarditis, and calcification may be apparent, depending on the causation.

- **Right atrial myxoma** should produce a prominent A wave in the venous pulse and requires echocardiographic exclusion.

- **Restrictive cardiomyopathy.** Restrictive physiology due to amyloid and endomyocardial fibrosis may mimic the hemodynamic findings of constrictive pericarditis. The presence of cardiac enlargement, prominent murmurs, and/or tricuspid regurgitation with prominent systolic V waves supports the diagnosis of restrictive cardiomyopathy. ECG findings may be similar in both conditions, but a pseudoinfarction pattern favors restrictive disease. Diagnosis can be difficult if pericardial calcification or pericardial thickening is not observed on echocardiography or computed tomography (CT) scan or in patients with left ventricular diastolic pressures equal to right ventricular diastolic pressures. Magnetic resonance imaging (MRI) may be helpful in identifying thickening of the pericardium. In patients with suspected myocardial disease, endomyocardial biopsy is desirable.

■ INVESTIGATIONS

A few or all of the following investigations may be required to be certain of the diagnosis:

- Chest x-ray may show pericardial calcification, especially of the apex and posteriorly, which is best seen on lateral views; the heart size is usually normal.
- ECG is virtually always abnormal but nonspecific and shows diffuse flat or inverted T waves in over 75% of patients; the depth of inversion of the T waves is usually proportional to the degree of pericardial adherence to the myocardium, which may make stripping difficult; low voltage is present in approximately 50% of cases, along with abnormal P waves and P-mitrale if in sinus rhythm. Atrial fibrillation is present in approximately 33% of patients.
- Echocardiography is of limited value in identifying thickened pericardium, unless calcification is present. Doppler echocardiography shows typical Doppler features in both mitral and hepatic vein flow in approximately 85% of patients with constriction amenable to surgery.
- Ultrafast cine-CT and/or MRI give fairly accurate assessment of pericardial thickness, pericardial impingement on the right ventricle, and the degree of dilation of the venae cavae and hepatic veins.
- Cardiac catheterization findings typically are elevation and equalization of all diastolic pressures and the dip and plateau (or square root sign), but these may be observed in some patients with restrictive cardiomyopathy; as outlined earlier, CT and MRI are useful in differentiating these two categories of patients.
- It is important to avoid diuretics prior to catheter studies, because sodium and water loss may cause equalization of left and right ventricular filling pressures in patients with restrictive cardiomyopathy.

■ THERAPY

Pericardiectomy is needed when medical therapy—the judicious use of diuretics and digoxin for control of the ventricular response in patients with atrial fibrillation—fails to reduce markedly elevated JVP and when symptoms are persistent and bothersome.

Cardiac tamponade may occur when pericardial fluid interferes with diastolic filling. The degree of tamponade and hemodynamic embarrassment is related to the rapidity of fluid accumulation and not the quantity of fluid. A large quantity of fluid may accumulate slowly with tuberculous or carcinomatous pericarditis without causing tamponade. The sudden accumulation of <200 ml of fluid, such as from trauma or infectious pericarditis, can cause tamponade. Severe impairment to diastolic filling of the ventricles occurs, and thus stroke volume is markedly reduced.

■ **PHONE CALL**

Questions

1. Does the patient have shortness of breath, and has the shortness of breath increased suddenly?
2. Is tightness or chest pain present?
3. Is the patient hypotensive?
4. Is the patient known to have acute pericarditis, or is this the second to fourth day after myocardial infarction (MI)?
5. Is there any traumatic injury to the chest?

Inform RN

"Will arrive at the bedside in . . . minutes."
This is a dire emergency requiring immediate assessment. Call a senior cardiology resident urgently if he or she has not already been notified by the RN.

■ **ELEVATOR THOUGHTS**

What are the causes of cardiac tamponade?
- Chest trauma: If the patient had recent chest trauma and has a sudden shock-like state with hypotension and increased jugular venous pressure (JVP), strongly consider cardiac tamponade.
- Acute MI with free-wall rupture
- Dissecting aneurysm (see Chapter 11)
- Underlying carcinoma

- Infectious pericarditis
- Uremic pericarditis

■ MAJOR THREAT TO LIFE

- Cardiac tamponade with cardiogenic shock.

■ BEDSIDE

Quick Look Test

Does the patient look sick (uncomfortable or distressed) or critical (about to die)?

If the patient's condition is critical, ask the nurse to prepare for immediate pericardiocentesis and request your resident to urgently perform this procedure. If the echocardiogram has not been done, have one done immediately; it should show diastolic collapse of the right ventricle and atrium.

Vital Signs

Reassess the vital signs.

Selective Physical Examination

What is the heart rate?

Sinus tachycardia is common with cardiac tamponade.

What is the blood pressure?

1. Mild to moderate hypotension is common. Assess the blood pressure (BP) and look for pulsus paradoxus.
2. Significant pulsus paradoxus is usually detectable but may be masked when severe hypotension is present, or if there is elevation of the diastolic pressure of either ventricle. Pulsus paradoxus is an exaggeration of the normal inspiratory fall in systolic BP that exceeds 10 mm Hg. First, determine the systolic BP by palpation, then inflate the BP cuff 30 mm Hg above the palpable systolic BP. Deflate the cuff slowly. Initially, the Korotkoff sounds are heard only on expiration; as the cuff pressure is slowly lowered, the sounds appear to double, because they now become audible in inspiration as well as expiration.
3. The difference in systolic BP recorded at the start of the Korotkoff sounds in inspiration and expiration is an estimate of pulsus paradoxus. If pulsus paradoxus is >12 mm Hg, it is significant; e.g., if the Korotkoff sounds are heard initially

at 140 mm Hg during expiration only and then appear to double at 120 mm Hg during inspiration, the pulsus paradoxus is 20 mm Hg. Pulsus paradoxus may be caused by other conditions such as status asthmaticus, massive pulmonary embolism, pneumothorax, constrictive pericarditis, and right ventricular infarction.

4. The JVP is often elevated to the angle of the jaw: a marked X descent may be seen in acute tamponade.

■ DIAGNOSTIC TESTING

Diagnostic Echocardiography

An early finding is diastolic right atrial collapse; it occurs in most cases except regional tamponade, in which right or left atrial collapse may be observed. Diastolic right ventricular collapse, **a swinging heart, and electrical alternans may occur (Fig. 10–1).**

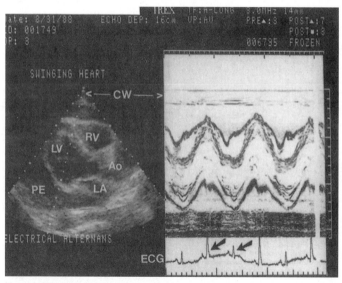

Figure 10–1 □ Cardiac tamponade in a patient with carcinoma of the lung. M-mode and two-dimensional echocardiogram reveal a large pericardial effusion (PE) with a swinging heart motion, diastolic collapse of the right ventricle and left atrium, and electrical alternans. Note in the M-mode tracing that when the cardiac wall swings anteriorly, the QRS voltage is high *(arrow)* and low *(arrow)* when it swings posteriorly. Ao = aorta; CW = chest wall; LA = left atrium; LV = left ventricle; RV = right ventricle. (From Gazes PC: Clinical Cardiology. Philadelphia, Lea & Febiger, 1990, p 374.)

■ MANAGEMENT

1. Maintain a preload adequate to generate stroke volume. Volume expansion with saline may provide hemodynamic stability until pericardiocentesis is completed. Volume expansion is essential to maintain right atrial pressure above intrapericardial pressure and thus prevent right atrial or ventricular collapse.

2. Pericardiocentesis should be performed by an experienced cardiologist under echocardiographic control or by a cardiothoracic surgeon.

3. In patients with underlying chronic disease, an indwelling pericardial catheter with multiple-sized holes should be used for drainage and for administration of antibiotics.

4. If cardiac tamponade recurs, a subxiphoid pericardial window should be performed by a cardiothoracic surgeon; this procedure provides adequate drainage.

11 | Aortic Dissection

The extremely high mortality rate from dissection of the ascending aorta (>50% of patients die in 15 minutes) calls for rapidity of diagnosis. Death often occurs within 1 to 6 hours of onset of symptoms. With dissection of the descending aorta, 2 to 12 hours is available for diagnostic workup.

■ PHONE CALL

Questions

1. Is the patient critically ill?
2. What are the patient's vital signs?
3. Is the patient's chest pain severe and persistent?
4. Has a transesophageal echocardiogram (TEE) been done to confirm the diagnosis?

Orders

1. Ask the RN to inform the senior cardiology resident and the on-call team if they have not already been notified.
2. If a TEE has not been requested, have one done immediately.

Inform RN

"Will arrive at the bedside immediately."

■ ELEVATOR THOUGHTS

These should be few, because you should hasten to the patient's bedside. Is it truly aortic dissection, or is it extensive myocardial infarction (MI) with mechanical complication or severe pulmonary embolism? Diagnostic confirmation by TEE or magnetic resonance imaging (MRI) scan within the hour, followed by surgical correction, offers the only means to survival for the patient.

■ BEDSIDE

Quick Look Test

Does the patient look sick (uncomfortable or distressed) or critical (about to die)?

Vital Signs

What is the blood pressure? Is hypotension present?

If the systolic blood pressure is >120 mm Hg, request a nitroprusside infusion. Prepare to administer a beta-blocking drug intravenously (IV) to decrease cardiac ejection velocity.

Selective History and Selective Physical Examination

1. Sudden onset of severe chest pain radiating to the back and the interscapular area, accompanied by a shock-like state with the patient cool, clammy, and vasoconstricted, even in the presence of a normal blood pressure, is a common feature of dissection.
2. Hypotension is an ominous sign.
3. Syncope may indicate rupture into the pericardial space with cardiac tamponade.
4. Listen for a loud aortic diastolic murmur, which may occur due to dissection involving the aortic valve. An aortic thrill may be present.
5. Assess for sternoclavicular joint pulsation.
6. Assess the pulses in the limbs; pulses may tend to come and go.
7. The blood pressure may be different in the arms if the left subclavian artery is affected.

■ DIAGNOSTIC TESTING

1. Assess the electrocardiogram (ECG). A lack of ST elevation or developing Q waves, in the presence of sudden severe chest pain with a shock-like state, suggests aortic dissection.
2. Obtain immediate estimation of hemoglobin, serum creatinine, and potassium.
3. Assess the chest x-ray.
4. A TEE done urgently in the emergency room or on the way to the operating room
5. An MRI scan is more accurate than a TEE. A computed tomographic (CT) scan is of little value and is not advisable.

■ MANAGEMENT

If the systolic blood pressure is >120 mm Hg, **nitroprusside 0.2 to 2 µg/kg/min IV** is given to decrease the afterload. A beta blocker such as **esmolol** is given, **infused IV at 3 to 6 mg over 1 minute;** the **maintenance dose is 1 to 5 mg/min** (maximum, 50 μg/kg/min). If hypotension is present or develops, decrease the maintenance dose to 1 to 3 mg/min.

With dissection of the descending aorta, diagnostic workup includes an aortic arteriogram. Elevated blood pressure is controlled with nitroprusside and a beta blocker. Surgery is not necessary in all cases, and if surgery is not urgently required, a followup examination with CT scans is indicated to assess for widening, which indicates the need for surgical intervention.

Study Section: Dissection of the Ascending Aorta

Dissection involving the ascending aorta has an extremely high mortality (up to 1% per minute, 60% in 60 minutes). Thus, time-consuming investigations that are not sufficiently sensitive or specific, such as CT scans, must be forsaken. Emergency surgery carries the only hope of survival for the patient with dissection of the ascending aorta, and immediate, accurate diagnosis is mandatory to guide interventional therapy. Presently, the quickest, most accurate diagnostic procedure is TEE, which can be performed at the bedside, in the intensive care unit (ICU), or in the operating room. A study by Nienaber and coworkers indicates a role for MRI as the noninvasive standard for the diagnosis.

Dissection involving the ascending aorta, type I of DeBakey, accounts for up to 66% of all aortic dissection. Usually, the intimal tear is located just above the aortic valve. It is very rare for the dissection to start or end in the transverse arch, so there is usually no need for arch repair, which requires hypothermic arrest and carries a high mortality. Also, it is important to know where the tear ends.

Type II of DeBakey may be regarded as a subgroup of type I, in which dissection is confined to the ascending aorta. Type III of DeBakey, in which the tear usually ends just distal to the left subclavian artery, accounts for up to 25% of all aortic dissections; the dissection is confined to the descending aorta, and rupture may occur into the left pleural space, causing a left hemothorax.

The Stanford classification system divides aortic dissections into two types:

- Type A dissection, when there is involvement of the ascending aorta regardless of the site of entry (DeBakey types I and II)
- Type B, which are distal dissections not involving the ascending aorta (DeBakey type III)

■ DIAGNOSTIC HALLMARKS

Diagnosis must be prompt. Clues include
- Sudden onset of severe chest and/or interscapular pain, like a "gunshot," whereas in acute MI, pain builds up gradually over several minutes
- Tearing, ripping pain
- Pain may spread to other areas as dissection advances
- A shock-like state: cool, clammy, and vasoconstricted; impaired sensorium, yet the blood pressure may be in the normal range. Occasionally, the blood pressure is high.
- Hypotension, an ominous sign, usually from external rupture
- Syncope, which usually indicates rupture into the pericardial space with cardiac tamponade; pericardial effusion heralds an extremely poor prognosis
- A new, loud aortic diastolic murmur
- An aortic thrill, if present, is a strong diagnostic point
- Sternoclavicular joint pulsation
- Loss of one or more pulses, or pulses that come and go
- Blood pressure difference in the arms if the left subclavian artery is affected
- Ischemic neuropathy due to ischemia of the limbs
- Signs of stroke
- Paraparesis or paraplegia may occur with marked decrease in blood supply to the spinal cord
- The scenario may mimic arterial embolism

When features are less typical in the presence of central chest pain, a diagnosis of MI is considered. The lack of developing Q waves and the absence of ST segment elevation in the majority of cases, especially in association with an elevated blood pressure in the presence of a shock-like state, should prompt the diagnosis of dissection. The early absence of an increase in creatine kinase (CK) and the CK-MB fraction does not exclude acute MI, and their estimation is not relevant for the urgent diagnosis of dissection.

■ PREDISPOSING FACTORS AND ASSOCIATIONS

The majority of patients with aortic dissection are hypertensive and older than 60 years of age. Hypertension coexists in up to 80% of patients and is more common in type B distal dissections. Hypertension accelerates the mild degree of aortic medial degeneration that occurs with normal aging. Normotensive younger patients usually have associated underlying disease of the aortic root. Marfan syndrome is the leading cause of aortic dissection in patients below the age of 40. Other causes include giant cell arteritis, lupus erythematosus, relapsing polychondritis, and Ehlers-Danlos, Turner's, and Noonan's syndromes. A congenital bicuspid valve appears to be present in up to 7% of patients with aortic dissection, versus 1.5% in the general adult population with a tricuspid aortic valve. The bicuspid valve is at least 5 times more common in patients with aortic dissection than in individuals with a tricuspid aortic valve.

Approximately 15% of patients with coarctation of the aorta die from aortic dissection.

■ INVESTIGATIONS

Investigations are limited to estimation of the hemoglobin, serum creatinine, and potassium; chest x-ray; and an ECG to exclude MI. There is no need to await CK-MB results.

TEE is done urgently, in the emergency room, ICU, or operating room suite prior to the surgical procedure. TEE has a sensitivity of about 99% and a specificity of 97%. CT scans have a sensitivity of only 60%.

In a series by Ballal and coworkers, TEE, compared with the diagnostic gold standard, aortography, correctly diagnosed aortic dissection in 33 of 34 patients. Nienaber's blinded study indicated a sensitivity of 96% for type A lesions but a specificity of only 77%, with six false-positive findings on TEE. The specificity of only 77% raises concern about the incidence of false positives. Nonetheless, because of its accuracy and speed at the bedside, further improvement in diagnostic features would likely establish TEE as the investigation of first choice, especially in patients who are unstable and in hospitals where MRI is not available. MRI has a role when patient access can be rapidly achieved.

■ THERAPY

For type A and B dissections, emergency surgery is a necessity if the patient's life is to be saved. Because it is extremely rare for the dissection to end or start in the transverse arch, there is usually no need for arch repair, which requires hypothermic arrest and is associated with an increase in surgical mortality. Short-term stabilization is attempted in the emergency room and in the operating room using beta blockade or nitroprusside.

1. **Nitroprusside. Dosage: IV 0.2–2 μg/kg/min**, i.e., 12 to 120

μg/min for a 60-kg patient. The aim is to reduce the blood pressure to the lowest possible level yet preserve cardiac, cerebral, and renal perfusion. An intra-arterial cannula is advisable to accurately monitor blood pressure.

2. **Beta-Adrenergic Blockers.** Beta-adrenergic blockade is of benefit because it decreases the velocity and force of myocardial contraction and reduces the rate of rise of aortic pressure, which is a major factor in determining extension of the dissection. Nitroprusside increases the velocity of ventricular contraction and the rate of pressure rise, hence the need for combination with a beta-adrenergic blocker.

   - **Esmolol. Dosage: IV infusion, 1.5 mg/kg bolus over 1 minute**, then an infusion of **0.15 to 0.3 mg/kg/min**. If hypotension is present or develops, decrease the maintenance dose to 1 to 3 mg/min.
   - **Metoprolol. Dosage: 1 mg/min at 5-minute intervals** to a maximum of 15 mg repeated every 6 to 8 hours.

12 | Hypotension and Cardiogenic Shock

Calls for the assessment of hypotension are common. Systolic blood pressure of <110 mm Hg, accompanied by symptoms and signs of hypoperfusion, requires prompt attention. Urgent stabilization of the blood pressure and a search for an underlying cause are necessary. Many young individuals have a systolic blood pressure normally in the range of 90 to 100 mm Hg. A systolic blood pressure of 105 to 120 mm Hg is not unusual in healthy, older individuals. In hypertensive patients, a sharp fall in blood pressure from values in the range of 150 to 200 mm Hg to <120 mm Hg may cause inadequate tissue perfusion.

Confusion, disorientation, loss of consciousness, and presence of angina and raised jugular venous pressure with oliguria are ominous symptoms and signs. When target tissue perfusion is inadequate to supply vital substrates and eliminate metabolic waste, shock is said to be present.

Target tissue perfusion may be inadequate because of pronounced reduction of cardiac output (CO), maldistribution of blood flow, or both.

Cardiogenic shock occurs when there is decreased ventricular systolic function secondary to complications of cardiac disorders, which results in a pronounced decrease in CO.

■ PHONE CALL

Questions

1. What is the patient's blood pressure?
2. Is the heart rate increased, suggesting that hypotension may be present?
3. Is the patient on medications that may cause lowering of blood pressure?
4. Is fever a prominent feature, suggesting impending septic shock?
5. What is the level of consciousness?
6. Is chest pain a prominent feature, suggesting myocardial infarction or aortic dissection with cardiogenic shock?
7. Is the patient bleeding, or is there evidence suggesting internal bleeding?

8. **Is the patient in the emergency room (ER), the intensive care unit (ICU), the ward, or the x-ray department?**

Orders

1. Obtain a large-bore 16-gauge needle IV to be inserted immediately for normal saline 0.9% infusion.
2. Place an arterial blood gas tray at bedside.
3. Administer oxygen by face mask.
4. If bleeding is suspected, crossmatch immediately for 2 to 4 units.
5. Obtain an electrocardiogram (ECG) immediately to exclude myocardial infarction or arrhythmia.

Inform RN

"Will arrive at the bedside immediately."

■ ELEVATOR THOUGHTS

What are the causes of hypotension?
Causes of hypotension include
- Hypovolemia
- Sepsis
- Anaphylaxis
  Consider anaphylaxis if antibiotics or contrast media were given recently.

What are the causes of cardiogenic shock?
- Myocardial infarction
- Severe valvular defects including acute mitral regurgitation
- Cardiac tamponade
- Aortic dissection
- Tachyarrhythmias
- Pulmonary embolism

■ MAJOR THREAT TO LIFE

Cardiogenic shock has a mortality rate exceeding 80%. If a right ventricular infarction is the underlying cause, coronary arteriography followed by coronary balloon angioplasty may be lifesaving (see Chapter 7).

■ BEDSIDE

Quick Look Test

Does the patient look sick (uncomfortable or distressed) or critical (about to die)?

Airway and Vital Signs

Is the airway clear?

Selective Physical Examination

Assess rapidly for
1. Severe hypotension, systolic pressure of <80 mm Hg without inotropic support, or systolic blood pressure of <90 mm Hg with inotropic support
2. Cool peripheries associated with diaphoresis
3. Clouding of consciousness

■ DIAGNOSTIC TESTING

Observe the ECG for sinus tachycardia that is associated with the hypotensive state and for tachyarrhythmias, such as atrial fibrillation with a rapid ventricular response, a ventricular rate of >150/min, supraventricular tachycardia, or ventricular tachycardia. If bradycardia is present, assess for complete heart block.

If the staff physician has not yet arrived, ask the registered nurse (RN) to call immediately.

■ MANAGEMENT

1. Have a cardiac arrest cart at bedside.
2. Ensure an adequate airway, and maintain a PaO_2 of 75 to 120 mm Hg. Use a well-fitting oxygen mask with a high flow rate of 10 to 15 L/min.
3. If the patient has clouding of consciousness or is in a coma, intubation is necessary. Arrange for the insertion of an indwelling arterial line, preferably femoral, for blood pressure and oximetric monitoring.
4. An indwelling catheter is necessary to monitor urinary output, which should be >30 ml/hr.
5. Measure the pulmonary capillary wedge pressure (PCWP). If this is <15 mm Hg, start a fluid challenge to bring the filling pressure of the left ventricle to about 18 mm Hg. If the PCWP is initially >18 mm Hg, discontinue the IV saline and replace with 5% dextrose in water (D5W). Obtain

measures of arterial blood gas (ABG), electrolytes, blood urea nitrogen (BUN), and creatinine. Arrange for a transesophageal echocardiogram (TEE) to exclude cardiac complications.

6. Nitroprusside is indicated for severe mitral regurgitation and mechanical complications of infarction for which afterload reduction is considered necessary. A combination of dobutamine and dopamine may be necessary to maintain a systolic blood pressure of >90 mm Hg. Inotropic drugs and vasopressors are of limited value. In patients with cardiogenic shock due to acute myocardial infarction (MI), coronary angioplasty has a role; discuss this with your resident. Ensure that the patient is not taking medications that would cause hypotension, e.g., angiotensin-converting enzyme (ACE) inhibitors, beta blockers, antiarrhythmics, and calcium antagonists.

7. Inotropic support is required to stabilize the patient for interventional procedures. **Dobutamine at a dosage of 2 to 10 μg/kg/min** is titrated to achieve a desired inotropic effect. If a dose of >6 μg/kg/min is required, add a dopamine infusion (see Appendix A).

8. **Dopamine dosage is 2.5 to 10 μg/kg/min via a central line.**

9. Nitroglycerin infusion may be required for patients who have associated pulmonary congestion and a PCWP of >22 mm Hg. Nitroglycerin may cause further hypotension, but it is safer than nitroprusside if ischemia is present. If hypotension is uncontrolled, if the patient requires interventional therapy, and if there is no limiting intercurrent illness, an intra-aortic balloon pump is advisable, to stabilize the patient during coronary arteriography, angioplasty, or surgery. Inotropic drugs may be required for temporary support, but they do not improve mortality.

10. Contraindications to the use of the intra-aortic balloon pump include
    - Aortic regurgitation
    - Aortic aneurysm
    - Contraindication to heparin therapy

11. Patients with shock caused by acute MI are best managed with percutaneous transluminal coronary angioplasty (PTCA) and stenting.

13 | Shortness of Breath

Shortness of breath, or dyspnea, is a common on-call problem. Dyspnea, by definition, is difficult breathing. The term is used synonymously with shortness of breath or breathlessness and may be expressed by individuals as follows: "I can't get enough air"; "I'm breathless or short of breath"; "I feel like I'm being smothered"; or "I'm out of breath, running after my breath." Because shortness of breath on exertion may be a normal phenomenon, it is necessary to make a careful assessment of the normal or altered lifestyle of the patient in relation to the degree of shortness of breath. For example, a change from a very active lifestyle, to a few years of sedentary life, then resumption of exercise or strenuous work may be the cause of shortness of breath. Increasing body weight and advancing or intercurrent illness may be important causal factors.

■ PHONE CALL

Questions

1. Is the shortness of breath mild, moderate, or severe?
2. Did it occur suddenly and become severe within minutes?

    This suggests pulmonary embolism, pneumothorax, or acute pulmonary edema.
3. How long has the patient been short of breath?
4. What is the admitting diagnosis, e.g., acute myocardial infarction (MI), congestive heart failure (CHF)?
5. What are the vital signs?

Orders

1. Give oxygen: start by nasal prongs at 2 to 4 L/min.
2. Determine arterial blood gasses (ABGs).

Inform RN

"Will arrive at the bedside immediately."

■ ELEVATOR THOUGHTS

What are the causes of dyspnea?
    The causes of dyspnea are given in Table 13–1.

Table 13–1 □ CAUSES OF SHORTNESS OF BREATH

Cause	Meaning or Association
Normal: to be expected because of relative age and lack of exercise, overweight	Excessive strenuous effort precipitates symptoms
Elevation of the diaphragm, e.g., pregnancy, ascites	Mechanical problem
Heart failure	Increased pulmonary venous pressure; interstitial pulmonary edema; frank pulmonary alveolar edema
Pericardial effusion	Restriction to ventricular filling
Angina equivalent of chest discomfort	LV dysfunction or discomfort appreciated as breathing with difficulty or suffocation
Pulmonary embolism	Apprehension, presyncope, pain
Pulmonary diseases	Pneumonia, asthma, pneumothorax, ARDS, pleural effusion, COPD, restrictive lung disease, lymphangitis carcinomatosa
Laryngeal stridor	Laryngotracheal obstruction
Thoracic defects	Neuromuscular or bony mechanical conditions
Decreased hemoglobin or available oxygen	Anemia, high altitude

LV = left ventricular; ARDS = adult respiratory distress syndrome; COPD = chronic obstructive pulmonary disease.

Pathophysiology of Dyspnea

Review briefly the pathophysiology of dyspnea.

1. An increase in the work of breathing due to changes in lung compliance or resistance, as occurs with interstitial pulmonary edema due to CHF or pulmonary fibrosis

    The respiratory center receives indirect stimuli via lung stretch (Hering-Breuer reflexes). Stretch receptors in the lung parenchyma relay information to the respiratory center, resulting directly or indirectly in dyspnea. Stretch receptors in respiratory muscles, irritant receptors, and juxtacapillary ("j") receptors are sensitive to congestion, vascular engorgement, and mechanical stimulation.

2. Shunting and other hypoxic stimulation to breathing, e.g., caused by adult respiratory distress syndrome (ARDS), pneumonia, pulmonary embolism, and right-to-left cardiac shunts

3. Airflow obstruction: chronic obstructive pulmonary disease (COPD), asthma, bronchiectasis

4. Mechanical limitation to ventilation: thoracic and neurologic abnormalities
5. Decrease in cardiac output
6. Decrease in hemoglobin (anemias)
7. High altitude

■ MAJOR THREAT TO LIFE

- Hypoxemia
- Left ventricular (LV) failure
- Pulmonary embolism

■ BEDSIDE

Does the patient look sick (uncomfortable or distressed) or critical (about to die)?

Airway and Vital Signs

- Make sure that the upper airway is clear.
- Determine the respiratory rate; if >20/min, consider hypoxemia, or anxiety and apprehension caused by pain and distress. Paradoxical abdominal and diaphragmatic movement during respiration indicates diaphragmatic fatigue or weakness; the presence of this sign is ominous, and some patients may require ventilator assistance. Discuss this problem immediately with your resident. A respiratory rate of <12/min indicates a central depression of ventilation caused by drugs or overdose, narcotics, or cerebrovascular accident.
- Assess the heart rate and the blood pressure. Hypotension suggests CHF caused by underlying cardiac disease or pulmonary embolism (check for pulsus paradoxus and cardiac tamponade) (see Chapters 4 and 10).

Selective History

It is necessary to listen intently to the patient's description before prompting for more specific descriptions. Often, errors in diagnosis and management occur because the patient's description is misunderstood.

Dyspnea

Dyspnea is the most common symptom of cardiac and respiratory disorders. It is often a difficult symptom to resolve, unless a clear description is obtained. It is necessary to exclude the following conditions, which are not truly dyspnea:

- Hyperventilation states caused by anxiety. The patient will refer to "feeling hungry for air."
- Sighing respirations, e.g., the sigh, "I feel like I need to take a deep breath."
- Splinting caused by pleuritic pain or rib or chest wall problems
- Laryngismus caused by hypocalcemia, which may occur because of hypoparathyroidism (occasionally surgically induced)

When it is determined that the patient is complaining of genuine shortness of breath, consider the following:

- Define what level of activity precipitated the shortness of breath, e.g., the number of stairs climbed, the number of steps taken, the number of blocks walked, the extent of the incline, the relation to various types of effort or exertion. Shortness of breath is abnormal when it occurs at rest or at a level of activity not expected to cause this situation.
- Duration: seconds, minutes, hours? If the sensation lasts <10 seconds, it is not true dyspnea.
- Is it occurring at rest? If so, determine the duration and what makes it better or worse.
- If it occurred suddenly and with the patient at rest, is it improving or getting worse?
- Is it accompanied by cough, wheeze, chest pain, palpitations, or edema?
- Is it worse on inspiration and accompanied by tracheal or laryngeal stridor? This indicates upper respiratory tract obstruction, which can be life threatening.
- Is it mainly with expiration? The patient has difficulty getting air out of the lungs because airflow is obstructed (a prolonged expiratory phase); this is usually due to an exacerbation of asthma or COPD.
- Is it worse only when lying down or when the trunk is immersed in water? This suggests diaphragmatic paresis or paralysis.

Orthopnea

Orthopnea is shortness of breath that occurs within minutes of lying down and is relieved within a few minutes (not a few seconds) of sitting upright or dangling the legs over the bedside. This symptom is not usually accompanied by wheezing or flatulence.

Orthopnea is usually caused by severe LV dysfunction, subtle LV failure, or increased pulmonary venous pressure, e.g., owing to mitral stenosis. In patients with poor LV function, blood returning to the heart from the lower limbs when the person is reclining is not ejected efficiently from the left ventricle. This results in an increase in left atrial and pulmonary venous pressures, causing increases in lung water and lung stiffness, which incite reflexes that trigger the sensation of shortness of breath. The upright position decreases venous return and improves the abnormal sensation within minutes. Orthopnea lasts from 1 to 5 minutes and does not usually exceed 10 minutes.

Warning: Shortness of breath of >10 minutes' duration while at rest is a life-threatening situation.

Paroxysmal Nocturnal Dyspnea

Paroxysmal nocturnal dyspnea is shortness of breath (a suffocating feeling) that occurs after the patient has been lying in bed for >1 hour. The patient usually awakens several hours after retiring, typically between 1 and 3 A.M., with severe shortness of breath. Relief is obtained only by getting out of bed, sitting in a chair, dangling the legs, or standing. Unlike with orthopnea, sitting up does not cause relief in 1 or 2 minutes. Shortness of breath usually lasts from 10 to 30 minutes. Paroxysmal nocturnal dyspnea is more common in patients with poor LV function who have peripheral edema. After the patient lies down for the night, it takes 1 to 3 hours for edema fluid from the lower limbs to return to the heart. An extra volume of sodium and water precipitates LV failure; this causes an increase in left atrial pressure, i.e., severe pulmonary venous hypertension that results in pulmonary edema. Cough is often associated with the feeling of suffocation and with the production of frothy, blood-tinged sputum.

Other Forms of Abnormal Breathing

- **Cheyne-Stokes respiration.** In this condition, the patient takes deep inspirations, the depth of inspiration increases with each consecutive breath for 1 to 2 minutes, and then there is cessation of breathing for 10 to 30 seconds, after which the patient resumes deep breathing. Cheyne-Stokes respiration is usually observed in patients with cerebrovascular accidents, in patients with head injury, and in patients with severe LV failure with coexisting cerebral disease.

- **Kussmaul breathing.** The patient takes deep breaths, with long inspiratory and expiratory phases, without wheezing and without the use of accessory muscles. The patient has no difficulty getting air into or out of the lungs and does not describe the sensation as a feeling of shortness of breath or breathlessness. This pattern of breathing is observed in patients with diabetic ketoacidosis, uremia, and salicylate overdose. Metabolic acidosis stimulates the respiratory center to produce this breathing pattern, which blows carbon dioxide out of the lungs and into the atmosphere. The loss of carbon dioxide causes a compensatory adjustment in blood pH. Unfortunately, the degree of acidosis is usually too intense to be completely corrected by ridding the lungs of carbon dioxide.

Selective Physical Examination

Inspection

1. Is the patient in distress, requiring being propped upright to ease difficult breathing?
2. Is the patient using accessory muscles of respiration?
3. Is cyanosis present?

   Do not forget that severe hypoxia may be present with no cyanosis apparent on observation. Different types of cyanosis are discussed in Chapter 4.
4. Is the patient wheezing, or is the patient a known asthmatic?

   Do not forget, "all that wheezes is not asthma"; patients with pulmonary embolism, pulmonary edema, and exacerbation of chronic bronchitis may exhibit audible wheezing.

Vital Signs

Repeat now and recheck patency of the airways. Sinus tachycardia is commonly caused by hypoxemia, pain, and anxiety. If the systolic blood pressure is <90 mm Hg with signs of hypoperfusion, begin measures for managing cardiogenic shock (see Chapter 12).

Cardiovascular System

1. The jugular venous pressure (JVP) should be elevated to >3 cm above the sternal angle in patients with CHF.

   Venous pressure may be markedly elevated, and the top of the blood column may be masked by the angle of the jaw. The ear lobes may pulsate in patients with markedly elevated JVP and tricuspid incompetence. Look tangentially across the neck for prominent venous waves (see Chapter 4, JVP and Venous Waves). The JVP is elevated in
   - CHF due to all causes
   - Cardiac tamponade
   - Superior vena cava obstruction

   A unilateral elevation of the JVP, which is nonpulsatile, is observed with superior vena cava obstruction. Watch for false elevation of the JVP in patients with an exacerbation of COPD. Venous pressure is elevated during the phase in which exhalation is difficult, and it falls during inspiration.
2. Listen for the presence of murmurs.

   A loud mitral systolic murmur with radiation to the left axilla or the spine may occur in patients with ruptured chordae or flail mitral valve leaflet. The murmur of aortic stenosis may be loud but, in the presence of a low cardiac output, may diminish in intensity and result in a misdiagnosis. The murmur of mitral regurgitation may be soft in patients with low cardiac output or a thick chest wall or concomitant COPD. *Patients with severe aortic stenosis may die during an episode of pulmonary edema.*

3. Listen carefully for a third heart sound, a gallop, which is commonly present if CHF is the cause of severe shortness of breath (see Chapter 4 for a description of gallop rhythms).

4. Is the heart clinically enlarged?

   Cardiomegaly may be mild and may be absent in patients with aortic stenosis or pure mitral stenosis.

5. Observe for abnormal pulsations including visible gallops.

   Abnormal dyskinetic myocardium may be visible just above the apex beat, in the region of the fourth interspace, caused by recurrent myocardial infarction or LV aneurysm, severe valvular defects, or cardiomyopathy.

6. Observe for bilateral ankle edema.

   Assess the extent of edema up to the knee and the degree of pitting. If shortness of breath was present for several days and the patient was confined to bed, check for presacral edema.

7. If CHF is present, verify the underlying cause of heart disease: valvular disease, coronary artery disease, congenital heart disease, hypertension, cardiomyopathy, and cor pulmonale.

8. Define a precipitating cause: recent MI or MI and mechanical defect, ruptured chordae tendineae, flail mitral valve, worsening of valvular defect, increased salt intake, and medications that precipitate CHF (beta blockers, calcium antagonists, and nonsteroidal anti-inflammatory drugs [NSAIDs]).

Respiratory System

1. Is the patient cyanotic?

   See Chapter 4 for a full discussion of cyanosis.

2. Is the trachea in the midline?

   A shift away from the side of the lesion is observed with pneumothorax and pleural effusion; a shift to the side of the lesion indicates atelectasis.

3. Is there dullness to percussion?

   Stony dullness is in keeping with pleural effusion. If there is mild impairment to percussion, consider consolidation.

4. Is there unilateral hyperresonance?

   Consider pneumothorax.

5. Auscultate for breath sounds.

   - Air entry: if air entry is decreased or absent over an area of dullness, with decreased bronchophony, consider pleural effusion; air entry absent over a hyperresonant area is diagnostic of pneumothorax.

- Quality of breath sounds: if bronchial breathing is present, consider consolidation.
- Added sounds: crackles (crepitations) over both lower lung fields associated with an increased JVP is diagnostic of CHF, but crackles may be maximal on one side.

■ DIAGNOSTIC TESTING

1. A chest x-ray confirms pulmonary edema or interstitial edema caused by heart failure (see Chapter 18).

   For pulmonary causes, a posteroanterior (PA) and left lateral film are essential: assess for pleural effusions, diaphragmatic paralysis, emphysema, tumors, and lymphangitis carcinomatosa. If emphysema or restrictive lung disease is suspected, a computed tomographic (CT) scan and gas transfer assessment are advisable.
2. An echocardiogram helps document the degree of valvular lesions, LV systolic function, ejection fraction, and pericardial effusion with tamponade.
3. Measures of ABGs assess hypoxemia and response to therapy.

■ MANAGEMENT

1. Dangle the patient's legs over the bedside and prop the patient upright as much as possible.
2. **Furosemide 80 mg IV immediately;** then, **oral furosemide 40 to 80 mg daily**. The infrequently used diuretic torsemide has recently been shown to be superior to furosemide for the management of CHF.
3. Oxygen by nasal prongs or mask 4 to 8 L/min until ABGs show the absence of hypoxemia and the underlying cause improves or is corrected (see Chapters 7, 17, and 18).

14 | Edema

Edema is an excessive accumulation of interstitial fluid in the subcutaneous tissue.

■ PHONE CALL

Questions

1. Does the patient complain that shoes feel tighter or that sock tops leave indentations as the day progresses?
2. Is the swelling more prominent at the end of the day?
3. Is the swelling unilateral or bilateral?
4. Is the swelling of recent onset, or is it recurrent?
5. Is the swelling associated with shortness of breath?

■ ELEVATOR THOUGHTS

What are the causes of edema?

Many patients are inappropriately treated with diuretics and digitalis for edema that is noncardiac in origin. A careful history and physical examination are necessary to accurately determine the cause (Table 14–1). Localization is determined mainly by gravity.

- Edema of cardiac origin involves both of the feet and ankles.
- Edema may involve the lower limbs, the trunk, the face, and the arms and may be associated with ascites and pleural effusions; this generalized edema is referred to as anasarca.
- Unilateral leg edema is typical of **venous and lymphatic** obstruction. **Venous edema is soft, pits easily, and spares the toes; lymphatic edema is firm, pits poorly, and involves the toes.** Patients with neurologic disease are commonly allowed to sit out of bed for prolonged periods; edema may worsen, because the leg muscles are not being used.
- Edema confined to the upper limbs and face occurs with superior vena cava obstruction.
- Edema of one arm may be due to venous occlusion or lymphatic obstruction, e.g., caused by breast cancer.

Bilateral edema of the lower limbs does not usually occur until >7 lb of fluid have accumulated. Weight gain of 5 to 10

Table 14–1 □ **EDEMA OF THE LOWER LIMBS**

Causes	Comments
Congestive heart failure	Symmetric, occurs before ascites
Constrictive pericarditis	Symmetric but occurs weeks after the occurrence of prominent ascites; high JVP
Cirrhosis	Ascites first, then leg edema; normal or slight increase of JVP
Venous obstruction	Commonly unilateral, one leg more than the other leg; **toes are spared**
Lymphatic obstruction	One side more than the other side; **toes involved**
Stasis	
Obesity	Dependent and stasis edema
Neurologic disorders; loss of muscle pump	Edema, mainly on the paralyzed side
Nephrotic syndrome	Edema commonly involves the face; JVP is normal with noncardiac causes
Pregnancy	Left leg more than right leg
Psychogenic factors	Young females during tension states: abnormal water tolerance
Heat edema	Due to aldosterone-mediated Na^+ and water retention
Drugs	Calcium antagonists, estrogens, NSAIDs, steroids

JVP = jugular venous pressure; NSAIDs = nonsteroidal anti-inflammatory drugs.

lb over a few days is a more reliable sign of intense sodium and water retention than is the demonstration of edema.

Edema in patients with heart failure occurs mainly when right-sided heart failure is present for several days. Acute left ventricular failure rarely causes significant leg edema. The most common cause of right-sided heart failure, however, is chronic left ventricular failure. Some degree of inappropriate shortness of breath is virtually always present when edema is caused by heart failure. Edema becomes more prominent if tricuspid regurgitation ensues.

The mechanism of edema formation is threefold.

- A decrease in cardiac output causes activation of the sympathetic and renin–angiotensin–aldosterone systems, which results in sodium and water retention and a high venous pressure. The jugular venous pressure (JVP) is always elevated in patients with heart failure who manifest edema. High systemic venous pressure increases the hydrostatic pressure at the venous end of capillaries, and sodium and water leak out into the subcutaneous tissue. The patient is not waterlogged but has an excess of brine (salt and water) in these tissues. In patients with nephrotic syndrome or cirrhosis, hypoalbuminemia causes a decrease in oncotic pressure, and fluid that exudes into the interstitial tissue is not able to regain entry into the vascular compartment. Because salt and water leave the vascular compartment, the decrease in effective vascular volume causes stimulation of the renin–angiotensin–aldosterone system. This results in retention of sodium and water by the kidney, and edema worsens.

- Edema of pregnancy is caused by activation of the renin–angiotensin system, which results in sodium and water retention; this increases blood volume. Approximately 8 L of water accumulates during normal pregnancy. Normally the common iliac artery partially compresses the left common iliac vein; this increases venous pressure in the left leg. In pregnancy, and in most individuals with edema, the left limb reveals edema before or of greater severity than that observed in the right leg.
- Lymphatic obstruction may be caused by inflammatory, parasitic, or neoplastic processes, resulting in unilateral or bilateral lower or upper limb edema.

Selective Physical Examination

1. Confirm that edema is unilateral or bilateral.
2. Test for pitting.

   Using two finger pads held about 1 cm apart, apply firm pressure to the lower tibial area. Press firmly for about 10 seconds. Edema leaves two pits, 0.5 to 2 cm deep, with a ridge in between. Observe the extent of edema: ankles only; to below the knee; or above the knee (presacral edema).

3. Is there associated swelling of the eyelids?
4. Assess the JVP; elevated to >3 cm bilaterally indicates congestive heart failure (CHF) (see Chapters 4 and 18).
5. Edema occurring weeks after the onset of ascites in a patient with a high JVP suggests constrictive pericarditis. If the JVP is not elevated, consider cirrhosis.
6. Is generalized edema, i.e., anasarca, present?

   This often occurs in patients with nephrotic syndrome but can occur with severe chronic CHF.

■ MANAGEMENT

Management of edema involves treatment of the underlying cause (see Table 14–1 and Chapter 18).

Symptomatic relief is obtained

- With the use of a diuretic: **furosemide 40 to 80 mg daily for a few days and then, for maintenance, 40 mg daily.**

- If CHF is the cause, usually treatment is with furosemide, angiotensin-converting enzyme (ACE) inhibitor, and digoxin.
- By treating the underlying cause of CHF.

If edema is chronic, furosemide may not cause complete clearing of edema. The addition of an aldosterone "antagonist," e.g., **spironolactone 25 mg or amiloride 5 mg daily,** is advisable. Furosemide may stimulate the renin–angiotensin–aldosterone system and is best used with amiloride or an ACE inhibitor. Moduretic, a hydrochlorothiazide-amiloride combination, is a suitable diuretic for this problem.

Cough is a common symptom of patients with cardiopulmonary disease. Cough is a defense mechanism that helps to protect the airways from the effects of irritant substances and to clear the airways of unwanted secretions.

■ PHONE CALL

Questions

1. Is the cough productive or nonproductive?
2. If productive, is the sputum blood-tinged or mucopurulent?
3. Is there associated shortness of breath or wheezing?
4. Is the patient's temperature elevated?

Orders

Ask the registered nurse (RN) to obtain sputum for culture and sensitivity if not already done.

Inform RN

If there is no shortness of breath and the vital signs are stable, see the patient within the next hour.

■ ELEVATOR THOUGHTS

What types of cough are associated with cardiopulmonary disease?

If cough is associated with hemoptysis and shortness of breath, consider left ventricular failure (LVF) and mitral stenosis. A brassy cough may indicate a thoracic aortic aneurysm.

■ BEDSIDE

Selective History and Selective Chart Review

Salient Features of Cough

1. Acute
   - Episodes lasting for several minutes suggest an irritating

phenomenon, mechanical or chemical; e.g., related to an allergic response or inhalation of smoke.

- Episodes lasting for several days with associated fever and evidence of upper respiratory tract infection suggest virus or laryngotracheobronchitis.
- Association with chills, rigors, weakness, or confusion suggests pneumonia.

2. Chronic
   - Coughing related to smoking suggests chronic bronchitis.
   - A change in character or pattern suggests carcinoma of the lung.
   - Weight loss, fever, and night sweats suggest tuberculosis.
   - Paroxysmal coughing, at nights or with exercise, with or without wheezing, suggests asthma.
   - Coughing precipitated by exercise or sexual intercourse may suggest tight mitral stenosis.
   - Paroxysmal "brassy" cough, often with stridor, suggests tracheal obstruction produced by an aortic aneurysm.

3. Productive of sputum
   - Purulent sputum associated with acute illness and fever suggests inflammatory conditions.
   - Purulent and chronic sputum, occurring especially in the early morning, suggests bronchiectasis.
   - Foul-smelling sputum suggests bronchoalveolar carcinoma.
   - Pink, foamy, and voluminous sputum with shortness of breath is typical of pulmonary edema.
   - Rusty "prune juice" sputum with fever and chills is diagnostic of pneumonia.

4. Nonproductive
   - This may result from a hyperactive cough reflex that responds to ordinary innocuous stimuli.
   - Several diseases may cause nonproductive cough, depending on the phase of the disease, notably cancer of the lung.
   - Sarcoidosis may cause cough with dyspnea and can be complicated by conduction disturbances including complete heart block.
   - Medications including angiotensin-converting enzyme (ACE) inhibitors, amiodarone, and methotrexate may be implicated.

5. Character
   - Barking or croupy due to laryngeal disease
   - Paroxysmal with whoops typical of whooping cough
   - Brassy from major airways

6. Time relationships
   - Nighttime, nonproductive, chronic, paroxysmal cough with wheeze suggests asthma.

- Nighttime cough, with orthopnea or paroxysmal nocturnal dyspnea, with or without wheeze, is typical of congestive heart failure (CHF).
- Cough occurring with meals may indicate gastroesophageal reflux or diverticulum.
- Cough on awakening, or with change of posture, is a hallmark of bronchiectasis; on awakening in a smoker, cough suggests chronic bronchitis or bronchogenic carcinoma.
- Intractable, chronic, but nonproductive cough suggests medications (especially ACE inhibitors and amiodarone).
7. Associations
  - Paroxysmal wheezing strongly suggests asthma.
  - Fever, chills, and rigors suggest pneumonia.
  - Stridor, which is a hallmark of involvement of the pharynx, larynx, extrathoracic trachea by foreign body, branchial cyst, acute epiglottitis, diphtheritic infection, or laryngeal edema caused by allergic reaction to drugs, such as ACE inhibitors, or other causes of angioneurotic edema.
  - Orthopnea suggests heart failure.
  - Weight loss, weakness, and night sweats suggest tuberculosis or carcinoma.
  - With particular occupations, consider restrictive lung disease.
  - Pleuritic chest pain: pneumonia, pulmonary embolism, and acute central chest pain suggest pulmonary embolism.

Cardiovascular Causes of Cough

1. Conditions that cause an increase in left atrial pressure: thus pulmonary venous hypertension that results in interstitial or pulmonary edema, LVF due to all causes, mitral stenosis, and left atrial myxoma
2. Pulmonary embolism
3. Compression of the tracheobronchial tree, as with aortic aneurysm
4. Compression of the recurrent laryngeal nerve caused by an aortic aneurysm, a greatly enlarged left atrium, or pulmonary artery can cause cough and hoarseness.
5. Congenital cyanotic heart disease, in particular Eisenmenger's syndrome

Hemoptysis

Determine if the sputum is
1. Blood-streaked: this can originate in the upper respiratory tract or bronchi and, although common in patients with chronic obstructive pulmonary disease (COPD), may be the only clue to bronchogenic carcinoma in a smoker.

2. Pink, frothy, voluminous, and associated with acute shortness of breath: these are hallmarks of pulmonary edema
3. Rusty, "prune juice" with fever and chills: these are typical of pneumonia
4. Frank blood, bright red or dark, suggests the following in the differential diagnosis: bronchogenic carcinoma, pulmonary embolism, aortic aneurysm, arteriovenous fistula, mitral stenosis, Goodpasture's syndrome, blood dyscrasias, and hereditary telangiectasia.

Determine whether the episodes of hemoptysis are associated with

1. Early-morning cough or cough with change in posture; this suggests bronchiectasis, chronic bronchitis, and bronchogenic carcinoma.
2. Dyspnea at rest, during effort, or during pregnancy; in this situation small amounts of rusty sputum or small amounts of bright red blood suggest mitral stenosis. Sudden increase in left atrial pressure during effort or pregnancy may cause rupture of small bronchopulmonary anastomosing veins. Severe dyspnea and blood-tinged sputum are typical of pulmonary edema caused by mitral stenosis or LVF.
3. Weight loss and night sweats; these suggest tuberculosis.
4. Pleuritic pain; this suggests pulmonary embolism.
5. Congenital heart disease and cyanosis; these suggest Eisenmenger's syndrome.

Selective Physical Examination

1. Assess vital signs.
2. Examine for the presence of LVF: crackles over the lower lung fields, gallop rhythm, and increased jugular venous pressure (JVP); valvular lesions, in particular mitral stenosis (see Chapter 4). Assess for consolidation caused by pneumonia.

■ DIAGNOSTIC TESTING

1. Chest x-ray
   Review posteroanterior and left lateral films with your resident; assess for lung lesions and subtle signs of LVF (see Chapter 18).

■ MANAGEMENT

1. Treat the underlying problem
   ▪ Cardiac

- Pulmonary
- Drugs causing cough
    Consider discontinuing drugs that cause cough, in particular ACE inhibitors and amiodarone.

2. Cough suppressants
    These are not recommended without considerable thought. Treatment of the underlying condition is recommended; if cough persists and is bothersome, preventing sleep, give a trial of dextromethorphan 15 mg at bedtime.

3. Cough expectorants
    These are not advisable, because they are ineffective. It is virtually impossible to liquefy thick, tenacious sputum. Ensure that the patient is well hydrated, and improve the humidity of the inspired air.

16 | Pulmonary Embolism

Pulmonary embolism (PE) is a common condition. The diagnosis of PE is often missed, however, because symptoms are not specific and investigations other than lung scan and angiography are nondiagnostic. The mortality rate of patients with massive pulmonary embolism is >40%.

■ PHONE CALL

Questions

1. Is the patient stable or in severe distress?
2. What are the vital signs?
3. Is acute dyspnea associated with central chest pain or pleuritic pain?
4. Is the patient tachypneic?
5. Did syncope, presyncope, or dizziness occur with the dyspnea?
6. Has the patient had surgery within past weeks?

Orders

1. Obtain arterial blood gas (ABG) results and an electrocardiogram (ECG) immediately.
2. Give oxygen at 5 to 10 L/min.
3. Call the medical resident if not already done.
4. Administer IV 0.9% saline to keep the vein open, and have heparin 5000 U available at bedside to be administered if there is no contraindication.

Inform RN

"Will be at the bedside in . . . minutes."

■ ELEVATOR THOUGHTS

What are the causes of pulmonary embolism?
Strongly consider PE if one or more of the following scenarios is present:
1. Acute, unexplained dyspnea lasting only a few minutes to several hours, i.e., sudden dyspnea, not due to

- An obvious cardiac cause
- An obvious pulmonary lesion

2. Acute cor pulmonale and cardiogenic shock
   - If >70% of the pulmonary vascular cross-sectional area is obliterated acutely by emboli, acute pulmonary hypertension at >40 mm Hg results. Right ventricular failure occurs, and death results often within the first hour of the onset of acute dyspnea or cardiogenic shock.
   - With massive PE, pain is usually central, oppressive, and nonpleuritic. Presyncope, syncope, **marked apprehension**, signs of cardiogenic shock, cough, and features that may simulate an acute exacerbation of chronic obstructive pulmonary disease (COPD) are hallmarks.

3. Chronic cor pulmonale in patients with recurrent PE
   - Increasing dyspnea due to pulmonary hypertension
   - Fatigue
   - Signs of right ventricular failure without an obvious cardiac cause

Probabilities

The trainee or physician must devise a system to evaluate the probability for the presence of PE based on a systematic clinical assessment that includes

1. A rapid but relevant history
2. Selective physical signs
3. Chest x-ray
4. ECG
5. Arterial blood gases

The analysis of these five assessments should result in a probability from clinical assessment (PCA). The PCA is useful in the construction of an algorithm for the diagnostic workup of PE (Fig. 16–1).

■ MAJOR THREAT TO LIFE

Massive or submassive PE poses an immediate threat to life.

■ BEDSIDE

Quick Look Test

Does the patient look relatively well, sick (uncomfortable or distressed), or critical (about to die)?

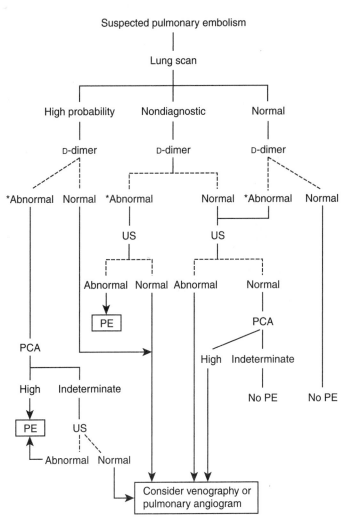

Figure 16–1 □ Algorithm for the diagnosis of suspected pulmonary embolism (PE). PCA = probability from clinical assessment; US = ultrasonography of the veins of the lower limbs.

* = exclude myocardial infarction, congestive heart failure, pneumonia, cancer, post surgery

Airway and Vital Signs

What is the blood pressure?

Cardiogenic shock may occur as a result of pulmonary embolism. The blood pressure (BP) may be in the normal range, however, with significant embolism.

What is the heart rate?

Tachycardia is common but is nonspecific.

Selective History

Rapidly assess
1. The quality of pain. Central chest pain with acute dyspnea, apprehension, and sinus tachycardia in the absence of pulmonary diseases, a history of unstable angina, and ECG signs of acute myocardial infarction (MI) suggests PE.
2. Pleuritic chest pain and hemoptysis in a patient without symptoms and signs of pneumonia or chest infection. If these symptoms are associated with an infiltrate or right-sided pleural effusion or with oligemic lung in a patient with a predisposing factor such as a postoperative state, then the PCA is high.
3. History of presyncope or syncope within the past few hours
4. Predisposing causes or **risk factors for thromboembolism**
   - Postorthopedic surgery; incidence of PE = 40 to 70%
   - All other surgical interventions with immobilization of >1 day; incidence of PE = 15 to 20%
   - Past history of thromboembolism or previous deep venous thrombosis (DVT)
   - Congestive heart failure (CHF)
   - Malignancy
   - Birth control pills in a smoker older than 25 years
   - Hypercoagulable diathesis

The presence of risk factors and unexplained chest pain, or unexplained dyspnea or syncope in a patient with a normal chest x-ray, strongly suggests a diagnosis of PE.

Selective Physical Examination

Clinical findings are nonspecific and require rapid documentation.
- Tachypnea and tachycardia are the most frequent signs.
- Increased P_2 sound
- Fourth heart sound gallop caused by right ventricular (RV) dysfunction
- A systolic murmur at the left lower sternal border that increases with inspiration indicates tricuspid regurgitation caused by acute pulmonary hypertension.

- Crackles (crepitations)
- Pleuritic friction rub over the area of pain
- DVT present

The differential diagnosis includes pneumonia, exacerbation of asthma or COPD, MI, pulmonary edema, anxiety, dissecting aneurysm, pericardial tamponade, pneumothorax, and musculoskeletal pain.

■ DIAGNOSTIC TESTING

Arterial Blood Gas

Findings are nonspecific. Acute respiratory alkalosis is the most common finding. Note that CO_2 retention may occur with massive PE. Therefore, the absence of acute respiratory alkalosis should not be taken as evidence against the diagnosis of PE. In medicine, a positive finding supports the diagnosis; a negative finding should not significantly alter diagnostic probabilities. The finding of hypoxemia and hypocapnia in the absence of conditions listed in the differential diagnosis with a normal chest x-ray increases the PCA, but these findings are nonspecific. **A normal blood gas result does not decrease the PCA.**

ELISA

Plasmin digests cross-linked fibrin from pulmonary emboli; degradation products containing D-dimers are released and can be detected in the plasma by monoclonal antibodies. A D-dimer enzyme-linked immunosorbent assay (ELISA) >500 ng/ml (500 µg/L) is abnormal and is present in >90% of patients with PE. The test is highly sensitive but not specific for the diagnosis of PE. Specificity is improved if other causes of abnormal results are **excluded: MI, CHF, pneumonia, cancer, and postsurgery. Most important, a normal D-dimer result gives reassurance in >90% of cases that PE is not present.** In one study using a whole-blood agglutination assay (SimpliRed), the test yielded a negative predictive value of 99%. A **rapid latex-agglutination test is not recommended** because it is inaccurate.

Chest X-Ray

The chest x-ray may be entirely normal. Subtle signs may be apparent on close scrutiny. The radiologic signs are nondiagnostic but can be used in conjunction with the clinical findings and ABG results to access the PCA (see Fig. 16–1).

- Atelectasis: plate-like or small segmental atelectases
- Pleural effusion

- "Infiltrate" or pleural-based consolidation; a peripheral wedge-shaped density above the diaphragm (Hampton's hump)
- Pulmonary artery enlargement and abrupt vessel cutoff
- An enlarged right descending pulmonary artery (Palla's sign)
- Oligemic, hyperlucent lung, distal to the abrupt cutoff of the pulmonary artery: focal oligemia (Westermark's sign)
- Elevated hemidiaphragm
- Dilatation of azygos vein

Electrocardiogram

The ECG may be entirely normal, but subtle abnormalities that are transient should alert suspicion.
- Sinus tachycardia without an obvious cause
- T wave inversion in leads V_1 to V_4 is one of the most common abnormalities (Fig. 5–56).
- S_1, S_2, S_3 heart sounds
- S_1, Q_3, T wave inversion in lead III with lead II ST segment and T wave normal and similar to lead I, rather than to lead III: i.e., finding is unlike that in acute MI (leads II, III, and aVF are involved with MI).
- Right ventricular strain pattern: T wave inversion in leads V_1 to V_3, S wave in leads V_5 and V_6 (see Fig. 5–56)
- Sudden right axis deviation compared with previous reading
- Transient right bundle branch block
- Nonspecific ST-T changes including T wave inversion in leads V_5 and V_6 occurring for a few hours only

Lung Scan

Request a ventilation-perfusion scan as soon as the clinical impression suggests a diagnosis of PE. A lung scan is the first-line investigation except for patients suspected of having a massive PE, which is indicated by acute cor pulmonale or cardiogenic shock. These patients require emergency pulmonary angiography.

A lung scan should be interpreted as one of the following:
- Normal
- **Nondiagnostic (intermediate and low-probability scans)**
- High probability

A normal scan in a patient with a normal D-dimer indicates an absence of PE in >99% of cases.

A high-probability scan is indicated by multiple, segmental perfusion defects without corresponding ventilation or chest x-ray abnormalities. A high-probability scan is 98% specific for PE but lacks sensitivity.

Echocardiogram

Right ventricular hypokinesis is present in approximately 40% of patients with PE; this finding is associated with a doubling of the mortality rate in 2 weeks, and it triples in 1 year. A typical feature is regional RV dysfunction in which apical wall motion remains normal despite hypokinesis of the free wall (McConnell's sign). **Diastolic and systolic bowing of the septum into the left ventricle reflects RV volume and pressure overload.**

Venous Ultrasonography

This test is accurate in patients with symptomatic DVT, but detection of DVT is much lower if symptoms and signs are absent; therefore, a normal result does not exclude DVT or PE. More than 20% of patients with normal ultrasonography have proven PE.

A combination of tests can resolve diagnostic difficulties: positive ultrasonography of the veins of the lower limbs and RV hypokinesis on echocardiogram is virtually diagnostic of PE. A normal lung scan and normal D-dimer virtually excludes PE.

Pulmonary Angiogram

Discuss the rationale for pulmonary angiography with your staff physician for the following scenarios:

- As an emergency procedure in patients suspected of having a massive embolism requiring immediate embolectomy
- In patients with nondiagnostic lung scan and a negative femoral venogram but a high PCA
- In patients with a high-probability scan and a high risk of bleeding

■ MANAGEMENT

1. Heparin
   If the PCA is high and there is no contraindication to heparin, start **heparin IV 5000 to 10,000 U-bolus** and a simultaneous infusion of **heparin 1520 U/hr** in patients without known risks of bleeding and **1200 U/hr** in those with risk of bleeding. Request the partial thromboplastin time (PTT) 6 hours later, and adjust the infusion to maintain a PTT of 1.5 to 2.3 times the patient control (see Table 26–2 and Chapter 26).
   Contraindications to heparin include
   - A bleeding disorder or a very low platelet count
   - Recent bleeding from a peptic ulcer
   - Recent intracranial bleeding

Heparin is advised for 5 to 7 days, depending on departmental policies. For submassive embolism, 5 days of heparin therapy should suffice. Assess platelet count on the third day of heparin therapy and then daily to detect heparin-induced thrombocytopenia (HIT). The complications of HIT may be life threatening.

2. Oral anticoagulants

Warfarin (Coumadin) 5 mg is started on the second day of heparin therapy. The initial dose should not exceed 5 mg. **A larger loading dose used to be recommended but may precipitate venous gangrene of the limbs, albeit rarely.** This dose is repeated the next day, and then the subsequent doses of warfarin depend on the International Normalized Ratio (INR) or prothrombin time (PT). Heparin is continued until the INR is in the desired range of 2 to 3 or PT is 1.3 to 1.5 times the control for at least 2 days. For submassive embolism, 5 days of IV heparin decreases hospital costs. Oral anticoagulants are continued for 3 to 6 months.

3. **Assess for hypercoaguable state in selected cases**. Test for
   - The factor V Leiden mutation
   - Hyperhomocysteinemia, if present, can be treated with B vitamins and folic acid.
   - The presence of antiphospholipid antibodies (lupus anticoagulant or anticardiolipin antibodies); this demands more intensive anticoagulation.

17 | Acute Pulmonary Edema

Acute pulmonary edema is a life-threatening situation and calls for immediate medical attention.

■ PHONE CALL

Questions

1. Why is the patient in the hospital?
2. What are the patient's vital signs?
3. Is the patient stable or unstable?

Orders

1. Give oxygen at a high flow rate of 6 to 10 L/min.
2. Give an IV of 5% dextrose in water immediately to keep the vein open.
3. Give morphine 4 mg IV immediately.

Inform RN

"Will arrive at the bedside immediately."

■ ELEVATOR THOUGHTS

What are the types and causes of acute pulmonary edema?
1. Cardiogenic; caused by
   - Severe left ventricular failure due to ischemic heart disease, tachyarrhythmias, hypertension, valvular lesions, and cardiomyopathy
   - Mitral stenosis or left atrial myxoma
2. Noncardiogenic; causes include
   - Adult respiratory distress syndrome
   - Others: drugs, uremia, neurogenic conditions, and lymphangitis carcinomatosa

■ MAJOR THREAT TO LIFE

Pulmonary edema caused by acute myocardial infarction (MI) poses a threat to life. Other causes of pulmonary edema require diligent management as soon as possible to prevent a fatal event; cardiogenic shock may ensue.

■ BEDSIDE

Quick Look Test

Does the patient look sick (uncomfortable or distressed) or critical (about to die)?

Airway and Vital Signs

Is the airway clear?

Is the patient's breathing severely compromised?

What is the patient's P_{O_2}?
   Assess the arterial blood gases (ABGs), and consider mechanical ventilation if the P_{O_2} is <50 mm Hg or P_{CO_2} is >50 mm Hg.

Selective Physical Examination

   Assess if the patient is using accessory muscles of respiration and if cyanosis is present (see Chapter 3 and Table 3–1). Check the jugular venous pressure; this is usually elevated. Auscultate the lung fields; usually with acute pulmonary edema, prominent crackles (crepitations) are heard over most of the lung fields. Occasionally, an added wheeze may be present. Assess the blood pressure (BP). If BP is >200 mm Hg systolic and if there is no evidence of acute MI, arrange for immediate reduction of blood pressure (see Chapter 22).

■ DIAGNOSTIC TESTING

Electrocardiogram

- Assess for the presence of acute MI (see Chapter 7).
- Assess for left ventricular hypertrophy and left atrial enlargement.
- Assess for arrhythmias, in particular atrial fibrillation with a fast ventricular response of >150 beats/min.

Chest X-Ray

   This should show the typical features of pulmonary edema (see Chapter 18).

■ MANAGEMENT

1. Maintain O_2 at a high flow rate of 6 to 10 L/min and assess ABGs.

2. Give **morphine 2 to 4 mg IV;** repeat if there is chest pain (see Chapter 7).

3. Give a **furosemide 80-mg IV bolus repeated in one-half to 1 hour** if shortness of breath and distress persist; **then 40 to 80 mg orally daily.**

4. Nitroglycerin is advisable if chest pain or ischemia is suspected. Dosage: **5 μg/min increased by 5 μg/min to a range of 50 to 200 μg/min,** to achieve blood pressure reduction and preload reduction.

5. Monitor cardiac rhythm and control arrhythmias. If atrial fibrillation with uncontrolled ventricular response is present, give **IV digoxin 0.5 mg immediately, then 0.25 mg in 2 hours;** further dosing depends on your assessment of the heart rate in 2 to 4 hours. Discuss this with your senior resident or staff physician.

6. If severe hypertension without ischemia is the cause of pulmonary edema, and systolic BP is >220 mm Hg or diastolic BP is >115 mm Hg, administer **nitroprusside IV infusion.** Start the infusion at **0.5 μg/kg/min, and adjust in increments of 0.2 μg/kg/min usually every 5 minutes** until the desired blood pressure reduction is obtained. **Dose range: 0.5 to 5 μg/kg/min.** As an alternative, **captopril 25 mg** could be tried.

7. Calcium antagonists, including nifedipine, are contraindicated if myocardial or cerebral ischemia is present.

8. If hypotension is present, a combination of small-dose dopamine and dobutamine is advisable. **Dopamine 2.5 to 10 μg/kg/min and dobutamine 2.5 to 10 μg/kg/min** (see Tables A–1, A–2).

Calls for the management of congestive heart failure (CHF) are frequent on cardiac wards.

■ PHONE CALL

Questions

1. Is shortness of breath mild, moderate, or severe?
2. What is the admitting diagnosis, i.e., acute myocardial infarction (MI), CHF, or cause to be determined?
3. Is atrial fibrillation present with a fast ventricular response of >150 beats/min?
4. What are the vital signs?

Orders

1. Keep the patient propped upright.
2. Start oxygen at 4 to 6 L/min by nasal prongs.
3. Order an IV of 5% dextrose in water to keep the vein open.

Inform RN

"Will arrive at the bedside in . . . minutes."

■ ELEVATOR THOUGHTS

What are the causes of congestive heart failure?
- Myocardial damage caused by ischemic heart disease and its complications, by myocarditis, and by cardiomyopathy
- Ventricular overload caused by pressure overload resulting from hypertension, from aortic stenosis, and from pulmonary stenosis
- Volume overload caused by mitral regurgitation, aortic regurgitation, ventricular septal defect, atrial septal defect, or patent ductus arteriosus
- Restriction and obstruction to ventricular filling caused by mitral stenosis, cardiac tamponade, constrictive pericarditis, restrictive cardiomyopathies, or atrial myxoma
- Cor pulmonale

- Other causes, including thyrotoxicosis and arteriovenous fistula

■ MAJOR THREAT TO LIFE

Underlying problems include acute MI, severe aortic stenosis, and development of cardiogenic shock.

■ BEDSIDE
Quick Look Test

Does the patient look sick (uncomfortable or distressed) or critical (about to die)?

Airway and Vital Signs

Is the airway clear?

Is the patient's breathing accompanied by severe distress?

Selective History

1. Determine the degree of shortness of breath (see Chapter 13) and assess for orthopnea and paroxysmal nocturnal dyspnea.
2. Document the history of acute MI, previous infarction or chronic ischemia, a past history of CHF, or known valvular lesions.
3. Ask if palpitations are bothersome and distressing.
4. If there is no evidence of the above-mentioned problems, ask about excessive alcohol consumption, which can cause heart failure.

Factors precipitating heart failure must be elucidated; these include

1. Reduction or discontinuation of medication, salt binge, and increased physical activity in patients with underlying cardiac disease
2. Increased cardiac output caused by severe hypertension, arrhythmia, or infection
3. Progression or complication of the basic underlying heart disease, i.e., ischemic heart disease, left ventricular aneurysm, or increasing valvular disease
4. Drugs that may precipitate cardiac failure, including nonsteroidal anti-inflammatory drugs (NSAIDs), beta blockers, corticosteroids, calcium antagonists, digitalis toxicity, and some antiarrhythmic agents, including disopyramide and procain-

amide. Also, chemotherapeutic agents may precipitate myocardial dysfunction and heart failure.

Selective Physical Examination

1. Cardiovascular system

Examine the cardiovascular system for increased jugular venous pressure (JVP). With CHF, the JVP is >2 cm above the sternal angle, with prominent V waves if tricuspid regurgitation is present. Note that the venous pressure may not be readily visible if it is markedly elevated to the angle of the jaw. Sit the patient upright and look for pulsation of the ear lobes; look tangentially across the neck for visible waves (see Chapter 3). Assess carefully for cardiomegaly with the patient in the left lateral position; assess thrills, murmurs, and gallop rhythms. An S_3 gallop is heard in most cases of CHF (see Chapter 4). An S_3 gallop or summation gallop (S_3 + S_4) is heard in virtually all patients with dilated cardiomyopathy; the sound is much louder than that heard with CHF due to ischemic or valvular heart disease.

2. Respiratory system

Assess for crackles (crepitations) over lung fields and for pleural effusion. Pleural effusion is much more common on the right side in patients with CHF.

Assess for bilateral pitting edema, and **in patients who have been confined to bed, check for presacral edema (see Chapter 14 and Table 14–1 for the differential diagnosis of edema).**

■ DIAGNOSTIC TESTING

Chest X-Ray

The radiologic signs of heart failure clinch the diagnosis, and it is important to learn to recognize these findings, which include

- Interstitial pulmonary edema; perihilar haze, pulmonary clouding, and Kerley B lines (septal lines at the bases that extend to the pleura and should not exceed 2 cm in length and 1 to 2 mm in width) are findings.
- Constriction of the lower lobe blood vessels and dilatation of the upper zone vessels, a sign of pulmonary venous hypertension; these findings may, however, occur in patients with mitral stenosis and severe chronic obstructive pulmonary disease and if the x-ray is taken with the patient in the supine position.
- Pleural effusions; blunting of the costophrenic angle, espe-

cially on the right side, which is greater than the left, is a common finding.

- Interlobar fissure thickening due to an accumulation of fluid; this is best seen in the lateral film.
- Dilatation of the central pulmonary arteries
- If left ventricular (LV) failure is severe, or if mitral stenosis is the cause, pulmonary edema may be severe, and a "butterfly" pattern becomes obvious.
- Heart size may be slightly increased, but in many types of heart failure, e.g., acute MI, mitral stenosis, aortic stenosis, and cor pulmonale, the heart size may remain within normal limits.

It is important to exclude radiologic mimics of heart failure; differential diagnosis includes viral and other pneumonias, allergic pulmonary edema caused by heroin and nitrofurantoin, lymphangitic carcinomatosis, high altitude, and alveolar proteinosis. Occasionally, uremia and inhalation of toxic substances and increase in cerebrospinal fluid pressure can cause radiologic changes.

Electrocardiogram

The electrocardiogram (ECG) may be normal in patients with heart failure. However, in most cases, the following subtle abnormalities may be detected:

- ST-T wave changes in keeping with ischemia
- Nonspecific ST-T wave changes
- Signs of acute infarction or previous infarction (see Chapter 5)
- Left atrial enlargement
- Left ventricular hypertrophy with strain pattern (see Chapter 5)
- Deep T wave inversion, Q waves, or conduction defects consistent with cardiomyopathy or specific heart muscle disease

Echocardiography

See the Study Section at the end of this chapter.

■ MANAGEMENT

1. Give oxygen during the first 24 hours and then only if hypoxemia is present. In general, oxygen is required for no more than 2 days.
2. Diuretics: **torsemide is more effective than furosemide in the prevention of recurrent CHF (see study section).** Furosemide, however, is used worldwide. **Furosemide 40 to 80 mg IV immediately, followed by 40 to 120 mg orally daily**

for several days, and then a **maintenance dose of 40 to 80 mg daily.**

3. Angiotensin-converting enzyme (ACE) inhibitors; captopril or enalapril should be started in most patients except those with valvular obstruction (aortic and mitral stenosis), and patients with relatively normal left ventricular function, e.g., patients with heart failure secondary to arrhythmias.

For those patients with aortic stenosis and mitral stenosis, after a test dose of 6.25 mg, if there is no hypotension within 2 hours, administer **captopril 12.5 mg 3 times per day, increasing to 25 to 50 mg 3 times per day**, depending on the patient's response and the level of systolic blood pressure (BP). Avoid dropping the systolic BP to <110 mm Hg or the diastolic BP to <65 mm Hg. The equivalent dose of **enalapril** is a test dose of 2.5 mg, with the BP checked within 4 hours, and then **5 to 10 mg once or twice daily**. An angiotensin II receptor blocker, such as **irbesartan (Avapro) 150 mg,** may be used if cough is a problem with ACE inhibitors. The angiotensin II receptor blockers have a significantly lower incidence of angioedema compared with ACE inhibitors, and this is a distinct advantage for physician and patient safety.

4. **Digoxin** is necessary in all patients with atrial fibrillation to control the ventricular response. If atrial fibrillation is not present and an S_3 gallop is present or the ejection fraction (EF) is <40%, digoxin should be administered. There is no longer a controversy as to the role of digoxin. This drug has been proven effective when given with a diuretic and an ACE inhibitor. This combination prevents recurrent heart failure and hospitalization and decreases mortality. Digoxin improves survival only in class IV patients and complements the salutary effects of spironolactone (see Study Section).

If a gallop rhythm is not present, digoxin is indicated if heart failure is recurrent or if left ventricular dysfunction is present. Left ventricular dysfunction is present if there are visible abnormal precordial pulsations indicating dyskinetic and akinetic areas of myocardium or if echocardiography reveals an EF <40%. The EF measured by echocardiography is sometimes misleading. Radionuclide EF is more accurate except in patients with atrial fibrillation and mitral regurgitation. Because the radionuclide scan is more costly and does not show valvular and other defects, the echocardiogram is preferred to radionuclide angiography when assessing patients with heart failure.

The **digoxin dose** should be **0.5 mg immediately, and then 0.25 mg daily**, preferably at bedtime so that when the digoxin level is assessed in a few months, it reflects a more accurate level. Patients with atrial fibrillation do not usually require a test of digoxin levels, because the dose is titrated to the ventricular response. Patients with an elevated creatinine level of >1.3 mg/dl (115 μmol/L), or most patients older than 70 years, should receive **a maintenance dose of 0.125 mg daily** except if atrial fibrillation is present with an uncontrolled response.

5. **Beta-blocker** therapy is strongly recommended for patients with class II or III CHF. Give **metoprolol succinate (controlled release) 12.5 mg once daily**, titrate slowly over 4 to 8 weeks to a target dose of 150 to 200 mg; or **carvedilol 3.125 mg once daily**, and titrate over weeks to 25 mg twice daily. (See Study Section for further details.)

6. **Spironolactone (Aldactone) 25 mg** is recommended for patients with class III or IV CHF along with the three agents noted earlier. Hyperkalemia may occur particularly when the drug is combined with an ACE inhibitor in patients with type 2 diabetes or renal dysfunction (creatinine >1.5 mg/dl [133 μmol/L]).

Refractory Heart Failure

Patients with heart failure refractory to the above measures should be assessed as follows:

- Salt intake may be higher than the patient relates; NSAIDs and other agents that cause sodium and water retention and that interact with furosemide and ACE inhibitors should be curtailed.

- Torsemide is superior to furosemide in this class of patients. Use of this diuretic can result in a decrease in hospitalization for CHF of 50%. Torsemide is completely absorbed and has high reliability and predictability compared with furosemide. Food markedly reduces absorption of furosemide, **and not many physicians, including cardiologists, recognize that this widely used drug must be taken on an empty stomach. Torsemide dosage is 2.5 to 20 mg orally once daily, or IV 50 mg**.

- If the furosemide dose has been divided to 40 mg twice daily, this should be given as **one dose of 80 mg in the morning, or a 200-mg dose is given as 120 mg in the morning and 80 mg at 2 P.M.** until the patient is stable enough to reduce the dose. The furosemide must be increased considerably if the serum creatinine level is >2.3 mg/dl (203 μmol/L). Thiazide diuretics are not used in patients with renal dysfunction, because they are ineffective if the glomerular filtration rate (GFR) is low.

- Metolazone is a unique thiazide that can be used in combination with furosemide in patients with refractory heart failure. **Dosage: 2.5 to 5 mg daily** is effective, whereas other thiazides are not effective when the GFR is <30 ml/min. A combination of metolazone and furosemide is useful in patients with refractory heart failure who fail to respond to doses of furosemide of >120 mg daily. Caution is required, however, because potassium loss may be considerable with this combination. The addition of an ACE inhibitor prevents potassium loss.

It is important to recognize that there is no first-line therapy in the management of severe heart failure and that combination therapy with diuretic, ACE inhibitor, and beta blocker is necessary. Digoxin has been shown to prevent hospitalization and to enhance the action of spironolactone and ACE inhibitors, and it is of value in patients with class III or IV CHF. Spironolactone is a major breakthrough in patients with refractory CHF.

Precautions for Digoxin

Conditions With Increased Sensitivity to Digoxin
1. Age >70 years
2. Hypokalemia
3. Hypoxemia
4. Acidosis
5. Acute MI
6. Hypomagnesemia
7. Myocarditis
8. Hypothyroidism

Causes of Digoxin Toxicity. Increased digoxin levels may occur when digoxin is combined with quinidine, verapamil, diltiazem, nicardipine, felodipine, amiodarone, or propafenone. If spironolactone is used concomitantly, digoxin levels may be falsely elevated. Levels of digoxin may be lowered with concomitant use of antacids, metoclopramide, cholestyramine, Metamucil, phenytoin, and salicylazosulfapyridine.

Digoxin toxicity is unusual if a careful physician assesses the serum creatinine level and relates this to the maintenance dose. Lean skeletal muscle mass is important, especially in the elderly, because digoxin binds to skeletal muscle. Thus, in an individual with lean skeletal muscle mass, more digoxin is available for myocardial binding. Hence, there is an increased incidence of toxicity in elderly patients with lean skeletal muscle mass. Also, in the elderly, mild renal dysfunction is a common scenario. Because the lean skeletal muscle mass decreases the level of serum creatinine, the level of serum creatinine cannot be used independently to gauge the maintenance dose of digoxin. In elderly patients without atrial fibrillation, it is advisable to test the digoxin level and the serum potassium level at least twice yearly. Levels of 1 to 2 ng/ml (1–2.3 nmol/L) are desirable and clinically effective.

Clinical Evidence of Toxicity
- Nausea, anorexia, vomiting, diarrhea, abdominal pain, and weight loss; visual hallucinations, blurring of vision, insom-

nia, and, rarely, mental confusion; cardiac arrhythmias may occur, in particular first-, second-, and third-degree AV block, sinus pauses, paroxysmal atrial tachycardia with block, multifocal ventricular premature beats, ventricular tachycardia, and ventricular fibrillation. Also, deterioration of heart failure may be caused by digoxin toxicity. Digoxin levels of >3 ng/ml (3.9 nmol/L) should be avoided, because this level virtually always causes clinically serious toxicity. Levels of <1.5 ng/ml (2 nmol/L), if drawn at an appropriate time when steady state is achieved, in particular if digoxin is given as a bedtime dose, are rarely associated with toxicity, except in patients with sensitivity as outlined earlier.

Management of Digoxin Toxicity
- Discontinue digoxin.
- Clarify conditions that increase sensitivity to digoxin, and ensure that renal dysfunction is not present.
- Give potassium if hypokalemia is present. Tachyarrhythmias, in particular multifocal ventricular premature beats or ventricular tachycardia, should be treated with lidocaine. The level of serum potassium must be corrected if hypokalemia is present. Lidocaine should be given only after correction of hypokalemia.
- Give **Digibind**; if digoxin toxicity is present clinically and there is ECG evidence of severe toxicity, e.g., second- or third-degree AV block, or ventricular tachycardia, digoxin immune Fab (Digibind) should be administered. **Dosage: 4 to 6 vials (160–240 mg) IV over 30 minutes** is adequate to reverse most cases of toxicity during chronic therapy. The dose can be given as an IV bolus if cardiac arrest is imminent.
- Hypokalemia should be anticipated and corrected after the administration of Digibind.

Other Precautions

When ACE inhibitors are used, interactions may occur with NSAIDs including aspirin and potassium-sparing diuretics; supplemental potassium should be avoided.

Weight reduction is necessary in patients with heart failure. The patient must be motivated to lose weight; this usually occurs if the patient is warned that he or she will require less medication if at least 10 to 20 lb are lost.

Alcohol intake should be discontinued or allowed only a few times a year. Patients with dilated cardiomyopathy should discontinue use of alcohol completely.

Study Section: Heart Failure

Heart failure is a syndrome identified by well-defined symptoms and hemodynamic findings caused by an abnormality of cardiac function that results in a relative decrease in cardiac output that triggers compensatory renal and neurohormonal changes (Fig. 18–1).

The management of heart failure requires the application of five basic principles to actuate a salutary effect:

- Ensure a correct diagnosis, excluding mimics of heart failure.
- Determine the underlying heart disease, if possible, and treat.
- Define precipitating factors, because heart failure can be a result of underlying disease and is often precipitated by conditions that can be prevented or easily corrected.
- Understand the pathophysiology of heart failure.
- Know the actions of the pharmacologic agents and their appropriate indications.

Symptoms, physical signs, and chest x-ray verification were discussed earlier in this chapter.

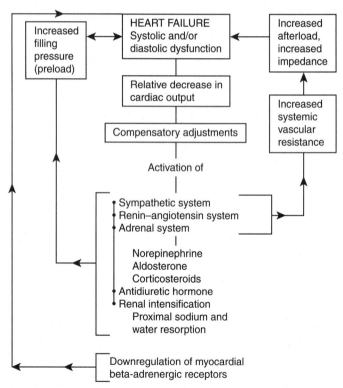

Figure 18–1 □ Pathophysiology of heart failure. (From Khan, M Gabriel: Heart failure. In: Heart Disease Diagnosis and Therapy: A Practical Approach. Baltimore, Williams & Wilkins, 1996, p 188.)

Echocardiography provides many diagnostic aids:

- Evidence of decreased systolic function: An ejection fraction (EF) <35% is often seen in patients with moderate heart failure. The EF may not be decreased in patients with heart failure caused by mitral regurgitation or ventricular septal defect and in patients with ventricular diastolic dysfunction. The radionuclide evaluation of EF is more accurate but more expensive than that of echocardiography, but the latter is superior in detecting the presence and significance of valvular lesions and specific chamber enlargement.
- Evidence of ventricular wall-motion abnormalities, global hypokinesia, and chamber enlargement
- Approximate assessment of pulmonary artery pressure can be made if tricuspid regurgitation is present
- Valvular abnormalities: reasonably accurate assessment of the severity of mitral regurgitation and obstructive lesions can be ascertained by continuous wave Doppler.
- Exclusion of cardiac tamponade
- Assessment of pericardial effusion and pericardial calcification
- Evidence of diastolic dysfunction abnormalities
- Assessment of left ventricular hypertrophy, left atrial enlargement, and right ventricular hypertrophy
- Essential for the diagnosis of hypertrophic, dilated, or restrictive cardiomyopathy

■ ASSESS FOR UNDERLYING CAUSE OF HEART FAILURE

A complete cure may be a rare reward if a surgically correctable lesion is uncovered.

- Left atrial myxoma
- Significant mitral regurgitation: may be missed because of the presence of a poorly audible murmur due to low cardiac output, thick chest wall, or chronic obstructive pulmonary disease
- Atrial septal defect
- Arteriovenous (AV) fistula
- Constrictive pericarditis
- Cardiac tamponade: may simulate heart failure and must be excluded because usual heart failure medications, diuretics, ACE inhibitors, or nitrates can cause marked hemodynamic deterioration in patients with tamponade
- Pulmonary edema or heart failure is not a complete diagnosis. The basic cause must be stated as part of the diagnosis and an associated precipitant must be defined, if present.

Approximately 60% of adult patients with heart failure have

severe LV dysfunction secondary to ischemic heart disease. Dilated cardiomyopathy accounts for approximately 18%, valvular heart disease for 12%, and hypertensive heart disease associated in some with ischemic heart disease for 10% of heart failure.

It is necessary to make a systematic search for the following basic causes of heart disease.

1. **Myocardial damage**
   a. **Ischemic heart disease and its complications**
   b. **Myocarditis**
   c. **Cardiomyopathy**
2. **Ventricular overload**
   a. **Pressure overload**
      (1) Systemic hypertension
      (2) Coarctation of the aorta
      (3) Aortic stenosis
      (4) Pulmonary hypertension
   b. **Volume overload**
      (1) Mitral regurgitation
      (2) Aortic regurgitation
      (3) Ventricular septal defect
      (4) Atrial septal defect
      (5) Patent ductus arteriosus
3. **Restriction and obstruction to ventricular filling**
   a. **Right ventricular infarction**
   b. **Constrictive pericarditis**
   c. **Cardiac tamponade (although not truly heart failure)**
   d. **Restrictive cardiomyopathies**
   e. **Specific heart muscle diseases**
   f. **Hypertensive, hypertrophic "cardiomyopathy" of the elderly**
   g. **Mitral stenosis and atrial myxoma**
4. **Others**
   a. **Cor pulmonale**
   b. **Thyrotoxicosis**
   c. **High-output failure**
      (1) AV fistula
      (2) peripartum cardiomyopathy
      (3) beriberi

■ PATHOPHYSIOLOGIC IMPLICATIONS

In the majority of patients with heart failure, cardiac output is reduced due to poor LV systolic function. However, LV systolic function may be relatively normal in some patients with valvular regurgitant lesions, hypertensive heart disease, and restrictive cardiomyopathy, in which diastolic dysfunction plays a major role in causing heart failure.

Improvement in cardiac output causes a favorable alteration of the compensatory responses of heart failure including the neurohormonal response. Cardiac output is the product of stroke volume and heart rate. Stroke volume is modulated by

- Preload
- Myocardial contractility
- Afterload

■ COMPENSATORY ADJUSTMENTS IN HEART FAILURE

1. The activation of the sympathetic system causes an increase in heart rate and in force and velocity of myocardial contraction in order to increase stroke volume and cardiac output. An increase in systemic vascular resistance occurs to maintain blood pressure. The body's homeostatic response is appropriate but is often not sufficient to compensate for the decrease in cardiac index and increased filling pressures. It is, in fact, counterproductive in some ways. Also, sympathetic stimulation causes sodium and water retention and an increase in venous tone in order to increase filling pressure that enhances preload, provided that there is no restriction to ventricular filling.

2. The renin–angiotensin system is stimulated. Patients with mild heart failure show little or no evidence of stimulation of the renin–angiotensin system. Stimulation of the system is observed in response to treatment with diuretics and is seen in untreated patients with more severe degrees of heart failure. The secretion of renin causes angiotensin I to be converted by angiotensin-converting enzyme to the vasoconstrictor angiotensin II. This action occurs in the circulation and in the tissues. Angiotensin II supports systemic blood pressure and cerebral, renal, and coronary perfusion through

    - Arteriolar vasoconstriction and an increase in systemic vascular resistance
    - Stimulation of central and peripheral effects of the sympathetic system
    - Marked resorption of sodium and water in the proximal nephron
    - Enhanced aldosterone secretion, which brings about sodium and water retention in the renal tubules, distal to the macula densa. Because the distal tubules handle only about 2% of the nephron's sodium load, this latter contribution is small, compared to proximal sodium resorption, but it is a final tuning of sodium balance.
    - Stimulating thirst and vasopressin release, thereby increasing total body water

3. Renal blood flow is preserved by selective vasoconstriction of postglomerular efferent arterioles.
4. **The adjustments made** to maintain blood pressure and cerebral, coronary, and renal perfusion **cause a marked increase in afterload**, which increases cardiac work and myocardial oxygen demand. Thus, heart failure may worsen (see Fig. 18–1).

The Renal Response

The renal homeostatic mechanisms are similar to those for heart failure, with a decrease in cardiac output, and for severe bleeding, which lowers blood pressure. The design of nature appears to protect systemic blood pressure in order to maintain adequate cerebral and renal perfusion in situations such as hemorrhage, in which this reaction is productive. Sodium and water retention occurs in the proximal tubule. The sensors that activate this response in heart failure are undetermined. Sensors are possibly linked to baroreceptors in the heart and to aortic arch and low-pressure sensors in the ventricle and atria, as well as at the level of the nephron and macula densa. Failure of the neurohumoral response and renal adjustment would result in a fall in blood pressure and deprivation of cerebral, coronary, and renal perfusion.

The compensatory neurohumoral response thus increases afterload to some extent in order to maintain adequate systemic blood pressure. The intense sodium and water retention and the increase in venous tone bring about an increase in filling pressure in an attempt to increase myocardial fiber stretch during diastole, i.e., **an increase in preload**.

■ DRUG THERAPY

Choice of Drug or Drug Combination

In clinical practice, an appropriate drug combination for patients with heart failure due to ventricular systolic dysfunction requires consideration of the patient's functional class. It is no longer acceptable to speak in terms of which drug is considered first-line therapy for heart failure. **The four agents—diuretics, digoxin, beta blockers, and ACE inhibitors—are complementary.** Digoxin or diuretics have not been shown to improve survival, but they prevent recurrence of heart failure and hospitalizations. ACE inhibitors have improved survival only in patients also treated with digoxin and diuretics. **Diuretics, particularly torsemide and spironolactone**, are a necessary part of symptomatic therapy and are more effective than ACE inhibitors in preventing hospitalizations or shortening hospital stay. Thus, we must desist from using the expressions "first-line," "second-line," or "stepped-care therapy" for heart failure. Recent clinical trials have shown that digoxin significantly reduces the recurrence of CHF and hospitalization, and it may improve survival in New York Heart Association (NYHA) class IV patients. Beta blockers significantly reduce mortality and the recurrence of CHF in patients with NYHA class II and III CHF.

NYHA Class IV Heart Failure. The Cooperative North Scandinavian Enalapril Survival Study (CONSENSUS) studied only NYHA class IV heart failure patients. In 253 randomized patients, the 6-month mortality was 44% in patients treated with diuretics and a digoxin combination and 26% in patients given enalapril in addition (P <0.002). Forty-two percent of the group treated with added ACE inhibitors showed an improvement in functional class, compared with 22% in the control group (P = .001). A significant reduction in mortality attributable to ACE inhibitor therapy was observed mainly during the first 6 months.

The CONSENSUS trial had too few patients in the placebo group between 6 months and 2 years to allow firm conclusions to be made regarding the beneficial effects of ACE inhibitors beyond 6 months in patients with class IV heart failure. The current recommendation to treat class IV heart failure patients with diuretics, digoxin, and an ACE inhibitor for life is appropriate.

NYHA Class II and III Heart Failure

- Clinical trials have confirmed that monotherapy with diuretics, digoxin, or ACE inhibitors is not satisfactory for NYHA class II patients in sinus rhythm who have an EF <35% and who have had overt heart failure.
- There are sufficient data that strongly indicate that these patients should be managed with triple therapy: diuretic, digoxin, and ACE inhibitor. It is this combination that has been shown in both the studies of LV dysfunction (SOLVD) and the Veterans Administration Cooperative Vasodilator Heart Failure Trial (VHeFT) II to improve survival, and in the SOLVD, significant reduction in hospitalization for recurrent heart failure **was achieved**.

■ MAJOR BREAKTHROUGHS IN THE MANAGEMENT OF HEART FAILURE

The management of CHF has drastically changed in the year 2001. More and more lives are being saved by the institution of more effective medical therapy that has recently evolved and has decreased the need for heart transplantation. **The addition of a**

beta blocker and spironolactone to the standard therapy with a diuretic, ACE inhibitor, and digoxin has resulted in a major and statistically significant decrease in mortality, reduction in hospitalization, and improved quality of life. **If physicians would change their prescribing habits and switch from the prevalent use of furosemide to torsemide**, a further significant reduction in hospitalization for recurrent CHF would emerge.

The following relevant points attest to the above recommendations.

1. **Beta blockers** are now recommended by the American College of Cardiology and virtually all cardiologists for the management of classes II and III heart failure. In these patients they have been shown to have a quantitatively greater effect on mortality reduction than ACE inhibitors. They should not be given, however, to patients with decompensated heart failure or to class IV patients. In the MERIT-HF trial total mortality or hospitalization for heart failure was significantly reduced, with a risk reduction of 31%. In patients with heart failure, beta blockers cause the ventricle to go from a more spheric shape to a more normal elliptic shape, and LV mass and end-diastolic volume decrease: **myocardial energetics and EF improve, and myocardial contractility and myocardial efficiency increase after 10 to 12 weeks of therapy.**

2. **Spironolactone (Aldactone) 25 mg** is strongly recommended in class III or IV patients because the drug caused a **30% reduction in the risk of death and hospitalization** in a recent clinical trial when used with a loop diuretic, digoxin, and an ACE inhibitor. Digoxin has a favorable interaction with spironolactone.

3. In a recent clinical trial, **torsemide was shown to be superior to furosemide** in preventing recurrent CHF and constitutes a major breakthrough in the management of recurrent CHF.

■ IMPORTANT UPDATE FROM THE ACC, MARCH 2001

The COPERNICUS study indicated that in patients on optimal therapy for severe chronic CHF, EF<25%, carvedilol judiciously titrated to 12.5 to 25 mg twice daily decreased mortality and hospitalizations for CHF significantly and improved quality of life.

Rapid heartbeats or an irregular cardiac rhythm may accompany most forms of heart disease. The process is often benign, but potentially lethal arrhythmias must be carefully assessed and treated to prevent cardiac events.

■ **PHONE CALL**

Questions

1. How fast is the heart rate?
2. Is the rhythm regular or irregular?
3. If the rhythm is irregular and there is documented atrial fibrillation, is the apical rate >150 beats/min?
4. What is the blood pressure? Is hypotension present?
5. What is the admitting diagnosis: acute myocardial infarction (MI), congestive heart failure (CHF), or arrhythmia?
6. Is presyncope or syncope associated with the feeling of palpitations?
7. Is there associated shortness of breath, chest pain, or clouding of consciousness?

Orders

1. Obtain an electrocardiogram (ECG) with a rhythm strip of leads II and V_1 immediately.
2. If ventricular tachycardia (VT) is suspected or if the patient is unstable, order a cardiac arrest cart to be placed at the bedside and attach the patient to the ECG for monitoring. A 12-lead ECG must be available for assessing the diagnosis.
3. If the heart rate is >150 beats/min and hypotension is present, order a large-bore (16-gauge) needle for IV immediately, and ask your senior resident or staff physician to assist with this emergency.

Inform RN

"Will be at the bedside in . . . minutes."

A patient with suspected VT or an unstable patient requires prompt attention.

■ ELEVATOR THOUGHTS

What are the four fundamental steps to consider in heart palpitations and arrhythmias?

1. Establish the ECG diagnosis (see Chapter 5).
2. Treat the unstable patient, often by direct current (DC) synchronized cardioversion.
3. Define and treat or remove precipitating factors.
   - CHF
   - Ischemia
   - Digitalis toxicity
   - Beta stimulants and theophylline
   - Sick sinus syndrome
   - Mobitz type II or third-degree atrioventricular (AV) block
   - Thyrotoxicosis
   - Hypokalemia
   - Hypomagnesemia
   - Hypoxemia
   - Acid–base imbalance
   - Chronic obstructive pulmonary disease (COPD)
   - Wolff-Parkinson-White (WPW) syndrome
   - Pulmonary embolism
   - Conditions as diverse as a ruptured esophagus
4. Define the mechanism of the arrhythmia
   - Disturbance of impulse generation; enhanced activity or ectopic
   - Disturbance of impulse conduction; reentrant arrhythmias; reentry is the major mechanism for VT.

■ MAJOR THREAT TO LIFE

- Hypotension leading to cardiogenic shock (see Chapter 12)
- Chest pain, angina progressing to MI (see Chapter 7)
- CHF

■ BEDSIDE

Quick Look Test

Does the patient look relatively well, sick (uncomfortable or distressed), or critical (about to die)?

Electrocardiographic Diagnosis

Carefully examine all 12 leads of the ECG and the rhythm strip of leads II and V_1. P waves are usually best seen in lead II. In patients with arrhythmias, the P wave position and morphology in leads II and V_1 provide crucial diagnostic information (see Chapter 5).

Divide tachyarrhythmias into

- Narrow or wide QRS complex tachycardias and
- Regular or irregular tachycardias

Narrow QRS Regular Tachycardia

1. Sinus tachycardia; if the rate is 100 to 140 beats/min, sinus tachycardia is the most common narrow QRS tachycardia.
2. AV nodal reentrant tachycardia (AVNRT); the rate is commonly 180 to 220 beats/min (see Figs. 5–62 and 5–64).
3. AV reentrant tachycardia (AVRT) WPW syndrome, causing circus movement; the rate is often 180 to 240 beats/min (see Figs. 5–62 and 5–70).
4. Atrial flutter; ventricular rate is commonly 150 beats/min with an atrial rate of 300 beats/min and a 2:1 AV conduction (see Fig. 5–72).
5. Atrial tachycardia (see Fig. 5–66).

Narrow QRS Irregular Tachycardia

1. Atrial fibrillation (see Fig. 5–74).
2. Atrial flutter, when AV conduction is variable (see Fig. 5–73).
3. Multifocal atrial tachycardia (see Fig. 5–67); there should be at least three different P wave morphologies recorded in one lead. The atrial rate is commonly 120 to 200 beats/min.

Wide QRS Regular Tachycardia

1. VT (see Figs. 5–79, 5–80, and 5–81).
2. Supraventricular tachycardia (SVT); with bundle branch block or functional bundle branch block.
3. WPW; using the accessory pathway for anterograde conduction, preexcited tachycardia with rates of >220 beats/min (see Fig. 5–83*B*).

Wide QRS Irregular Tachycardia

1. Atrial fibrillation, with intraventricular conduction delay.
2. WPW antidromic tachycardia; anterograde conduction over the accessory pathway, causing atrial fibrillation and preexcited tachycardia at fast rates (see Fig. 5–83*A*).
3. Torsades de pointes (see Fig. 5–82).

Selective History and Physical Examination

1. Verify the patient's degree of distress and the presence or absence of chest pain or clouding of consciousness.
2. Verify the blood pressure. Patients with hypotension caused by tachycardia look sick or critical. Most patients with SVT and nonsustained VT maintain their blood pressure and may not look very distressed.

3. Assess the jugular venous pressure and for crackles over the lower lung fields to exclude CHF.
4. If the rhythm is irregular, assess if this is regularly irregular due to premature beats or completely irregular (irregularly irregular) due to atrial fibrillation.
5. If atrial fibrillation is present, recheck the apical rate and the pulse rate. A pulse deficit is usually present.
6. With atrial flutter, the heart rate may be regular or irregular.
7. If there is a regular fast rhythm and SVT is suspected, check for carotid bruits and a history of stroke or transient ischemic attack (TIA) before considering carotid sinus massage.

■ MANAGEMENT

Definitions of Patient Instability
- Presence of chest pain
- Hypotension (BP <100 mm Hg)
- Presence of severe shortness of breath or CHF
- Syncope or presyncope
- Clouding of consciousness

If the patient is unstable, immediate synchronized cardioversion is necessary for the patient to revert to a normal sinus rhythm.

Orders
- Ask the RN to call for the staff physician if not already done.
- Place a cardiac arrest cart at the bedside; hook up the patient to the cardiac monitor if not already done.
- Determine if oxygen is at a high flow rate (6–10 L/min).
- Give diazepam 10 mg IV at bedside.
- With a large-bore needle, give an IV of 5% dextrose in water to keep the vein open.

Management of Narrow QRS Regular Tachycardia

Sinus Tachycardia. Sinus tachycardia is the most common cause of narrow QRS regular tachycardia and should be suspected if the rate is 100 to 140 beats/min. Verify the ECG diagnosis. Causes of sinus tachycardia, as follows, should be assessed and treated:
- Acute MI
- Hypovolemia
- Hypotension due to cardiogenic and noncardiogenic causes (see Chapter 12)
- Hypoxemia caused by CHF, pulmonary infections, pneumothorax, or atelectasis

- Pyrexia, pain, and anxiety
- Drugs, in particular beta stimulants, including albuterol (salbutamol) and terbutaline, commonly used on wards
- Thyrotoxicosis

Atrioventricular Nodal Reentrant Tachycardia. If the patient is stable and there is no evidence of cerebrovascular insufficiency, TIAs, or carotid bruits, try carotid sinus massage. This will cause conversion to sinus rhythm or have no effect (see Chapter 5).

If there is no response from sinus massage, drug therapy is indicated. An algorithm for the management of AVNRT is given in Figure 19–1.

ADENOSINE. Adenosine (Adenocard) is a relatively safe agent for the termination of AVNRT. Adenosine has replaced verapamil where rapid conversion of the tachyarrhythmia is required, in particular when heart failure or hemodynamic compromise is present, and avoids DC cardioversion in many individuals. Adenosine is safer than verapamil because it does not cause CHF or severe hypotension and does not pose a threat in patients with WPW orthodromic tachycardia. In patients with SVT with aberration, no harm occurs if the diagnosis is VT, whereas the use of verapamil is detrimental. The drug's short half-life of <2 seconds allows for rapid dose titration and rapid disappearance of minor side effects, which include facial flushing, dyspnea, chest pain, and bronchospasm. Avoid the drug in patients with asthma.

Dosage: An **IV bolus of 6 mg (0.05–0.25 mg/kg) over 2 seconds**, directly into a peripheral vein; if given into an IV line, it should be followed by a rapid saline flush. (The solution must be clear at the time of use.) This dose usually causes reversion to sinus rhythm in 1 minute. The arrhythmia recurs in approximately 25% of cases. A second bolus injection of 12 mg usually causes sustained reversion.

The effects of adenosine are enhanced by dipyridamole and antagonized by theophylline. Adenosine should be used with caution in patients with acute MI, asthma, and unstable COPD.

VERAPAMIL. Verapamil has been proven effective for causing reversion in >90% of cases. It does not have the undesirable adverse effects of chest discomfort, facial flushing, and wheezing. Also, the drug is inexpensive compared with adenosine. Verapamil remains useful where cost consideration exists and is used in some countries. This agent should be considered **in patients with asthma and in patients without the following complications**:

- Hypotension
- Acute MI, CHF, or cardiomegaly
- WPW syndrome
- Wide QRS tachycardia
- Beta blocker use within the past 24 hours

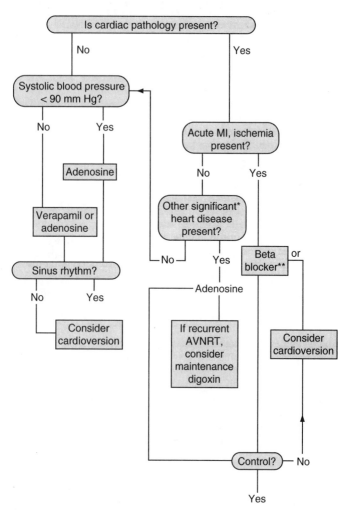

Figure 19–1 □ Algorithm for the management of atrioventricular (AV) nodal reentrant tachycardia. AVNRT = AV nodal reentrant tachycardia; MI = myocardial infarction.

  * = e.g., heart failure, cardiomegaly

  ** = if heart failure is not present

(Redrawn from Khan, M Gabriel: Cardiac Drug Therapy, 5th ed. London, WB Saunders, 2000, p 255.)

In patients with these complications, verapamil is contraindicated and adenosine is the drug of choice.

Dosage: 0.075 to 0.15 mg/kg IV; a 5-mg bolus given slowly over 1 to 2 minutes, followed, if needed, by a 10-mg bolus. In elderly patients, a 2.5-mg bolus should be tried. The second bolus is usually given if Valsalva's maneuver fails to produce reversion to sinus rhythm. The second dose, not exceeding 5 mg, may be considered after 30 minutes.

DIGOXIN.   Because of digoxin's slow onset of action, the drug is not recommended except in patients with concomitant CHF and left ventricular dysfunction.

PROCAINAMIDE.   Procainamide is the drug of choice.

Dosage: A 100-mg bolus at a rate of 20 mg/min, then 10 to 20 mg/min to a maximum of 1 g over the first hour.

Hypotension may occur. Failure to respond to procainamide is an indication for synchronized DC cardioversion.

Atrial Flutter.   Atrial flutter tends to be unstable and may degenerate to atrial fibrillation or revert to sinus rhythm over 24 hours. Structural disease is usually present. Underlying heart disease, hypoxemia due to pneumothorax, and atelectasis should be excluded.

DILTIAZEM.   If the patient is hemodynamically stable, with a ventricular response of >150 beats/min, diltiazem IV may be used to slow the ventricular response.

Dosage: 20 mg (0.25 mg/kg) over 2 minutes.

If response is inadequate, wait 15 minutes and give a **repeat bolus of 25 mg (0.35 mg/kg over 2 minutes, or infusion of 5 or 10 mg over 1 hour, to a maximum of 15 mg/hr)**. A beta blocker such as esmolol or metoprolol may be used.

DIGOXIN.   Digoxin is indicated in patients with CHF or left ventricular dysfunction. Removal of the underlying cause may be followed by spontaneous reversion to sinus rhythm.

PROPAFENONE AND FLECAINIDE.   Propafenone and flecainide have been shown to convert atrial flutter to sinus rhythm in approximately 25% of patients. Atrial flutter is easily converted to sinus rhythm by synchronized DC shock using low energies of 25 to 50 joules. This is usually necessary only in patients who are hemodynamically compromised and unstable, or if WPW is suspected. Dixogin, verapamil, and beta blockers are contraindicated in patients with WPW who present with atrial flutter or fibrillation. These agents may accelerate the ventricular response and precipitate ventricular fibrillation.

Atrioventricular Reentrant Tachycardia (AVRT). WPW syndrome, causing circus movement tachycardia (see Figs. 5–62 and 5–70).

Management of Narrow QRS Irregular Tachycardia

Atrial Fibrillation. In most patients, a drug that controls the ventricular response to <90 beats/min provides beneficial effects. Digoxin is indicated if CHF, ventricular dysfunction, cardiomegaly, or aortic stenosis is present. An algorithm for the management of atrial fibrillation is given in Figure 19–2.

If atrial fibrillation is acute, define the underlying cause. If the cause is cardiac, heparin IV should be started. More than 75% of patients revert to sinus rhythm over 24 to 48 hours; if there are no contraindications, slowing of the ventricular response with diltiazem or a beta-blocking drug should suffice until sinus rhythm resumes naturally. If atrial fibrillation persists for >3 days and there is no significant valvular disease, antiarrhythmic therapy with sotalol or ibutilide (Corvert) may be tried to convert the patient to sinus rhythm; sotalol is useful to maintain sinus rhythm. If atrial fibrillation is >3 days in duration, in particular if valve disease is present, 3 weeks of warfarin therapy is instituted followed by synchronized DC cardioversion if there are no limiting circumstances.

In patients with chronic atrial fibrillation of >1 year in duration but with a fast ventricular response, echocardiography is useful for making further decisions (see Fig. 19–2). Digoxin is commonly used and is effective in controlling the ventricular response, in particular in patients with CHF or left ventricular dysfunction. If CHF or left ventricular dysfunction is not present, a beta blocker alone should suffice, and in some, a combination of digoxin and a beta blocker may be required, because digoxin may not control the ventricular rate during exercise or other activities in very active individuals.

SOTALOL. If atrial fibrillation is paroxysmal, sotalol is the drug of choice (see Fig. 19–2). In patients with chronic atrial fibrillation, sotalol should not be used solely to control the ventricular rate because of the risk of torsades de pointes with this agent; any other beta blocker should be used. Sotalol is advisable in patients with paroxysmal atrial fibrillation, with the hope that sinus rhythm may be maintained, and in patients after conversion, to maintain sinus rhythm. **Sotalol, 160 to 240 mg daily**, appears to be as effective as quinidine for the maintenance of sinus rhythm. Some reports indicate that quinidine is more effective, but this drug carries the risk of precipitating ventricular arrhythmias and cardiac events.

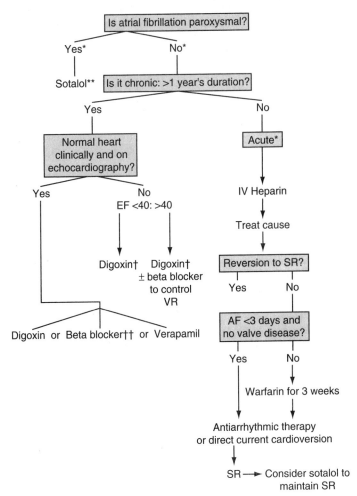

Figure 19–2 □ Algorithm for the management of atrial fibrillation (AF). EF = ejection fraction; IV = intravenous; SR = sinus rhythm; VR = ventricular response during activities or exercise (some patients may need beta blocker or verapamil).

* = slow the ventricular rate with diltiazem or beta blocker; if hemo-
    dynamic compromise or ventricular rate >240 beats/min, consider
    urgent cardioversion

** = see text for dosage and cautions

† = not in obstructive cardiomyopathy, suspected Wolff-Parkinson-
    White syndrome, or sick sinus syndrome

†† = not sotalol; preferably metoprolol or atenolol to control rate and
    to avoid risk of torsades de pointes

(Modified from Khan, M Gabriel: Cardiac Drug Therapy, 5th ed. London, WB Saunders Co., 2000, p 262.)

In patients with atrial fibrillation with or without underlying cardiac disease, **thyroid function should always be assessed** to exclude a treatable thyrotoxic cause.

DIGOXIN. **Dosage: 0.5 mg immediately, and then, in 6 hours, 0.25 mg**. Further doses of digoxin should be given only after determining the apical rate clinically or from a rhythm strip. Usually, a further dose of **0.25 is given 12 hours later, then a 0.25-mg maintenance dose daily**. In some patients if the ventricular rate remains at >110 beats/min, the dosage can be increased to 0.375 mg daily. In patients older than 70 years, or in those with renal dysfunction, i.e., a creatinine level of >1.3 mg/dl (115 μmol/L), the dose of digoxin should be reduced to 0.125 mg daily, with close assessment of the apical response. Digoxin levels are not usually required in patients with atrial fibrillation, because the dose can be titrated to the ventricular rate. Nonetheless, a test of the level is advisable in a few weeks, and then every 4 months **if renal dysfunction is present.**

DILTIAZEM. Diltiazem IV is useful to reduce a fast ventricular rate except in patients with WPW syndrome; see previous discussion under Atrial Flutter.

IBUTILIDE (CORVERT). **Ibutilide IV infusion 0.010 to 0.025 mg/ kg over 10 minutes** is useful for conversion to sinus rhythm; see product monograph for warnings (hospitalization required).

METOPROLOL. **Metoprolol 5 mg IV at a rate of 1 mg/min; 5 minutes later, a second bolus of 5 mg; a third bolus of 5 mg** may be required if the ventricular rate is >120 beats/min. Then give a **maintenance dose of 25 to 50 mg twice daily**, and this can be increased over the ensuing months to **50 to 100 mg twice a day**.

ANTICOAGULANTS. If atrial fibrillation is chronic and valvular heart disease is present, anticoagulation with warfarin to maintain an International Normalized Ratio of 2 to 3 is advisable. If valvular heart disease is not present but the patient is determined to be at high risk because of age older than 70 years, presence of CHF with left ventricular dysfunction, or prior thromboembolism, anticoagulation is recommended. Patients at low risk, i.e., those younger than age 65 with a normal heart clinically and a normal echocardiogram, may be treated with **enteric-coated aspirin 325 mg once daily**. Future clinical trials will determine if this low-risk group should be treated with oral anticoagulants or aspirin.

Multifocal Atrial Tachycardia. Treatment of the underlying cause (COPD, electrolyte or acid–base imbalance, theophylline toxicity) should suffice. If the ventricular rate is rapid, verapamil is usually effective. Magnesium sulfate may cause a salutary response; adenosine is ineffective.

Management of Ventricular Premature Beats

Ventricular premature beats (VPBs) are usually benign, and treatment is not warranted in most patients. Consideration for treatment may be given in patients with

- Multifocal VPBs
- Salvos of three, recurring over hours (in patients with ischemia or considered at risk)
- Multifocal VPBs or salvos associated with hypotension, lightheadedness, or presyncope

  There is no evidence that suppression of VPBs reduces the incidence of sudden death. VPBs occurring during acute MI do not usually require treatment (see Chapter 7). Drugs used to suppress VPBs often have proarrhythmic effects and cause arrhythmias that are life threatening. The dangers of flecainide, encainide, and moricizine have been documented by the Cardiac Arrhythmia Suppression Trial (CAST). Bothersome VPBs in the presence of ischemia or acute MI are best controlled with the use of a beta-blocking drug. These agents are lifesaving, and although their effects are modest, they should be used as the first choice. Arrhythmias are controlled in particular when induced by increased catecholamine secretion or in the presence of ischemia.

METOPROLOL. Metoprolol **50 to 100 mg twice daily** may be given a trial; **then give Toprol XL 50 to 100 mg once daily**. Sotalol should not be used for the treatment of VPBs, because this is the only beta blocker that may precipitate torsades de pointes; sotalol should be reserved for the management of VT or life-threatening arrhythmias.

Management of Wide QRS Regular Tachycardia

Ventricular Tachycardia. Consider all wide regular QRS tachycardia as VT unless there is strong evidence to the contrary. Cardioversion is frequently used, in particular in patients with acute MI or when the rate is >200 beats/min or in patients who are unstable. If drug therapy is used, cardioversion should be available immediately for drug failures. An algorithm for the management of sustained VT is given in Figure 19–3. First-line drugs are as follows.

LIDOCAINE (LIGNOCAINE). **Dosage: An IV bolus of 75 to 100 mg (1–1.5 mg/kg). After 5 minutes, administer a second bolus of 75 to 100 mg. A simultaneous infusion is started within 2 minutes of the first injection; infuse 2 mg/min. A third bolus of 75 mg should be tried before increasing the rate to 3 mg/min and a maximum of 4 mg/min.** VT due to digitalis intoxication,

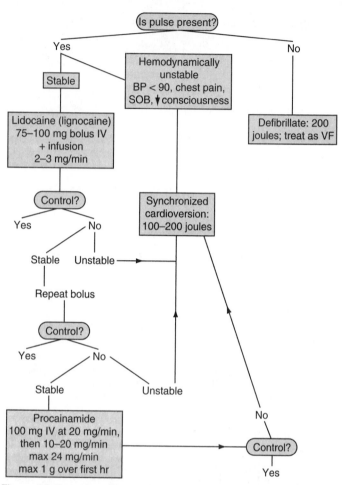

Figure 19–3 □ Algorithm for the management of sustained ventricular tachycardia. (Sustained = VT for >30 seconds or unstable signs.) BP = blood pressure; IV = intravenous; SOB = shortness of breath; VF = ventricular fibrillation; VT = ventricular tachycardia. (Redrawn from Khan, M Gabriel: Heart Disease Diagnosis and Therapy: A Practical Approach. Baltimore, Williams & Wilkins, 1996, p 258.)

phenothiazines, or tricyclic antidepressants usually responds to lidocaine therapy.

PROCAINAMIDE. **Dosage: An IV bolus of 100 mg at a rate of 20 mg/min, and then 10 to 20 mg/min.** Do not exceed 1 g over the first hour. If sinus rhythm occurs, start **oral dosing at 500 mg, then 375 to 500 mg every 3 hours for 24 to 48 hours, and then approximately 500 mg every 6 hours for a patient weighing 60 kg.** Oral use is limited to a maximum of 6 months because of the occasional occurrence of lupus, leukopenia, or agranulocytosis. Procainamide may cause severe hypotension; the drug has a negative inotropic effect, and heart failure may be precipitated. This drug is advisable for patients with lidocaine failure.

Management of Wide QRS Irregular Tachycardia

Torsades de Pointes. This life-threatening arrhythmia is a particular type of VT. ECG shows a typical twisting of the QRS complexes (see Fig. 5–82 and Chapter 5). The arrhythmia is usually precipitated by drugs that prolong the QT interval. Precipitants of torsades de pointes include

- Antiarrhythmic agents that prolong the QT interval, including quinidine, procainamide, disopyramide, amiodarone, and sotalol
- Tricyclic antidepressants and phenothiazines
- Electrolyte imbalance, in particular hypokalemia and hypomagnesemia
- Histamine H_1 blockers, e.g., astemizole and terfenadine
- Pentamidine, erythromycin, and antifungal agents
- Congenital QT prolongation syndrome
- Subarachnoid hemorrhage
- Liquid protein diet

Increasing the heart rate is the simplest and quickest method to shorten the QT interval, and it often results in control of the arrhythmia.

MAGNESIUM SULFATE. **A bolus injection of 2 g (10 ml of a 2% solution over 1 minute)** should be tried and causes reversion to sinus rhythm in patients with acquired torsades de pointes.

If magnesium sulfate fails, temporary atrial or ventricular pacing is indicated. Call your resident to discuss and manage the case. While considering pacing, a trial of isoproterenol IV infusion of 2 to 8 µg/min may prove effective over a few minutes. Isoproterenol should not be used in patients with acute MI, angina, or uncontrolled hypertension.

BETA BLOCKERS. In patients with prolonged QT syndrome, beta blockers are of proven value. Precipitating factors should be clarified, and drugs that cause QT syndrome prolongation must be discontinued; the patient should be given a card stating the effects.

WPW Antidromic Tachycardia (see Fig. 5–83). This requires therapeutic catheter ablation.

Study Section: Arrhythmias

■ DIAGNOSTIC GUIDELINES

Accurate differentiation of ventricular and supraventricular tachycardia is essential for appropriate management. It is important to designate the tachycardia as narrow QRS or wide QRS and to determine whether the rhythm is regular or irregular.

The differential diagnosis of wide QRS complex tachycardia includes

- Ventricular tachycardia (coronary and noncoronary)
- Supraventricular tachycardia (SVT) with preexisting bundle branch block
- SVT with functional aberrant conduction
- Preexcited tachycardia, SVT with anterograde conduction over an accessory pathway

The severity of the underlying diseases, particularly the degree of left ventricular (LV) dysfunction, may dictate the choice of antiarrhythmic agent and the outcome. The prognosis of ventricular arrhythmias is closely linked to the degree of LV dysfunction: an ejection fraction (EF) >50% carries an excellent prognosis; an EF of 40 to 50% carries a fair prognosis and is commonly associated with benign arrhythmias; an EF of 25 to 30% is often associated with potentially lethal arrhythmias; and an EF <25% indicates a poor prognosis.

Adverse effects of drug therapy are clearly related to the degree of LV dysfunction. Determining the EF is essential to the management of ventricular arrhythmias.

The emergency management of arrhythmias calls for a quick assessment of the

- Hemodynamic status: Is the blood pressure <90 mm Hg and are there signs of peripheral hypoperfusion?
- Symptomatic status: chest pain, shortness of breath, presyncope, syncope, or clouding of consciousness
- Cardiac decompensation: signs of heart failure

An essential step in the management of arrhythmia is to rapidly define the clinical setting and correct a precipitating cause, in order to obviate the need for antiarrhythmic therapy and to appraise and prevent deleterious proarrhythmic effects of these agents, if administered.

Precipitating factors and/or clinical settings include

- Acute MI or ischemia
- Those characterized by myocardial reperfusion: e.g., post-thrombolytic therapy in acute MI, balloon deflation during coronary angioplasty, release of coronary artery spasm
- Hypotension
- Sick sinus syndrome or AV block

- Heart failure
- Hypokalemia, hypomagnesemia, hyperkalemia
- Alkalemia: may develop rapidly in ventilated patients
- Acidemia
- Hypoxemia
- Pulmonary disease, e.g., cor pulmonale, atelectasis, pneumothorax, and carcinoma of the lung: may precipitate atrial flutter or atrial fibrillation
- Infection
- Fluctuations in autonomic tone
- Acute blood loss
- Thyrotoxicosis
- Digoxin toxicity
- Proarrhythmic effects of antiarrhythmic drugs: Quinidine and other class IA drugs may cause torsades de pointes; they are also rarely caused by class III agents and sotalol, and extremely rarely caused by amiodarone. More typical monomorphic VT and other lethal arrhythmias may be initiated by antiarrhythmic drugs.
- Beta agonists
- Theophylline
- Ruptured esophagus: may initiate atrial flutter or atrial fibrillation

■ SUPRAVENTRICULAR ARRHYTHMIAS

AV Nodal Reentrant Tachycardia

Paroxysmal supraventricular tachycardia (PSVT) is most often due to AVNRT and is one of the most frequently encountered arrhythmias in clinical practice. In patients younger than 35 years, PSVT usually occurs in an otherwise normal heart and has a good prognosis. However, AVNRT is not uncommon with organic heart disease that is due to ischemic, rheumatic, or other valvular heart disease, and rarely it can be life threatening. The onset and termination are abrupt; heart rate varies from 140 to 220 beats/min.

ECG hallmarks include

- The impulse circulates within the AV node. The ventricles are activated from the anterograde path of the circuit and the atria are activated retrogradely.
- In the commonest form, >50% of AVNRT, the P waves are hidden within the QRS complex (see Fig. 5–62).
- The P wave, when visible, is inverted. In approximately 40% the P wave distorts the terminal QRS causing a pseudo-S wave in leads II and III and a pseudo-r' in lead V_1 (see Fig. 5–64), whereas in the common-type Wolff-Parkinson-White

(WPW) orthodromic circus movement tachycardia, the P wave can be observed separate from the QRS in leads II, III, aVF, and aVL.

- In <5% of cases the P wave occurs at the onset of the QRS and may be observed as pseudo-q waves in leads II, III, and aVF.
- In about 5% of cases the P wave is negative in leads II, III, and aVF and follows the QRS with an RP ≥ PR; this form of AVNRT cannot be differentiated clinically from the rare type WPW, i.e., orthodromic circus movement tachycardia that uses the retrograde slowly conducting accessory pathway to activate the atria resulting in a long RP interval.

Therapy

Carefully instituted, **carotid sinus massage with the patient rhythm-monitored** is an excellent diagnostic maneuver and may result in termination of AVNRT and circus movement tachycardia.

- Carotid sinus massage is not recommended in the elderly or in patients with known or highly suspected carotid disease or digitalis toxicity. Before attempting massage, assess for transient ischemic attacks and carotid artery stenosis.
- Response is either reversion to sinus rhythm or no effect at all, in contrast to atrial flutter, in which slowing of heart rate virtually always occurs and atrial activity is exposed, thus confirming the diagnosis of flutter.
- With the patient supine (head slightly hyperextended, turned a little toward the opposite side), locate the right carotid sinus at the angle of the jaw. Apply firm pressure in a circular or massage fashion for 2 to 6 seconds, using the first and second fingers. It is necessary to monitor the cardiac rhythm and gauge exactly when to stop massage because asystole, although rare, can occur. If unsuccessful, massage the left carotid sinus after an interval of 2 minutes to allow acetylcholine to be manufactured in the AV node. (If asystole occurs during the procedure, ask the patient to cough and/or give the patient one or more light chest thumps, which usually reverses transient asystole.)

Caution: Never massage for more than 10 seconds.

Other vagal maneuvers include Valsalva's maneuver or squatting and the Valsalva maneuver, putting a finger into the throat to initiate a gag reflex, immersion of the face in cold water, taking a drink of cold water, or elevating the legs against a wall. The Valsalva maneuver is effective in approximately 50% of patients with AVNRT.

Caution: Never apply eyeball pressure because **retinal detachment may occur.**

Atrial Tachycardia

Atrial tachycardia can be paroxysmal (PAT), nonparoxysmal, "incessant," or multifocal. The ECG hallmarks include

- The atrial rate is generally 150 to 200 beats/min. The P wave precedes the QRS; the P wave polarity depends on the site of origin in the atrium (see Fig. 5–62). A positive P wave in leads II, III, and aVF excludes AVNRT or WPW circus movement tachycardia.
- Rhythm is regular but beats may be grouped in pairs (bigeminy) causing some irregularity.
- AV conduction may vary 1:1, 2:1, or 3:2.

Paroxysmal Atrial Tachycardia With Block.   ECG hallmarks include

- Isoelectric intervals can be observed between P waves and the QRS. Assess the T waves for the hidden P waves.
- An atrial rate <240 beats/min excludes atrial flutter.

If the heart rate is 90 to 120 beats/min with a normal serum potassium count and symptoms of angina and dyspnea are absent, no immediate treatment is required. If the serum potassium level is <3.5 mEq (mmol)/L and a high degree of AV block is absent, give **potassium chloride IV (60 mEq) in 1 L normal saline over 5 hours.** In recent years with more intelligent use of digoxin, this arrhythmia has become uncommon with digoxin use. "PAT with block" is not always caused by digitalis toxicity.

Persistent ("Incessant") Atrial Tachycardia.   The rhythm is regular, with P waves in front of the QRS. Carotid sinus massage increases the AV block. This very rare persistent arrhythmia of unknown mechanism may cause dilated cardiomyopathy; removal of the area of impulse formation is curative.

Multifocal Atrial Tachycardia.   ECG hallmarks include

- The rhythm is an irregular, chaotic atrial rhythm.
- At least three different P wave morphologies should be recognized in one lead. The PR interval is variable.

Multifocal atrial tachycardia (MAT) and other ectopic atrial tachycardias are usually seen in patients with chronic lung disease, hypoxemia, theophylline toxicity, ischemic heart disease, and myocarditis.

Therapy

The therapy should be directed at the underlying cause. If tachycardia is symptomatic or causes cardiac embarrassment, give **verapamil (2.5 to 5 mg IV, repeated in 30 minutes).** IV verapamil is usually successful and **80 mg orally 3 or 4 times daily** can be administered until the underlying problem resolves. Often, the arrhythmia causes no hemodynamic disturbances, especially at heart rates of 100 to 130 beats/min, and requires no drug therapy, or the initial dose of verapamil can be given orally. Magnesium sulfate is effective in some patients. Arrhythmias due to triggered activity or increased automaticity appear to be partly due to potassium flux from cells; magnesium has a direct effect on potassium channels and increases intracellular potassium.

A beta blocker, especially metoprolol (IV, then orally), is more effective than verapamil, but caution is necessary to avoid the use of beta blockers in patients with COPD. In patients in whom arrhythmia is not terminated by a beta blocker, verapamil, or treatment of the underlying cause and remains bothersome, amiodarone orally may prove effective after a few weeks of administration. **Caution:** Amiodarone is not generally recommended for non–life-threatening arrhythmias.

Atrial Flutter

ECG hallmarks include
- Rhythm is regular if there is a fixed AV conduction ratio and irregular if there is variable AV conduction; the term "AV block" should be avoided in this context.
- "Sawtooth" pattern of flutter (F) waves in leads II, III, and aVF. Positive P-like waves are seen in lead V_1, but they may be negative in leads V_5 and V_6, with nearly no atrial activity in lead I (see Fig. 5–73).
- The heart rate is often 150 beats/min, because the atrial rate is commonly 300 beats/min with 2:1 conduction. Conduction ratios of 2:1 and 4:1 occur commonly.
- T waves may distort the F wave pattern.
- If the diagnosis is not obvious, flutter waves can be made visible with carotid sinus massage or adenosine, which slows AV conduction.

Atrial flutter is usually due to underlying cardiac pathology, particularly ischemic heart disease, MI, and valvular heart disease. Noncardiac disturbances may initiate atrial flutter: hypoxemia caused by pulmonary embolism, pneumothorax, chronic lung disease, and thyrotoxicosis. Removal of the underlying cause may be followed by spontaneous reversion to sinus rhythm. The mechanism of this arrhythmia is still not clarified. A reentrant mechanism in the right atrium is the currently accepted mechanism for the common (type 1) atrial flutter.

Therapy

Atrial flutter is easily converted to sinus rhythm by synchronized DC shock, 20 joules increased to 50 joules, if required. This should be carried out early if the patient is hemodynamically compromised, has symptoms or signs of ischemia or a ventricular response >200 beats/min, or is known or suspected of having

WPW syndrome. For patients with a ventricular rate <200 beats/min, esmolol, propranolol, or metoprolol may be used to slow the ventricular response. Digoxin often converts atrial flutter to atrial fibrillation and slows the ventricular response. Verapamil may reduce the ventricular response, but conversion to sinus rhythm rarely occurs. Verapamil, digoxin, and beta blockers are contraindicated in patients with WPW presenting with atrial flutter or atrial fibrillation. In this setting, verapamil or digoxin may precipitate ventricular fibrillation (VF). Rapid atrial pacing is effective in terminating atrial flutter, but in drug-refractory cases, cardioversion is usually employed.

Chronic Atrial Flutter. If the arrhythmia is resistant to pharmacologic therapy or synchronized DC shock, digoxin is indicated to control the ventricular response, especially if structural heart disease or chronic lung disease is present. Anticoagulants are not indicated for patients with atrial flutter undergoing cardioversion or in those with chronic atrial flutter because cardiac systemic thromboembolism usually does not occur.

Atrial Fibrillation

Atrial fibrillation is the most common sustained arrhythmia observed in clinical practice.

ECG hallmarks include

- The rhythm is completely irregular. RR intervals are irregularly irregular.
- Depending on the degree of AV conduction, the ventricular response is described as controlled if the heart rate is <100 beats/min, and uncontrolled or fast ventricular response if the rate exceeds 120 beats/min. The atrial rate varies from 350 to 500 beats/min, and variable AV conduction causes a chaotic ventricular response.
- P waves are not visible. Irregular undulation of the baseline may be gross and distinct, but barely perceptible or invisible in lead V_1 where undulations are best visualized.
- A slow regular ventricular response in a patient with known atrial fibrillation on digoxin indicates complete AV dissociation caused by digitalis toxicity.

In patients with cardiac pathology, the overall prevalence rate of atrial fibrillation is 4%. Atrial fibrillation is present in >50% of patients with mitral stenosis or heart failure. Causes of atrial fibrillation include other valvular heart disease, hypertension, ischemic heart disease, rheumatic cardiomyopathies, cor pulmonale, pulmonary embolism, thyrotoxicosis, sick sinus syndrome producing tachyarrhythmias and bradyarrhythmias, WPW syndrome, alcohol abuse, postthoracotomy, esophagojejunostomy, ruptured esophagus, carbon monoxide poisoning, and idiopathic.

Investigations should include an echocardiogram to confirm underlying structural heart disease and evaluate left atrial size. Two-dimensional echocardiography may miss atrial thrombus detected by transesophageal echocardiography (TEE).

Caution: Atrial fibrillation with a fast ventricular rate >240 beats/minute, often with wide QRS complex, occurs in up to 10% of patients with WPW syndrome. In this subset of patients, digoxin, beta blockers, and calcium antagonists and lidocaine are contraindicated because VF may be precipitated (see later discussion of WPW syndrome).

Therapy

- Digoxin is used in the majority of patients, particularly in those with heart failure, to control the ventricular response, except when the ventricular rate is >220 beats/min and WPW syndrome is suspected. Digoxin has a role, especially if heart failure requires digitalis therapy on a chronic basis. In symptomatic patients with ventricular rate of 150 to 220 beats/min: give **digoxin IV 0.5 mg slowly under ECG monitoring, followed by 0.25 mg IV every 2 hours** to control the ventricular response. A **total dose of 1 to 1.25 mg** is usually necessary if the patient has not taken digoxin in the past 2 weeks. For patients who have taken digoxin within 1 week, a **dose of 0.125 mg IV should be tried, followed by an additional 0.125 mg after 2 hours if needed, followed by maintenance doses (0.25 to 0.375 mg daily)**. In the elderly or in patients with mild renal dysfunction, give **0.125 mg daily**. This dose is stabilized using the apical rate as a guide and not resorting to the inappropriate use of digoxin serum levels. Digoxin does not cause reversion to sinus rhythm; spontaneous reversion may occur. In some patients, digoxin fails to prevent activity-induced tachycardia and a small dose of a beta blocker, e.g., **atenolol 25 mg daily**, usually causes a satisfactory reduction of fast heart rates.

- Diltiazem IV is useful for the control of fast ventricular rates in patients without heart failure and in the absence of significant LV dysfunction. The drug has replaced verapamil, which causes a high incidence of heart failure. Also, a therapeutic response is observed in 3 minutes vs. 7 minutes for verapamil. **Caution**: Hypotension may ensue. **Dosage: IV initial bolus 0.25 mg/kg over 2 minutes; rebolus 0.35 mg/kg over 2 minutes given 15 minutes later if necessary**. IV continuous infusion should be given under medical supervision: 10 mg/hr may be started after the bolus dose to maintain response for 24 hours; increase to 15 mg/hr if needed. Repeat bolus and infusion sequence if response is lost.

- Esmolol slows the rate adequately over 20 minutes and sinus rhythm may ensue. The drug causes hypotension in up to

40% of patients. The combination of esmolol and digoxin is effective, and hypotension is much less common than when esmolol alone is used. Digoxin appears to protect from hypotension.

Conversion to Sinus Rhythm. Conversion may be achieved in some patients if it is believed to be desirable: conversion may be achieved after full digitalization and control of ventricular response by adding quinidine (200–300 mg) every 6 hours, or if ventricular function is unimpaired, disopyramide may be used instead of quinidine. Maintenance of sinus rhythm may be difficult, and quinidine increases mortality. In view of the hazards associated with these agents, sotalol is as effective (see Fig. 19–2). Conversion to sinus rhythm is achieved in about 50% of patients. DC cardioversion should be used in individuals with suspected WPW syndrome or heart rate >220 beats/min, in unstable patients, and in patients with acute MI with hemodynamic compromise. DC conversion is also deemed necessary in patients with severe aortic stenosis or cardiomyopathy in whom atrial transport function is of great importance. Amiodarone has a role in the latter subset of patients and in others with failed drug therapy or poor LV function.

- Ibutilide (Corvert) has been shown to convert up to 48% of patients with atrial fibrillation of recent onset (1 to 90 days) to sinus rhythm. **Dosage: IV infusion 1 to 2 mg** (0.015–0.025 mg/kg) **over 10 minutes. Caution: torsades de pointes**.
- Flecainide IV is more effective than a combination of digoxin and quinidine in converting paroxysmal atrial fibrillation to sinus rhythm. The drug is effective mainly in patients with atrial fibrillation of recent onset (<6 weeks) or in patients with small atria (<4 cm). The drug is not approved by the Food and Drug Administration (FDA) for the management of atrial fibrillation. **Dosage: IV bolus 2 mg/kg over 10 minutes**, followed by **oral** treatment **200 to 300 mg daily, maximum 400 mg daily**. Flecainide given orally is useful in preventing recurrence of paroxysmal atrial fibrillation, but the drug's use may be hazardous and caution is required. The manufacturers no longer recommend the drug for benign or potentially lethal arrhythmias, and its use is restricted to the management of patients with postcardiac surgical atrial fibrillation in an intensive care setting. The CAST initiated this recommendation. The drug must not be used in patients with heart failure, poor ventricular function, and/or conduction defects.
- It is advisable to combine a class IC or IA agent with digoxin when attempting to convert paroxysmal atrial fibrillation because failure to slow conduction in the AV node may precipitate rapid life-threatening tachycardia. Fatalities have been reported with the use of class IA or IC drugs when used

without prior administration of digoxin. It is well established that quinidine must not be used alone to convert atrial fibrillation because atrial flutter with 1:1 AV conduction may supervene, resulting in hazardous ventricular rates exceeding 240 beats/min.

Synchronized DC Cardioversion.   Electrical conversion requires careful consideration in properly selected patients. Immediate DC cardioversion is indicated for patients who are hemodynamically unstable.

- DC cardioversion is usually contraindicated in chronic atrial fibrillation of >1 year in duration because sinus rhythm is usually not maintained (see Fig. 19–2). Less than 60% and 33% of patients remain in sinus rhythm 1 week or 1 year postconversion, respectively. Conversion, however, is often attempted when heart failure or other symptoms of low cardiac output warrant an aggressive approach.
- Patients with atrial fibrillation <1 week in duration usually regain atrial function after conversion.
- If the patient is hemodynamically stable and there is no underlying structural heart disease, a trial of reversion is not indicated because about 60% revert spontaneously over 1 to 3 days. Control of the ventricular response is readily achieved with the administration of IV esmolol, metoprolol, or diltiazem.
- Embolization occurs in about 2% of patients.
- DC conversion is not advisable in patients with suspected digitalis toxicity because of the risk of precipitating VF, but titrated energy doses are permissible in addition to other measures, such as potassium administration.
- Patients with sick sinus syndrome may develop prolonged postconversion pauses, which often can be terminated by a series of chest thumps.
- In patients with left atrial size >5 cm, sinus rhythm is usually not maintained. A report, however, indicates that left atrial size >5 cm does not appear to be a major determinant of failure to maintain sinus rhythm postconversion. Again, the decision depends on the importance of restoring sinus rhythm.
- Amiodarone has been shown to cause reversion and maintenance of sinus rhythm for up to 3 months in approximately 60% of patients with atrial size <6 cm.
- For DC conversion, anticoagulants are not generally used if atrial fibrillation is <24 hours' duration, because approximately 14% of patients with acute atrial fibrillation reportedly have left atrial thrombus compared with 27% in patients with chronic atrial fibrillation. Anticoagulation or TEE is advisable in acute atrial fibrillation, particularly in patients with valvular heart disease prior to cardioversion.

- If atrial fibrillation is >24 hours' duration and conversion is necessary, oral anticoagulants are given. In patients with duration slightly over 24 hours, IV heparin for 72 hours or TEE may be an acceptable compromise. Embolization has been reported postconversion, however, in patients with no visible thrombi on TEE. In a study by Arnold and coworkers in 454 patients undergoing direct current cardioversion, the incidence rate of embolism in nonanticoagulated patients with atrial fibrillation average duration 6 ± 4 days was 1.32% (six patients), compared with no embolic complications in patients who received oral anticoagulants to maintain a prothrombin time ≥15 seconds. Nonanticoagulated patients with atrial flutter undergoing cardioversion did not have embolic complications, which supports the standard recommendation that patients with atrial flutter do not require anticoagulants during conversion or for long-term therapy. When anticoagulants are commenced in patients with atrial fibrillation undergoing cardioversion, these agents should be continued for at least 3 weeks postconversion because mechanical atrial systole with peak A wave velocity returns only after about 3 weeks postconversion to sinus rhythm.
- Digoxin is maintained for the period before conversion and is interrupted 24 to 48 hours prior to conversion.
- Light anesthesia (IV diazepam, midazolam, or thiopental) with a standby anesthesiologist is necessary.

Quinidine or disopyramide given immediately after conversion and continued in order to increase the chance of perpetuating sinus rhythm is not of proven value. In addition, quinidine is associated with a threefold increase in mortality.

Sotalol is as effective as quinidine in prevention of recurrent atrial fibrillation and for the maintenance of sinus rhythm. This unique beta-blocking drug is useful for the management of paroxysmal atrial fibrillation because it is more effective than other beta blockers for maintaining sinus rhythm and for reversion. Postcardioversion the drug has a definite role; approval by the FDA for these indications is expected. This agent is widely used outside of the United States. For the control of fast ventricular rates sotalol should not be used because all other beta blockers are as effective and do not carry the rare risk of torsades de pointes. Patients administered sotalol should not be given potassium-losing diuretics.

Amiodarone is reserved for patients with EF <30% in whom the maintenance of sinus rhythm is considered essential.

Chronic Atrial Fibrillation. Slowing of the heart rate with digitalis suffices in many. Younger patients, and all patients who have a fast ventricular response during daily activities or on exercise, are controlled with a one-a-day beta blocker, e.g., **atenolol 25 to 50 mg daily**.

Role of Anticoagulants. Patients with paroxysmal atrial fibrillation should be anticoagulated if there is no contraindication in order to prevent embolization. In patients with chronic atrial fibrillation and structural heart disease, systemic embolization is expected in >33% of patients over a period of 5 years. Risk of embolization is about 20% higher in patients with rheumatic heart disease and congestive cardiomyopathy; thus, anticoagulation is strongly recommended in patients with structural heart disease.

In patients younger than 60 years of age who have lone atrial fibrillation (absence of cardiopulmonary disease or hypertension), the risk of stroke is <0.5% per year; if hypertension is included, as in the Framingham study, the risk of stroke increases to 2.6% per year in older patients (mean age: 70 years).

In the Copenhagen Atrial Fibrillation, Aspirin, Anticoagulant (AFASAK) study of 1000 patients with nonrheumatic atrial fibrillation, the stroke reduction risk was 58% for oral anticoagulants and only 16% for aspirin. In the Stroke Prevention in Atrial Fibrillation (SPAF) study, stroke risk reduction was 67% for anticoagulants and 42% for aspirin, but this was an interrupted study and a direct comparison of warfarin and aspirin was not done; aspirin reduced the stroke rate mainly in younger patients (<60 years). **Aspirin (162–325 mg daily)** has a role in patients less than age 70 with lone atrial fibrillation if relative contraindications to anticoagulants exist; a **165-mg enteric-coated tablet** is available in the United States. Ongoing studies will clarify guidelines for therapy of lone atrial fibrillation.

Wolff-Parkinson-White Syndrome

The WPW syndrome is discussed in Chapter 5. See also Figures 5–62, 5–65, 5–68, 5–69, 5–70, and 5–71.

Therapy. In the management of AVRT in patients with WPW, adenosine rapid-bolus injection is indicated (see previous section regarding management of AVNRT). A ventricular response >240 beats/min should be managed with IV procainamide. **Caution:** Avoid adenosine in patients with hypertrophic cardiomyopathy. In tachycardia, which could be preexcited, e.g., atrial fibrillation or flutter, procainamide **up to 10 mg/kg IV over 30 minutes, maximum 1 g in 1 hour** is advisable, provided that the patient is not hypotensive and does not develop hypotension. Failure to convert the arrhythmia or hemodynamic deterioration is an indication for prompt electrical conversion. Patients with the rare-type orthodromic or antidromic circus movement tachycardia require ablation therapy.

■ VENTRICULAR ARRHYTHMIAS

The following grades of ventricular arrhythmia determine outcomes from low risk to high risk: benign arrhythmias to potentially lethal and lethal arrhythmias. This grading is important for decision making concerning appropriate therapy.

- Ventricular premature beats (VPBs): unifocal
- VPBs: multifocal
- VPBs: couplets, runs, or salvos, 3 to 5 consecutive beats
- Nonsustained ventricular tachycardia (VT): A run of three or more consecutive beats lasting <30 seconds and not associated with hemodynamic deterioration
- Sustained VT: Runs ≥30 seconds or associated with unstable cardiovascular symptoms or signs (chest pain, shortness of breath, syncope, or clouding of consciousness); sustained VT is considered potentially lethal.
- Ventricular fibrillation or resuscitation from cardiac arrest: lethal arrhythmias

The outcome and prognosis of ventricular arrhythmias are clearly related to EF. An arrhythmia associated with an EF <30% has a poor prognosis compared with the same arrhythmia and an EF of >50%.

The differentiation of VT and wide QRS forms of SVT can be difficult. A long rhythm strip using lead II is inadequate. A 12-lead tracing is necessary because the precordial leads show distinctive features of VT (see Fig. 5–81).

ECG findings that are diagnostic of VT include

- A totally negative precordial concordance is always VT because WPW circus movement tachycardia never causes negative precordial concordance.
- Predominantly negative QRS complexes in leads V_4 to V_6 or in one or more of leads V_2 to V_6

WPW can cause a wide QRS complex and positive concordance (see Fig. 5–83): atrial flutter with antidromic circus movement should be considered if the patient is known to have WPW syndrome.

Calls related to slow heart rates are uncommon compared with calls for fast heart rates and irregular rhythms.

■ PHONE CALL

Questions

1. **Is the heart rate <45 beats/min?**
   A heart rate of 45 to 59 beats/min usually causes no symptoms and requires no therapy except for controlling underlying problems and discontinuing offending medications.
2. **Is the patient taking a beta blocker, verapamil, diltiazem, digoxin, or other antiarrhythmic agent that slows the heart rate?**
3. **What is the blood pressure (BP)?**
4. **What is the admitting diagnosis—acute myocardial infarction (MI), or investigation of syncope or bradycardia?**

Orders

1. If the patient is symptomatic or hypotensive with a BP <95 mm Hg, give an IV of 5% dextrose in water immediately to keep the vein open.
2. If the heart rate is <42 beats/min, have atropine 0.6 mg at the bedside, to be used after assessment of the patient.
3. Order an electrocardiogram (ECG) and a rhythm strip immediately.
4. If the patient is hypotensive and the pulse rate is <42 beats/min, have the cardiac arrest cart placed at the bedside and hook up the patient to the ECG monitor; call the senior resident or staff physician for assistance if this has not already been done.

Inform RN

"Will arrive at the bedside in . . . minutes."

Rates of <42 beats/min with hypotension require immediate attention.

■ ELEVATOR THOUGHTS

What are the causes of bradycardia?
Causes of a slow heart rate include
- Acute inferior MI
- Drugs, e.g., beta blockers, verapamil, diltiazem, digoxin, morphine, amiodarone, or a combination of these agents
- Sick sinus syndrome
- Complete heart block
- Atrial fibrillation with a slow ventricular response (often caused by digitalis toxicity)
- Hypothyroidism
- Normal state in healthy athletes
- Increased intracranial pressure
- Obstructive jaundice

■ MAJOR THREAT TO LIFE

- Complete heart block or Mobitz type II block
- Acute MI with Mobitz type II block or complete heart block
- Hypotension: cardiogenic shock may ensue

■ BEDSIDE

Quick Look Test

Does the patient look well (comfortable), sick (uncomfortable or distressed), or critical (about to die)?

Airway and Vital Signs

What is the heart rate?
Assess the ECG, and verify the cause of the abnormal heart rhythm (see Chapter 5). If the patient is hypotensive, with a pulse rate of <42 beats/min, or the ECG appears to show Mobitz type II or complete atrioventricular (AV) block, ask your staff physician or cardiology resident for help immediately.

■ MANAGEMENT

1. Sinus bradycardia
   Bradycardia is not usually symptomatic until the heart rate falls to <42 beats/min (seven small squares on an ECG tracing). Blood pressure may fall, and dizziness, presyncope, or syncope may occur. Stop all offending drugs that cause bradycardia. If the heart rate is <42 beats/min or hypoten-

sion is associated, administer **atropine 0.5 or 0.6 mg IV,** then repeat if needed in 5 to 10 minutes to increase the heart rate to approximately >50 beats/min but not to >80 beats/min. The maximum dose of atropine, given in 4 divided doses over a period of approximately 1 hour, should not be >2.4 mg. If bradycardia fails to respond to this dose, call your staff physician or seek further advice.

2. AV block (see Chapter 5 for ECG diagnosis)
   - First-degree AV block. This requires no treatment. Discontinue or reduce the dose of offending drugs (e.g., digoxin, beta blockers, verapamil, diltiazem, and amiodarone). First-degree AV block usually does not progress to symptomatic advanced AV block. Added right or left bundle branch block of recent onset usually indicates infra His conduction delay, and a permanent pacemaker may be advisable if there are symptoms or an intermittent complete AV block; discuss this scenario with your resident.
   - Second-degree AV block: Mobitz type I (Wenckebach) (see Fig. 5–84 and Chapter 5). The block is above the His bundle. This is a benign condition that usually resolves spontaneously when the underlying cause is eliminated. Search for reversible causes, i.e., use of beta blockers, diltiazem, or calcium antagonists; acute inferior MI is a common cause of bradycardia and Wenckebach, but the condition usually resolves over a period of 1 to 3 days and pacing is not required.
   - Mobitz type II (see Fig. 5–85 and Chapter 5). Because the block is below the level of the His bundle, severe bradycardia or complete heart block may ensue. Even in asymptomatic individuals, progression to symptomatic severe bradycardias usually occurs, and thus, pacing is indicated. Stokes-Adams attacks may occur. During acute MI, Mobitz type II block may proceed to complete AV block, and temporary pacing is indicated. If AV block persists beyond 3 weeks, a permanent pacemaker may be required. Mobitz type II block unrelated to antiarrhythmic drug therapy is an indication for permanent cardiac pacing.
   - Complete (third-degree AV block) (see Fig. 5–86 and Chapter 5). Patients may present with presyncope or Stokes-Adams attacks, i.e., sudden loss of consciousness without warning, during which the patient becomes very pale and during recovery from which the face becomes flushed as the circulation is restored. At times, AV block may be asymptomatic, transient, or due to reversible factors. Search for underlying causes of complete AV block:
     - Drugs
     - Acute MI and degenerative disease of the electrical system

- □ Sarcoidosis
- □ Hemochromatosis
- □ Paget's disease
- Atrial fibrillation with slow ventricular response. In patients with atrial fibrillation with a ventricular rate of <50 beats/min, consider digitalis toxicity; at times, the irregular rhythm may become somewhat more regular; a regular rhythm with no P waves suggests a diagnosis of slow junctional rhythm with AV dissociation. Stop digoxin, and call your resident for assistance.
- Sick sinus syndrome. Patients with sick sinus syndrome may present with marked sinus bradycardia with rates of <42 beats/min, sinus arrest, paroxysmal atrial tachyarrhythmias, or a combination of bradycardia and tachyarrhythmia. In the same individual over several days, the ECG may show atrial flutter, atrial fibrillation, or atrial tachycardia or bradycardia. Because approximately 33% of patients with sick sinus syndrome have a conduction defect involving the AV node and bundle branches, consideration should be given to the type of pacemaker used. Discuss this with your resident and staff cardiologist. Because of the intermittent nature of arrhythmias in patients with sick sinus syndrome, correlation of symptoms with a specific arrhythmia is essential. If symptoms are present, a permanent pacemaker is indicated. Asymptomatic sinus bradycardia, sinus pauses, and sinoatrial exit block are not indications for a permanent pacemaker. Sinus pauses of ≥3 seconds that are symptomatic are an indication for permanent pacing. In patients with bradycardias, before pacemaker implantation, it is necessary to verify that symptoms are related to a specific bradyarrhythmia.

Fever With Valve Murmur: Endocarditis

All patients with a valvular heart murmur and a fever of unknown origin (FUO) should be considered as having infective endocarditis until proven otherwise.

■ PHONE CALL

Questions

1. Has the patient been admitted for investigation of intermittent fever or FUO?
2. Is the patient known to have valvular heart disease?
3. Does the patient have a prosthetic heart valve?
4. Is there a history of dental work, genitourinary instrumentation, or other surgical intervention in recent months?
5. Is the patient a known or suspected drug addict?

Orders

Take four blood cultures over 1 hour. One culture bottle should be sent for anaerobic culture.

Inform RN

"Will arrive at the bedside in . . . minutes."

■ ELEVATOR THOUGHTS

What are the causative organisms of endocarditis?
1. Causative organisms are usually a wide range of bacteria, but fungi, *Coxiella* species, or *Chlamydia* species may be implicated.
2. Strongly consider acute endocarditis, in particular if pyrexia is prominent for 3 to 7 days and if the patient looks ill.

3. Although infection usually involves damaged heart valves, infection may occur in patients with bicuspid aortic valves, ventricular septal defect, coarctation of the aorta, patent ductus arteriosus, and aneurysm.

4. Although controversial, the type of presentation may be helpful in decision making. Subacute bacterial endocarditis (SBE) is commonly caused by *Streptococcus viridans* and *Streptococcus faecalis*. In elderly patients with valvular heart disease, *S. faecalis* is commonly the offending agent, but *S. viridans* is implicated in about 50% of cases.

5. If the patient has a prosthetic heart valve, consider *Staphylococcus aureus* or *Staphylococcus epidermidis* if the timing is early postoperative. For late postoperative patients, the organism is similar to those seen in SBE or acute endocarditis.

6. If the presentation is that of acute bacterial endocarditis, the organism is usually *S. aureus.*

7. If the patient is a drug addict, consider right-sided endocarditis; the organism is commonly *S. aureus, Pseudomonas* species, or *Serratia* species.

8. Remember to consider culture-negative endocarditis if previous antibiotics have been used. Slow-growing penicillin-sensitive streptococci that have fastidious nutritional requirements may fail to grow on culture; and the culture may be negative if the infection is caused by *Coxiella* species or *Chlamydia* species.

9. Dental work, even as long as 4 months earlier, should be considered as a precipitating factor. If dental work is implicated, the organism is commonly *S. viridans,* or rarely, *S. faecalis* and *Fusobacterium* species.

■ MAJOR THREAT TO LIFE

- Rupture of a valve cusp leading to hypotension and cardiogenic shock
- Embolization

■ BEDSIDE

Quick Look Test

Does the patient look well (comfortable), sick (uncomfortable or distressed), or critical (about to die)?

Selective History and Chart Review

1. Review the precipitating and predisposing factors.
2. Has the patient had chills or rigors?

Selective Physical Examination

Look for
- Finger clubbing and Osler nodes
- Anemia
- Splinter hemorrhages; if they occur, trauma may be the cause; count the number of splinter hemorrhages and compare in the ensuing days
- Roth's spots of the retina
- Intensity of heart murmurs, which may change over a period of days (see Chapter 4)
- Splenomegaly

■ DIAGNOSTIC TESTING

1. Blood cultures must be incubated, both aerobically and anaerobically. One of four cultures should be anaerobic to assess for *Bacteroides* species and anaerobic streptococci. If SBE is suspected because of a prolonged course over weeks, four cultures can be taken over 24 hours from separate venipuncture sites and antibiotics started within 12 hours of culture. If the presentation is one of acute endocarditis, cultures should be taken over 1 hour and antibiotics should be started within the hour.
2. Echocardiogram: two-dimensional echocardiography detects approximately 60% of vegetations. Some organisms, in particular *S. aureus* and streptococci, may produce small lesions of <5 mm, however, and these are poorly detectable by transthoracic echocardiography. Transesophageal echocardiography (TEE) is a superior technique, and vegetations are detected in >90% of cases. TEE can be crucial to the management of endocarditis. TEE is a semi-invasive procedure, however, and should be used if transthoracic echocardiography fails to show vegetations in a patient strongly suspected of having endocarditis. Also, in patients with a prosthetic heart valve, TEE is strongly recommended. Complications with TEE include bronchospasm, pharyngeal bleeding, and arrhythmias.

■ MANAGEMENT

Prior to Obtaining Culture Results

1. For patients with infective endocarditis and not allergic to penicillin: give **nafcillin or cloxacillin 2 g every 4 hours,**

Text continued on page 307

Table 21-1 □ CARDIAC CONDITIONS ASSOCIATED WITH ENDOCARDITIS

Endocarditis Prophylaxis Recommended

High-Risk Category

Prosthetic cardiac valves, including bioprosthetic and homograft valves

Previous bacterial endocarditis

Complex cyanotic congenital heart disease (e.g., single ventricle states, transposition of the great arteries, tetralogy of Fallot)

Surgically constructed systemic pulmonary shunts or conduits

Moderate-Risk Category

Most other congenital cardiac malformations (other than above and below)

Acquired valvar dysfunction (e.g., rheumatic heart disease)

Hypertrophic cardiomyopathy

Mitral valve prolapse with valvar regurgitation and/or thickened leaflets*

Endocarditis Prophylaxis Not Recommended

Negligible-risk category (no greater risk than the general population)

Isolated secundum atrial septal defect

Surgical repair of atrial septal defect, ventricular septal defect, or patent ductus arteriosus (without residua beyond 6 months)

Previous coronary artery bypass graft surgery

Mitral valve prolapse without valvar regurgitation*

Physiologic, functional, or innocent heart murmurs*

Previous Kawasaki disease without valvar dysfunction

Previous rheumatic fever without valvar dysfunction

Cardiac pacemakers (intravascular and epicardial) and implanted defibrillators

---

Modified from Dajani AS, Taubert KA, Wilson W, et al: Prevention of bacterial endocarditis: Recommendations by the American Heart Association. JAMA 1997; 277:1794–1801. Copyright 1997, American Medical Association.

*Mitral valve prolapse on auscultation or echocardiography, and/or thickened leaflets.

Table 21-2 □ DENTAL PROCEDURES AND ENDOCARDITIS PROPHYLAXIS

Endocarditis Prophylaxis Recommended*

Dental extractions
Periodontal procedures including surgery, scaling and root planing, probing, and recall maintenance
Dental implant placement and reimplantation of avulsed teeth
Endodontic (root canal) instrumentation or surgery only beyond the apex
Subgingival placement of antibiotic fibers or strips
Initial placement or orthodontic bands but not brackets
Intraligamentary local anesthetic injections
Prophylactic cleaning of teeth or implants where bleeding is anticipated

Endocarditis Prophylaxis Not Recommended

Restorative dentistry† (operative and prosthodontic) with or without retraction cord‡
Local anesthetic injections (nonintraligamentary)
Intracanal endodontic treatment; post placement and buildup
Placement of rubber dams
Placement of removable prosthodontic or orthodontic appliances
Postoperative suture removal
Taking of oral impressions
Fluoride treatments
Taking of oral radiographs
Orthodontic appliance adjustment
Shedding of primary teeth

Modified from Dajani AS, Taubert KA, Wilson W, et al: Prevention of bacterial endocarditis: Recommendations by the American Heart Association. JAMA 1997;277:1794–1801. Copyright 1997, American Medical Association.

*Prophylaxis is recommended for patients with high- and moderate-risk cardiac conditions.

†This includes restoration of decayed teeth (filling cavities) and replacement of missing teeth.

‡Clinical judgment may indicate antibiotic use in selected circumstances that may create significant bleeding.

Table 21–3 □ OTHER PROCEDURES AND ENDOCARDITIS PROPHYLAXIS

Endocarditis Prophylaxis Recommended

Respiratory Tract

Tonsillectomy and/or adenoidectomy
Surgical operations that involve respiratory mucosa
Bronchoscopy with a rigid bronchoscope

Gastrointestinal Tract *

Sclerotherapy for esophageal varices
Esophageal stricture dilation
Endoscopic retrograde cholangiography with biliary obstruction
Biliary tract surgery
Surgical operations that involve intestinal mucosa

Genitourinary Tract

Prostatic surgery
Cystoscopy
Urethral dilation

Endocarditis Prophylaxis Not Recommended

Respiratory Tract

Endotracheal intubation
Bronchoscopy with a flexible bronchoscope, with or without biopsy†
Tympanostomy tube insertion

Gastrointestinal Tract

Transesophageal echocardiography†
Endoscopy with or without gastrointestinal biopsy†

Genitourinary Tract

Vaginal hysterectomy†
Vaginal delivery†
Cesarean section
In uninfected tissue:
  Urethral catheterization
  Uterine dilatation and curettage
  Therapeutic abortion
  Sterilization procedures
  Insertion or removal of intrauterine devices

Other

Cardiac catheterization, including balloon angioplasty
Implanted cardiac pacemakers, implanted defibrillators, and coronary stents
Incision or biopsy or surgically scrubbed skin
Circumcision

Modified from Dajani AS, Taubert KA, Wilson W, et al: Prevention of bacterial endocarditis: Recommendations by the American Heart Association. JAMA 1997;277:1794–1801. Copyright 1997, American Medical Association.
  *Prophylaxis is recommended for high-risk patients; optional for medium-risk patients.
  †Prophylaxis is optional for high-risk patients.

Table 21-4 □ PROPHYLACTIC REGIMENS FOR DENTAL, ORAL, RESPIRATORY TRACT, OR ESOPHAGEAL PROCEDURES

Situation	Agent	Regimen*
Standard general prophylaxis	Amoxicillin	Adults: 2.0 g; children: 50 mg/kg orally 1 hr before procedure
Unable to take oral medications	Ampicillin	Adults: 2.0 g intramuscularly (IM) or intravenously (IV); children: 50 mg/kg IM or IV within 30 min before procedure
Allergic to penicillin	Clindamycin or	Adults: 600 mg; children: 20 mg/kg orally 1 hr before procedure
	Cephalexin† or cefadroxil† or	Adults: 2.0 g; children: 50 mg/kg orally 1 hr before procedure
	Azithromycin or clarithromycin	Adults: 500 mg; children: 15 mg/kg orally 1 hr before procedure
Allergic to penicillin and unable to take oral medications	Clindamycin or	Adults: 600 mg; children: 20 mg/kg IV within 30 min before procedure
	Cefazolin	Adults: 1.0 g; children: 25 mg/kg IM or IV within 30 min before procedure

Modified from Dajani AS, Taubert KA, Wilson W, et al: Prevention of bacterial endocarditis: Recommendations by the American Heart Association. JAMA 1997;277:1794–1801. Copyright 1997, American Medical Association.

*Total children's dose should not exceed adult dose.

†Cephalosporins should not be used in individuals with immediate-type hypersensitivity reaction (urticaria, angioedema, or anaphylaxis) to penicillins.

plus ampicillin 2 g every 4 hours, plus gentamicin 1 to 1.4 mg/kg every 8 hours. Caution is used to avoid gentamicin toxicity, in particular in patients older than 65 years and in those with impaired renal function.

2. For patients allergic to penicillin: Administer **vancomycin 15 mg/kg IV every 12 hours.**

After Obtaining Culture Results

1. For *S. viridans* and *Streptococcus bovis,* "susceptible" organisms sensitive to penicillin, in patients with native valve endocarditis:

   ▪ Administer **penicillin 2 to 3 million U every 4 hours, plus gentamicin 1 to 1.2 mg/kg every 8 hours, for 2 weeks.** This therapy should suffice in >98% of patients with sensitive strains of *S. viridans* and *S. bovis.* In patients older than 65 years and in those with renal impairment, gentamicin therapy for 1 week should suffice, but the dose interval should be titrated to the creatinine clearance and to the gentamicin levels; caution is necessary.

   ▪ In patients with a risk of aminoglycoside toxicity, in the presence of sensitive organisms, penicillin alone for 4 weeks should suffice.

   ▪ **Ceftriaxone IV or IM once daily for 4 weeks** has been shown to be as effective as penicillin and gentamicin in a multicenter study. **Ceftriaxone 2 g IV or IM once daily for 2 weeks, followed if needed by oral amoxicillin 1 g four times per day for 2 weeks** was shown to be effective in a small open Argentinian study. These and other studies have documented the efficacy of this therapy, which saves on expensive hospitalization. In the **United States, ceftriaxone is commonly recommended for the treatment** of these patients. Ceftriaxone IM is painful.

2. For more resistant *S. viridans:*
   ▪ Give both penicillin and gentamicin for 4 weeks.

3. For patients with prosthetic valve endocarditis due to *S. viridans* or *S. bovis* infection: penicillin and gentamicin for 2 weeks, followed by penicillin IV for a further 2 weeks.

4. Enterococcal endocarditis caused by *S. faecalis, Streptococcus faecium,* or *Streptococcus durans* presents major difficulties, because these organisms are relatively resistant to most antibiotics. Thus, antibiotic combinations are necessary. It is advisable to use a combination of **penicillin at a high dose and gentamicin 1 mg/kg every 8 hours for 4 weeks.** In some patients, 6 weeks of therapy may be necessary, in particular in patients who have had infections for >3 months.

5. For *S. aureus* on native valve: **Cloxacillin or nafcillin IV for 4 to 6 weeks plus optional gentamicin for 5 days.** If methicillin resistant, administer vancomycin for 4 to 6 weeks.

6. *S. epidermidis* commonly causes prosthetic valve endocardi-

Table 21-5 □ PROPHYLACTIC REGIMENS FOR GENITOURINARY GASTROINTESTINAL (EXCLUDING ESOPHAGEAL) PROCEDURES

Situation	Agent	Regimen*
High-risk patients	Ampicillin + gentamicin	Adults: ampicillin 2.0 g intravenously (IV) plus gentamicin 1.5 mg/kg (not to exceed 120 mg) within 30 min of starting procedure; 6 hr later, ampicillin 1 g IV or amoxicillin 1 g orally Children: ampicillin 50 mg/kg IV (not to exceed 2.0 g) plus gentamicin 1.5 mg/kg within 30 min of starting procedure; 6 hr later, ampicillin 25 mg/kg IV or amoxicillin 25 mg/kg orally
High-risk patients allergic to ampicillin/amoxicillin	Vancomycin + gentamicin	Adults: vancomycin 1.0 g IV over 1–2 hr plus gentamicin 1.5 mg/kg IV (not to exceed 120 mg); complete injection/infusion within 30 min of starting procedure Children: vancomycin 20 mg/kg IV over 1–2 hr plus gentamicin 1.5 mg/kg IV; complete injection/infusion within 30 min of starting procedure

| Moderate-risk patients | Amoxicillin or ampicillin | Adults: amoxicillin 2.0 g orally 1 hr before procedure, or ampicillin 2.0 g IV within 30 min of starting procedure
Children: amoxicillin 50 mg/kg orally 1 hr before procedure, or ampicillin 50 mg/kg IV within 30 min of starting procedure |
| Moderate-risk patients allergic to ampicillin/amoxicillin | Vancomycin | Adults: vancomycin 1.0 g IV over 1–2 hr; complete infusion within 30 min of starting procedure
Children: vancomycin 20 mg/kg IV over 1–2 hr; complete infusion within 30 min of starting the procedure |

Modified from Dajani AS, Taubert KA, Wilson W, et al: Prevention of bacterial endocarditis: Recommendations by the American Heart Association. JAMA 1997;277:1794–1801. Copyright 1997, American Medical Association.
*Total children's dose should not exceed adult dose.
†No second dose of vancomycin or gentamicin is recommended.

tis. Because the organism is often methicillin resistant, administer a combination of vancomycin and rifampin for 4 weeks and gentamicin for 2 weeks. If the strain is methicillin sensitive, substitute cloxacillin for vancomycin.

7. For patients with right-sided endocarditis (usually drug addicts): administer cloxacillin and gentamicin until sensitivities are identified.

8. Indications for surgical interventions:
   - Patients who have deterioration causing congestive heart failure (CHF)
   - Patients with marked worsening of aortic and mitral regurgitation with precipitation of CHF
   - Patients with prosthetic valve endocarditis after the infection has been brought under control

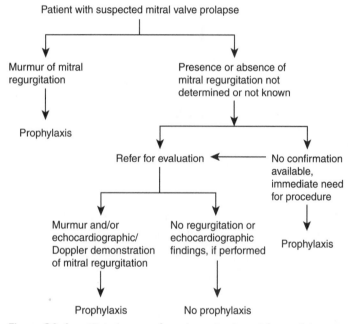

Figure 21–1 □ Clinical approach to determination of the need for prophylaxis in patients with suspected mitral valve prolapse. For more details on the role of echocardiography in the diagnosis of mitral valve prolapse, see the text and the 1997 American College of Cardiology/American Heart Association guidelines for the clinical application of echocardiography. (From Dajani AS, Taubert KA, Wilson W, et al: Prevention of bacterial endocarditis. Recommendations by the American Heart Association. JAMA 1997;277:1794–1801. Copyright 1997, American Medical Association.)

- Patients with fungal infection (difficult to eradicate medically in a prosthetic valve)
- Patients who relapse after 6 weeks of medical therapy
- Patients with complications, including aneurysm of the sinus of Valsalva, septal or valve ring abcesses, and repeated embolization. Patients with right-sided endocarditis have a 75% incidence of pulmonary embolism, but this is not an indication for surgery.

Endocarditis Prophylaxis

It is difficult to prevent endocarditis; the American Heart Association and British Society recommendations change every 3 to 5 years. Current recommendations are given in Tables 21–1 through 21–5. **Recommendations for suspected mitral valve prolapse are indicated in Figure 21–1.**

22 | Hypertensive Emergencies

Hypertensive emergencies may pose an immediate threat to life, and they require prompt attention.

■ PHONE CALL

Questions

1. Is the diastolic blood pressure (BP) >125 mm Hg? Is the systolic BP >225 mm Hg, with a diastolic BP >110 mm Hg?
2. Why is the patient in the hospital or the emergency room?
3. Is chest and back pain a feature, suggesting aortic dissection?
4. Is shortness of breath severe, suggesting pulmonary edema?
5. Is there a history of vomiting, confusion, or seizures, suggesting hypertensive encephalopathy?
6. Are there headaches, confusion, and neck stiffness, suggesting subarachnoid hemorrhage?

Orders

If any of the above symptoms are present, order an IV of 5% dextrose in water to keep the vein open.

Inform RN

"Will arrive at the bedside in . . . minutes."

■ ELEVATOR THOUGHTS

What are the causes of hypertensive emergencies?
1. **True hypertensive emergencies are conditions that pose an immediate threat to life and require immediate IV therapy to reduce BP within minutes,** even though the initial BP may not be alarmingly high. For example, with aortic dissection, a BP of 165/90 mm Hg **must be reduced. Most important, with many emergencies, only a small reduction of BP is required.**

- Severe hypertension causing pulmonary edema
- Aortic dissection (see Chapter 11)
- Hypertensive encephalopathy
- Eclampsia
- Malignant hypertension: systolic and diastolic pressures usually exceed 220/125 mm Hg, and constitute an emergency if associated with papilledema, renal failure, microangiopathic hemolytic anemia, or encephalopathy.

2. **Hypertensive urgencies: BP may be much higher than with emergencies, but there is no acute progressive organ damage or immediate threat to life imposed by the elevated BP.** The BP can usually be reduced with oral medications over a day or two. Important causes of hypertensive urgencies that require therapy within hours to days include

- Pheochromocytoma and other catecholamine-induced hypertension, such as that caused by cocaine or amphetamine abuse
- Severe hypertension associated with subarachnoid hemorrhage, cerebral hemorrhage, or thrombotic stroke
- Withdrawal of some antihypertensive agents, i.e., sudden discontinuation of clonidine, guanfacine, methyldopa, nifedipine, and other dihydropyridines, but rarely beta blockers and angiotensin-converting enzyme (ACE) inhibitors

■ MAJOR THREAT TO LIFE

A marked elevation of BP, associated with aortic dissection, pulmonary edema, myocardial ischemia, hypertensive encephalopathy, and eclampsia, poses a threat to life.

■ BEDSIDE

Quick Look Test

Does the patient look sick (uncomfortable or distressed), or critical (about to die)?
Pulmonary edema is manifested by a marked shortness of breath and a cough, often with production of frothy pink sputum and crackles (crepitations) over the lung fields.

Airway and Vital Signs

What is the BP?
Assess the BP in both arms. With aortic dissection, the BP may be lower in the left arm.

Selective History and Selective Physical Examination

Assess the following:
1. Chest pain: Is there a pattern of myocardial infarction (MI) or aortic dissection?
2. Marked shortness of breath due to the presence of pulmonary edema
3. Quality, severity, and rapid or slow onset of headaches
4. Neck stiffness
5. Neurologic deficit
   - Fundi for papilledema; this sign may be present in patients with malignant hypertension or hypertensive encephalopathy, but it is not essential for the diagnosis
   - Hemorrhages and exudates
6. Chest: Are there widespread crackles, indicating pulmonary edema?
7. Cardiovascular system
   - The jugular venous pressure is elevated and an S_3 or an S_3 plus S_4 summation gallop is expected in some patients with congestive heart failure (CHF)
   - The absence of pulse in an arm or the limbs or a new aortic diastolic murmur may indicate aortic dissection
8. Central nervous system: confusion, agitation, and possibly focal deficits

■ MANAGEMENT

For patients with conditions that pose an immediate threat to life, i.e., pulmonary edema, aortic dissection, hypertensive encephalopathy, myocardial ischemia, and eclampsia, **the goal is to produce an immediate but modest reduction in BP:**
   - A 20% reduction from baseline of the mean arterial pressure or
   - A reduction in the diastolic pressure to about 110 mm Hg, and no less than 100 mm Hg, over a period of several minutes.

The BP is maintained at this level for a further 12 to 24 hours, at which time a further lowering should be carefully considered.

Hypertensive Emergencies

Drugs and dosages for hypertensive emergencies are given in Table 22–1.
1. Aortic dissection
   The above guidelines must be modified in patients with aortic dissection. In this setting, further reduction of BP is

Table 22–1 □ DRUGS AND DOSAGES
FOR HYPERTENSIVE EMERGENCIES*

Nitroprusside	IV 0.5–8 μg/kg/min
	    Average dose: 3 μg/kg/min (see Table A–5
	    in Appendix)

Labetalol	IV 20–160 mg/hr; 0.5–2 mg/min infusion
Fenoldopam	0.1–0.3 μg/kg/min

Hydralazine	IV 5–10 mg test dose over 1–2 min; or IV
	    infusion 5–15 mg/hr plus furosemide 40 mg
	    daily

Methyldopa	IV 250 mg in 100 mg 5% dextrose in water over 60 min, repeated every 4 or 6 hr

Metoprolol	Oral: 50–100 mg every 12 hr, often in
	    combination with nifedipine (if renal failure is
	    present, add furosemide 80 mg)

Captopril	Oral: 25-mg test dose, then 25–50 mg every
	    8 hr; if response is partial, add furosemide
	    40–80 mg every 12–24 hr

Magnesium sulfate	IV 4 g diluted in 100–200 ml IV solution over 20 min, then 1–2 g/hr
Urapidil	12.5–25 mg bolus IV, then infusions 5–40 mg/hr

*Appropriate oral agents must be started to prevent resurgence of the severely hypertensive state.

usually required, as well as the addition of a beta-blocking drug to reduce the rate of rise of aortic pressure (see Chapter 11).

2. Pulmonary edema
   Ensure that severe hypertension is present and that ischemia or infarction has been excluded (see Chapter 17).
   - If ischemia is present, use a **nitroglycerin infusion (see Table A–4). Furosemide** is commonly added, **40 to 80 mg IV immediately** with monitoring of serum potassium. Torsemide is more effective than furosemide particularly for prevention of recurrent CHF (see Chapter 18).
   - If ischemia or infarction is absent, start **nitroprusside 0.5 to 8 μg/kg/min** (see Table A–5). The dose of nitroprusside is titrated to decrease intra-arterial BP 25% and diastolic BP to <110 mm Hg but >100 mm Hg. If nitroprusside is not available, **fenoldopam 0.1 to 0.3 μg/ kg/min** can be used, except in patients with glaucoma. **Urapidil, an alpha blocker with central serotonin-agonist activity, is commonly used in Europe: 12.5- to 25-mg bolus followed by infusion of 5 to 40 mg/hr;** action occurs in 3 to 5 minutes, with a duration of action

of 4 to 6 hours. The drug does not influence heart rate or myocardial oxygen consumption. Labetalol has a negative inotropic effect and should be avoided in patients with CHF or asthma. Nifedipine has a mild negative inotropic effect; the drug can cause uncontrolled lowering of BP in some patients; myocardial ischemia or cerebral hypoperfusion may be precipitated.

3. Hypertensive encephalopathy

The drug of choice is **nitroprusside 0.5 to 8 μg/kg/min** to decrease mean arterial pressure approximately 25% from the baseline, or the diastolic pressure to <110 mm Hg. If nitroprusside is not available, **fenoldopam, labetalol, or urapidil** can be tried (see Table 22–1). **Diazoxide should be avoided** because a dangerous crash in BP may occur; **the drug is considered obsolete.**

4. Eclampsia

After discussion with the obstetrician, the usual measures are

- **Magnesium sulfate 4 g diluted in 100 to 200 ml of IV solution given over 20 minutes;** a maintenance dose is 2 g/hr with careful monitoring of BP and urine output.

  Caution: Magnesium sulfate is contraindicated in patients with renal failure and hepatic dysfunction and should not be used with calcium antagonists, because severe hypotension may occur. The drug does not cause significant lowering of BP and is used mainly to prevent seizures. The drug remains the most useful agent in the prevention of seizures associated with severe preeclampsia.

- BP may be lowered with careful titration of labetalol (see Table 22–1).

- Hydralazine may be used if labetalol is not available.

5. Malignant hypertension

A malignant phase of essential hypertension is now uncommon because of better control of severe hypertension. First, exclude the withdrawal of drugs that cause rebound hypertension, i.e., clonidine, guanfacine, beta blockers, calcium antagonists, and rarely, ACE inhibitors.

If papilledema, hemorrhages, or exudates are present, treat urgently with nitroprusside, fenoldopam, or labetalol IV. **Sublingual nifedipine must not be used and the 10-mg oral dose also may cause a dangerous crash of the BP. Many strokes have been caused by this method of therapy, although many physicians have used it successfully.** A sudden fall in systolic BP, from 240 to 90 mm Hg, can occur, albeit rarely; this precipitous drop may cause cerebral infarction or MI. Sublingual nifedipine has been used in many countries for >15 years, but this therapy is not approved by the Food and Drug Administration (FDA).

One dose of **furosemide 40 mg** may be given if fluid retention is a feature. Sodium and water retention occurs commonly in patients with volume overload due to renal failure or in patients treated with methyldopa, clonidine, and alpha blockers. The addition of **metoprolol 50 to 100 mg every 12 hours** usually results in control of BP. Further reduction may be obtained by the addition of furosemide or a thiazide diuretic. Alternatives include the use of captopril or another ACE inhibitor, complemented by **hydrochlorothiazide 25 to 50 mg daily.**

Caution: Do not administer nifedipine if there are signs of cerebral or myocardial ischemia, because a stroke or MI may be precipitated. The patient's prior medications should be reviewed; discuss the maintenance therapy with your resident.

6. Renal failure

   Sudden severe elevations of BP may occur because of volume overload, which is always a prominent feature of uncontrolled or progressive hypertension in patients with renal failure. The sudden increase in the size of an atheromatous plaque in the renal artery may cause elevation of BP.

   Emergency management often requires the use of three agents.

   - **Furosemide** at high doses: **80 to 160 mg IV immediately, then every 12 hours;** a high dose is required because of the low glomerular filtration rate.
   - **Nifedipine, 10-mg oral capsules immediately, then 10 to 20 mg every 4 or 6 hours.**
   - Failure of nifedipine should prompt the use of labetalol IV if beta blockers are not contraindicated. As an alternative, urapidil may be tried. The addition of **metoprolol 100 mg every 12 hours** can be rewarding. Do not use atenolol, nadolol, or sotalol, because their elimination is renal.

7. Cerebral hemorrhage

   BP elevation may fluctuate widely in patients with cerebral damage. Attempts to lower the BP should be considered only after assessing BP readings over several hours. Abrupt reduction of BP must be avoided. **If the BP is <180/105 mm Hg, do not attempt reduction, because it will stabilize naturally to a lower level within hours.** If the BP is >220/130 mm Hg, decrease this slowly to 180/105 mm Hg. **Reduction should not exceed 20% of pretreatment BP level. Choose nitroprusside, fenoldopam, labetalol, or urapidil.** Discuss the problem with your neurologic team. If the patient can take oral medication and there is no contraindication to a beta-blocking drug, administer **metoprolol 50 to 100 mg every 12 hours.** These agents given orally cause mild, slow lowering of BP, and postural hypotension does not occur except with labetalol, which has added alpha-blocking properties.

Consider **methyldopa 250 mg diluted in 5% dextrose in water given every 4 to 6 hours.** IV therapy is still used in some countries where newer agents are not available. The drug may cause some sedation, and this is a mild disadvantage. It is an otherwise safe therapy for IV use, because it causes only a mild reduction in BP. Drugs that cause marked unpredictable lowering of BP should be avoided. Labetalol IV causes postural hypotension and should be used only if the systolic BP is >220 mm Hg or the diastolic BP is >120 mm Hg. Labetalol can cause a precipitous fall in BP, but in most patients the drug allows a titrated reduction in BP. If an arterial line is in place, nitroprusside is the most satisfactory agent for titrated reduction in BP; this agent, however, is rarely required for the management of hypertension in the setting of cerebral hemorrhage. **For acute ischemic strokes: Lowering of BP is not recommended unless BP is >230/120 mm Hg and persists for several hours. Use nitroprusside or fenoldopam: slowly reduce to the target level of 180/105 mm Hg.**

8. Subarachnoid hemorrhage

Nimodipine improves the outcome of patients and is widely used. The combination of **metoprolol 50 to 100 mg every 12 hours and nimodipine** should suffice to control BP.

Caution:
- Diazoxide is contraindicated in patients with cerebral hemorrhage and with many other conditions.
- **Labetalol is a beta blocker and an alpha blocker; therefore, do not use it in asthmatic patients or in patients with CHF.**
- **Nitroprusside is very useful for perioperative hypertension and particularly with clipping of aneurysms; a sudden increase in BP may burst the clip.**

9. Pheochromocytoma

Clinical suspicion of this diagnosis should peak if the following symptoms and signs occur in the absence of other causes of severe hypertension:
- Severe headaches
- Profuse sweating
- Palpitations
- Sudden pallor
- Labile hypertension and postural hypotension
- History of marked fluctuation in BP, with marked eleva-

tion during anesthesia, or with antihistamine, phenothiazine, or tricyclic antidepressant use.

If the BP is dangerously elevated, phentolamine IV may be required. Discuss this drug with your resident, because it is expensive and difficult to obtain in large quantities. Phentolamine (Regitine; in Canada and the United Kingdom, Rogitine) is a direct alpha blocker and may precipitate tachyarrhythmias.

Dosage: 2.5 to 5 mg IV over 5 minutes, then 5 to 60 mg over 15 to 30 minutes (0.1–2 mg/min); or an infusion of 10 to 20 μg/kg/min.

If the drug causes tachyarrhythmias, a beta blocker is administered, if not contraindicated because of CHF or asthma. A beta blocker should not be used before alpha blockade, because unopposed stimulation of alpha receptors can cause a marked increase in BP. **The combination of nitroprusside with beta blockers is useful.**

10. Other catecholamine-induced hypertension
    - Cocaine can cause marked elevation in BP, myocardial ischemia, and MI. Administer a benzodiazepine for sedation and nitroglycerin IV to control BP if myocardial ischemia is present; a calcium antagonist such as **nifedipine 10 mg every 4 hours as needed** to control severe hypertension may be used if myocardial ischemia is not present. Beta blockers should be avoided.

Amphetamines: administer **chlorpromazine 1 mg/kg IM.**

23 | Hypertension

A patient may be admitted for the control of severe hypertension (see Chapter 22), or you may be called to see a patient who has an elevated blood pressure (BP) or an uncontrolled BP preoperatively, or you may be called to advise on BP medications before the patient's discharge from the hospital.

■ PHONE CALL

Questions

1. How high is the BP?
2. Why is the patient in the hospital?
3. Is the patient pregnant?
4. Are there features of hypertensive emergencies? (See Chapter 22.)

Orders

If there are symptoms or signs of a hypertensive emergency, order an IV of 5% dextrose in water to keep the vein open.

Inform RN

"Will be at the bedside in 15 to 30 minutes."

■ ELEVATOR THOUGHTS

What are the primary and secondary causes of hypertension?

Systolic hypertension is as important as diastolic hypertension. In more than 95% of cases no cause for the hypertension can be identified. A secondary cause prevails in only 5% of patients with hypertension, and it is important to exclude the following causes:

- Renal parenchymal disease: can be identified in 3%
- Renovascular disease: can be identified in 1%
- Pheochromocytoma: can be identified in 0.1%
- Cushing's syndrome: can be identified in 0.1%
- Primary hyperaldosteronism syndrome: can be identified in 0.1%
- Estrogens: can be identified in 0.4%
- Alcohol: can be identified in >0.2%

The Sixth Joint National Committee on Prevention, Detection, Evaluation, and Treatment of High Blood Pressure (JNC VI) has reclassified hypertension into three stages (Table 23–1). When systolic and diastolic pressures fall into different categories, the higher category should be used to classify the patient's BP status.

■ BEDSIDE

Quick Look Test

Does the patient look well (comfortable) or sick (uncomfortable or distressed)?

Vital Signs

What is the BP?
Assess the BP in both arms.

Table 23–1 □ CLASSIFICATION OF BLOOD PRESSURE FOR ADULTS AGED 18 YEARS AND OLDER*

Category	Blood pressure (mm Hg)		
	Systolic		*Diastolic*
Optimal†	<120	and	<80
Normal	<130	and	<85
High normal	130–139	or	85–89
Hypertension‡			
Stage 1	140–159	or	90–99
Stage 2	160–179	or	100–109
Stage 3	≥180	or	≥110

From the Sixth Report of the Joint National Committee on Prevention, Detection, Evaluation, and Treatment of High Blood Pressure. Arch Intern Med 1997;157:2413–2446.

*Not taking antihypertensive drugs and not acutely ill. When systolic and diastolic blood pressures fall into different categories, the higher category should be selected to classify the individual's blood pressure status. For example, 160/92 mm Hg should be classified as stage 2 hypertension, and 174/120 mm Hg as stage 3 hypertension. Isolated systolic hypertension is defined as systolic blood pressure ≥140 mm Hg and diastolic blood pressure <90 mm Hg and staged appropriately (e.g., 170/82 mm Hg is defined as stage 2 isolated systolic hypertension). In addition to classifying stages of hypertension on the basis of average blood pressure levels, clinicians should specify presence or absence of target organ disease and additional risk factors. This specificity is important for risk classification and treatment (see Table 23–2).

†Optimal blood pressure with respect to cardiovascular risk is <120/80 mm Hg. However, unusually low readings should be evaluated for clinical significance.

‡Based on the average of two or more readings taken at each of two or more visits after an initial screening.

Selective History and Chart Review

1. List the medications taken previously by the patient, and ascertain if adverse effects were caused by any of these medications.
2. A beta-blocking drug cannot be used if the patient has asthma or severe bronchitis, so it is important to identify these conditions.
3. Has the patient discontinued medication that can cause rebound hypertension, i.e., clonidine, guanfacine, methyldopa, and occasionally, beta blockers, calcium antagonists, angiotensin-converting enzyme (ACE) inhibitors?
4. Is the patient on medication that may interact with antihypertensive agents, e.g., nonsteroidal anti-inflammatory drugs and nasal decongestants?
5. Is there a history of drug abuse, e.g., cocaine or amphetamines?
6. Is there a past history of renal failure? Volume overload in patients with renal failure may be the cause of resistant or accelerated hypertension. If renal failure is present and the serum creatinine level is >2.3 mg/dl (203 μmol/L), use furosemide and not hydrochlorothiazide, because the latter drug is ineffective in patients with a lowered glomerular filtration rate. In patients with a history of angina, palpitations, or previous myocardial infarction, a beta-blocking drug would be a good choice, used either alone or in combination with an ACE inhibitor to maximize cardioprotection. Inquire about uncontrolled diabetes or about hypoglycemic episodes, which would contraindicate the use of a beta-blocking drug.

Selective Physical Examination

1. Assess for left ventricular hypertrophy; an S_4 gallop is commonly present; an aortic diastolic murmur may occur with severe hypertension.
2. Palpate the femoral pulses, and if these appear low, take the BP in the arms and legs and assess for coarctation of the aorta.
3. Palpate the kidneys for enlargement, which may indicate polycystic kidney or unilateral kidney disease.
4. Listen for renal bruits.
5. Check the fundi for exudates, hemorrhages, papilledema, arterial narrowing, and arteriovenous nicking.
6. Assess the thyroid; patients with thyrotoxicosis may have systolic hypertension.
7. Cushing's syndrome is manifested by truncal obesity, prominent purple-red striae over the abdomen, and weakness of

the quadriceps muscles; the patient has difficulty standing quickly from a squatting position and may have a history of difficulty climbing stairs.

■ MANAGEMENT

1. If the patient is not being advised about salt restriction by a dietitian, request a consultation with a dietitian for briefing on foods that contain hidden sodium. It is surprising how many patients claim to use little salt, but use garlic salt, meat tenderizer, canned foods, dill pickles, and other foods that have a high sodium content.
2. Assess the electrocardiogram for left ventricular hypertrophy, ventricular strain, and left atrial enlargement (see Figs. 5–25 and 5–26); if this is present, more aggressive therapy is required.
3. Check the levels of serum potassium and creatinine, the level of cholesterol, and the levels of low- and high-density lipoproteins.
4. The JNC VI guidelines for drug therapy specify the importance of defining the presence of target organ damage, coexisting disease, and risk factors (Table 23–2). Initial therapy with a diuretic or a beta blocker is further endorsed. If a diuretic is not chosen as initial therapy, it should be the second-choice drug.

Antihypertensive Drugs of Choice

Beta Blockers. Use a beta-blocking drug as first choice in most patients, if this has not been done and if there is no contraindication to the use of these agents. Beta blockers decrease BP, but most important, they reduce cardiac ejection velocity and protect the arteries and the heart. The beneficial effects of beta-blocking drugs on the arterial tree become obvious when the physician recognizes that, in patients with aortic dissection, the BP must be lowered by nitroprusside or a similar agent, but that a beta-blocking drug is necessary even if the systolic BP is <110 mm Hg. The beta-blocking drug used in this context prevents further dissection. In all patients with moderate or severe hypertension, beta-blocking drugs can prevent further damage to the arteries, propropagation or rupture of atheromatous plaques in the renal and coronary arteries, and aneurysmal dilation of the aorta.

The beta-blocking drug of choice is usually **metoprolol 50 to 100 mg every 12 hours or metoprolol succinate (Toprol XL) 50 to 100 mg once daily;** this preparation lowers BP for 24 hours and is a most convenient formulation. Alternatives are **acebutolol 100 to 200 mg twice daily, timolol 5 to 10 mg twice daily, or**

Table 23-2 □ RISK STRATIFICATION AND TREATMENT*

Blood Pressure Stages (mm Hg)	Risk Group A (no risk factors; no TOD/CCD†)	Risk Group B (at least 1 risk factor, not including diabetes; no TOD/CCD)	Risk Group C (TOD/CCD and/or diabetes, with or without other risk factors)
High-normal (130-139/85-89)	Lifestyle modification	Lifestyle modification	Drug therapy§
Stage 1 (140-159/90-99)	Lifestyle modification (up to 12 mo)	Lifestyle modification‡ (up to 6 mo)	Drug therapy
Stages 2 and 3 (≥160/≥100)	Drug therapy	Drug therapy	Drug therapy

From the Sixth Report of the Joint National Committee on Prevention, Detection, Evaluation, and Treatment of High Blood Pressure. Arch Intern Med 1997;157:2413-2446.

*For example, a patient with diabetes and a blood pressure of 142/94 mm Hg plus left ventricular hypertrophy should be classified as having stage 1 hypertension with target organ disease (left ventricular hypertrophy) and with another major risk factor (diabetes). This patient would be categorized as stage 1, risk group C and recommended for immediate initiation of pharmacologic treatment. Lifestyle modification should be adjunctive therapy for all patients recommended for pharmacologic therapy.

†TOD/CCD indicates target organ disease/clinical cardiovascular disease.

‡For patients with multiple risk factors, clinicians should consider drugs as initial therapy plus lifestyle modifications.

§For those with heart failure, renal insufficiency, or diabetes.

atenolol 50 to 100 mg once daily. The antihypertensive effects of beta blockers are excellent in white patients of all ages. They are more effective than calcium antagonists and ACE inhibitors in older white patients. They are also fairly effective in young black patients and are superior to ACE inhibitors in this group. Only calcium antagonists appear to be more effective than beta blockers in younger black patients. Beta blockers are not recommended in older black patients, because they are not usually effective. In this subset of patients, a diuretic or a calcium antagonist is superior to beta blockers and ACE inhibitors. **Thus, beta blockers are recommended as initial therapy in all patients except in elderly black patients.** If fatigue, marked tiredness, or sexual dysfunction occurs, albeit rarely, the beta blocker should be replaced; note that the incidence of these three adverse effects is similar for diuretics, and sexual dysfunction is even greater with diuretics.

The antihypertensive effects of beta blockers are complemented by calcium antagonists; thus, the combination of a beta blocker with amlodipine (Norvasc) or nifedipine (Procardia XL or Adalat XL) constitutes appropriate therapy when a combination is required. Also, the addition of a diuretic to a beta blocker provides adequate antihypertensive effects in most patients with moderate hypertension. I highly recommend the combination of a very small dose of a beta blocker and a diuretic, which also is endorsed by the JNC VI; an appropriate agent, **Ziac (bisoprolol 5–10 mg + hydrochlorothiazide [HCTZ] 6.25 mg)** is approved by the Food and Drug Administration (FDA) as first-line therapy for hypertension.

In general it is advisable to use combinations with small doses of two drugs rather than exposing the patient to the risk of adverse effects from high doses of a single agent. Always, each agent of a combination drug should be tried before the selection of the combination.

The combination of a beta blocker, a calcium antagonist, and a diuretic is often effective in patients with severe hypertension.

Diuretics. The JNC VI advises a diuretic as first choice in patients without ischemic heart disease and in patients with coexisting disease or organ damage that does not dictate the use of other agents. In this large subset of patients (except in elderly black people), I prefer a small dose of a beta blocker as first choice, e.g., **Toprol XL 50 mg,** or **atenolol 25 mg (maximum 50 mg);** if BP reduction is not excellent or if fatigue and other adverse effects occur, a diuretic should replace the beta blocker. A diuretic such as **HCTZ 12.5 mg, to a maximum of 25 mg daily,** or a preparation that retains potassium, e.g., Moduretic (a combination of HCTZ and amiloride) half a tablet daily should suffice in most patients with mild hypertension in whom a beta blocker is contraindicated. A diuretic is more effective in black patients age 65 to 75 years than in whites of the same age. Diuretics may, however, cause frequency of micturition, which can be bothersome in older men with prostatic enlargement and men and women with contracted bladder or with stress incontinence. Small-dose diuretics, however, remain extremely useful when combined with other agents, in particular beta blockers and ACE inhibitors. A diuretic is always required when an alpha blocker or a centrally acting drug such as methyldopa is administered; these agents virtually always cause sodium and water retention, which leads to diminution of antihypertensive effects.

ACE Inhibitors. These are excellent antihypertensive agents that can be used as monotherapy; their effects are considerably enhanced by diuretics. ACE inhibitors have been shown to be effective in white patients below age 65, and they have significant antihypertensive effects in whites older than 65. **They are, however, not sufficiently effective in black patients of any age, and their use should be discouraged except in diabetics with proteinuria.** ACE inhibitors are equally effective in whites at all ages.

Commonly used ACE inhibitors include
1. **Captopril (Capoten) 25 to 50 mg twice daily**
2. **Enalapril (Vasotec) 5 to 20 mg once daily with occasional twice-daily use**
3. **Lisinopril (Prinivil and Zestril) 5 to 30 mg once daily**
4. **Lotensin (Benazepril) 5 to 20 mg once daily**
5. **Cilazapril (Inhibace) 1 to 5 mg once daily**
6. **Fosinopril (Monopril) 10 to 40 mg once daily**
7. **Perindopril (Coversyl) 2 to 8 mg once daily**
8. **Quinapril (Accupril) 5 to 40 mg once daily**
9. **Ramipril (Altace) 2.5 to 15 mg once daily**

Angiotensin II Receptor Blockers. These agents specifically block the angiotensin II receptor AT_1, which causes blockade of circulating angiotensin II and of that produced by tissues; they have been shown to have antihypertensive effects equal to or slightly greater than that of ACE inhibitors. **The major advantage of these agents is that they do not cause cough, and angioedema occurs rarely compared with ACE inhibitors.** Available agents include
1. **Losartan (Cozaar) 50 to 100 mg once daily** (in elderly patients, 25 mg once daily). Losartan is eliminated by the kidney and bile; it has a short half-life of 6 to 9 hours. It is the only AT_1 receptor blocker that increases uric acid excretion. Hyzaar is a combination of losartan 50 mg and HCTZ 25 mg, and dosage is 1 tablet daily.
2. **Candesartan (Atacand, Amias) 4 to 16 mg once daily (maximum 32 mg).** Renal elimination is 60%; bile elimination, 40%. It has a medium half-life of 3 to 11 hours.
3. **Eprosartan (Teveten) 200 to 400 mg twice daily.** Bile elimination, 90%; it has a short half-life of 5 to 7 hours.

4. **Irbesartan (Avapro, Aprovel) 75 to 300 mg once daily.** Bile elimination, 80%; it has a half-life of 11 to 15 hours.
5. **Telmisartan (Micardis) 20 to 80 mg once daily.** Elimination in the feces, 98%; it has a long half-life of 24 hours.
6. **Valsartan (Diovan) 40 to 160 mg once daily (maximum 320 mg).** Bile elimination, 70%; half-life is 9 hours.

Calcium Antagonists. These agents are effective in patients with all grades of hypertension; the higher the BP, the greater the reduction obtained with calcium antagonists. They are especially effective in blacks of all ages; they are superior to all other agents in this group. In older black patients, a combination of a calcium antagonist and a small dose of diuretic is especially effective. Calcium antagonists are also effective in older white patients; the antihypertensive effects are equal to that of beta blockers in older white patients. They are less effective, however, than beta blockers or ACE inhibitors in younger white patients.

Commonly used calcium antagonists include

1. **Amlodipine (Norvasc) 5 to 10 mg once daily**
2. **Diltiazem (Cardizem CD) 120 to 300 mg once daily**
3. **Nifedipine (Procardia XL and Adalat XL) 30 to 60 mg once daily**
4. **Verapamil (Isoptin SR) 120 to 240 mg once daily; half of the 240-mg tablet is often effective for the control of mild hypertension, especially in blacks, but constipation may be a bothersome adverse effect. Verapamil (Covera-HS, Chronovera)** is an extended-release formulation designed to provide extra reduction of BP and heart rate in the morning relative to other times, but this strategy is of doubtful value. **Dosage: 180 to 360 mg at bedtime.**

The short-acting rapid-release preparations, i.e., nifedipine capsules and diltiazem and verapamil tablets, are not recommended for the management of hypertension or angina, because of controversies relating to the safety of some of these rapid-acting formulations.

Alpha Blockers. These agents do not protect from the development of left ventricular hypertrophy; *they increase the size of aneurysms and are contraindicated if aneurysms develop.* They increase cardiac ejection velocity and may cause palpitations or significant increase in heart rate; these effects, as well as retention of sodium and water, are major disadvantages of alpha blockers. *The JNC VI has inappropriately recommended alpha blockers as first-line therapy.* In the second edition of *Cardiac Drug Therapy 1988,* I warned against their use. **Recently the ACC has recommended that their use be curtailed** because they have been shown to increase cardiac events, particurlarly CHF. Labetalol has both alpha- and beta-blocking properties and is the only beta-blocking drug that causes postural hypotension. This agent has also been reported to cause life-threatening hepatic necrosis and has no advantage over a pure beta blocker.

Hypertension and Pregnancy

Most drugs, including antihypertensive agents, are contraindicated during the first 14 weeks of pregnancy. Several agents used during the second and third trimesters may affect growth and functional development of the fetus or cause toxic effects on fetal tissues. Some agents may cause adverse effects on labor or may affect the newborn.

Agents that can be used from the 16th week to delivery include
- Beta blockers; **atenolol 25 to 50 mg once daily or metoprolol 50 to 100 mg twice daily. During lactation propranolol is the best choice, because the concentration in breast milk is comparatively low.**
- **Methyldopa 250 mg twice daily (a maximum of 500 mg twice daily);** assess for orthostatic hypotension and depression.
- **Hydralazine 25 mg twice daily, increasing to 50 mg 3 times daily if needed.** The addition of a beta blocker to hydralazine 25 mg three times daily should suffice in most patients. Hydralazine may cause dizziness, postural hypotension, and palpitations, and if used for more than several months, a lupus syndrome can occur; fetal thrombocytopenia has been reported.

Agents that have been used in the past but that are not presently favored include thiazide diuretics. Thiazides may cause neonatal thrombocytopenia. Because preeclampsia is associated with reduced plasma volume, diuretics are contraindicated. Furosemide is contraindicated during pregnancy.

Nifedipine has been used successfully to lower BP 4 to 6 weeks before delivery in patients with severe hypertension that is resistant to therapy.

Caution: The combination of nifedipine and magnesium sulfate may cause marked lowering of BP, and the combination should be avoided.

Nifedipine 10 mg 3 times daily or Procardia XL (or Adalat XL) 30 to 60 mg once daily should suffice in many patients during the few weeks before labor.

Agents contraindicated in pregnancy include ACE inhibitors, nitroprusside, furosemide, diltiazem, verapamil, and reserpine.

Study Section: Drug Therapy for Hypertension

Strive for monotherapy in the treatment of systolic or diastolic hypertension whenever possible. The ideal choice is a drug that is effective for 24 hours when given once daily and that produces few or no adverse effects.

Each of the four classes of drugs recommended for initial therapy has unique pharmacologic properties that can be tailored to the hemodynamic, neurohormonal, and volume-related factors and the concomitant diseases that may exist in certain subsets of hypertensive patients.

- White patients up to age 75 and blacks below age 65 respond well to beta blockers.
- Diuretics have been shown in many studies to be effective in white and black patients older than age 60.
- Calcium antagonists are effective in older whites and blacks at all ages.
- ACE inhibitors are effective in young whites and moderately effective in older whites but are not effective in blacks at any age.

■ BETA BLOCKERS

A hallmark study by Materson and coworkers comparing six antihypertensive agents indicates that

- Beta blockers are effective in young and older white patients. They are particularly more effective than diuretics and calcium antagonists in younger patients and just as effective as calcium antagonists in older white patients.
- Beta blockers are effective in younger blacks.
- Only elderly black patients do not qualify for a trial of a beta-blocking drug because at this age, diuretics or calcium antagonists are more effective.

Beta blockers are considered first-choice therapy for the management of hypertension in several subsets of patients in whom no contraindications to beta blockade exist.

Indications

- In white patients up to age 75, these agents are effective in >65%, and in younger blacks atenolol was shown by Materson and coworkers to be effective in 47% of patients.
- They are indicated in elderly patients with hypertensive, hypertrophic "cardiomyopathy" with impaired ventricular relaxation, because diuretics and ACE inhibitors are contraindicated in these patients.
- Beta blockers are first choice in patients with ischemic heart disease manifested by angina or silent ischemia and following myocardial infarction, and in individuals at high risk for the occurrence or complications of ischemic heart disease.

- They are first-choice agents in patients with supraventricular or ventricular arrhythmias. Beta blockers are the only category of antihypertensive agent that decreases the rate and force of myocardial contraction and ejection velocity. This effect has been shown to decrease the rate of aneurysmal dilatation in patients with Marfan syndrome. Beta blockers are an essential part of the treatment of patients with dissecting aneurysm. The beneficial effects of beta blockers in arteries prone to rupture logically dictate that these agents may be useful in decreasing the risk of cerebral hemorrhage and other complications of cardiovascular disease.
- Patients with left ventricular hypertrophy are at high risk for sudden death; beta blockers are the only antihypertensive agents that have the potential to prevent sudden death in this subset of patients. ACE inhibitors prevent left ventricular hypertrophy but have not been shown to prevent sudden death.
- They are of particular value in patients with increased adrenergic activity, including the younger age group, who often have high plasma norepinephrine levels, and in patients with hyperkinetic heart syndrome, alcohol withdrawal hypertension, or the hyperdynamic beta-adrenergic circulatory state, with labile or elevated blood pressure and palpitations.
- They are indicated in patients with migraine and hypertension.
- Orthostatic hypertension—i.e., exaggerated increase in diastolic pressure on standing—usually indicates increased adrenergic tone, and beta blockers produce a salutary effect in these patients.
- Patients prone to postural hypotension may benefit because these agents, unlike all other antihypertensives, do not usually decrease systemic vascular resistance.
- Beta blockers are first choice for patients with aneurysms.
- In females over age 55, beta blockers are a rational choice because the incidence of myocardial rupture is high in hypertensive women who sustain a first infarction. Beta blockers protect sufficiently from myocardial rupture to warrant their use in patients considered at risk. The combination of a beta-blocking agent and low-dose diuretics is advisable if prevention of osteoporosis also requires therapeutic consideration.

Dosage

See Appendix Table C–4.

Choosing a Beta Blocker

The beta-blocking drugs have important subtle differences in pharmacologic and adverse effect profiles that may dictate which beta blocker is best for a given clinical situation. Also, switching from one beta-blocking agent to another may result in the disappearance of adverse effects and/or improvement of salutary effects. The following guidelines are suggested:

- Depression with propranolol: switch to metoprolol, acebutolol, atenolol, or timolol; however, depression can occur rarely with all beta blockers, including atenolol, which attains low brain concentration.
- Mild memory impairment with propranolol: switch to metoprolol, acebutolol, or timolol.
- Insomnia with propranolol or pindolol: switch to atenolol or timolol.
- Refractory smoker: switch from propranolol to metoprolol, acebutolol, or timolol, to ensure salutary effects including prolongation of life.
- Vivid dreams with lipophilic beta blocker: switch to timolol or acebutolol.
- Decreased ability to perform complex tasks with atenolol: switch to metoprolol: Toprol XL has a 24-hour duration of action.
- Marked fatigue with atenolol or sotalol: switch to acebutolol, metoprolol, or timolol.
- Sedation with atenolol: change to metoprolol or timolol.
- Symptomatic sinus bradycardia with propranolol or other beta blocker: switch to acebutolol.
- Moderate hyperlipidemia, total cholesterol >240 mg/dl (6.2 mmol/L), LDL cholesterol >160 mg/dl (4 mmol/L), HDL <35/mg dl (0.9 mmol/L): avoid propranolol; switch to acebutolol plus drug therapy for hypercholesterolemia.
- Renal failure, serum creatinine >2.3 mg/dl (203 μmol/L): extend the dosing interval of hydrophilic renal-excreted agents, i.e., atenolol, nadolol, and sotalol, to alternate-day or change to acebutolol, metoprolol, or timolol.

The above points indicate that metoprolol is the beta blocker of choice.

■ ANGIOTENSIN-CONVERTING ENZYME INHIBITORS

Angiotensin-converting enzyme (ACE) inhibitors have provided a major advance in the management of hypertension. They are useful agents for initial therapy in some subsets of hypertensive patients. These inhibitors of ACE prevent the conversion of angiotensin I to the potent vasoconstrictor angiotensin II. This action causes arteriolar dilatation and a fall in total systemic vascular resistance; diminished sympathetic activity, causing vasodilatation (but heart rate does not increase as with other vasodilators); and reduction in aldosterone secretion, promoting sodium excretion and potassium retention.

Indications

- ACE inhibitors are most effective in patients with high renin hypertension and especially in white patients below age 65. Materson and associates showed a 55% antihypertensive response in younger and older whites, but a poor effect in young or old blacks.
- ACE inhibitors are indicated in hypertensive patients with left ventricular dysfunction or heart failure
- ACE inhibitors are indicated in diabetic patients with hypertension of all grades. Mild hypertension (systolic CBP 140–160 mm Hg, diastolic BP 90–95 mm Hg) in diabetic individuals must be aggressively treated, preferably with an ACE inhibitor.

Advantages

- ACE inhibitors have been shown to cause regression and prevention of left ventricular hypertrophy. Other vasodilators may not prevent the development of hypertrophy, presumably because they cause sympathetic stimulation, which results in an increase in heart rate and increased myocardial oxygen requirement.
- These agents have been shown to reduce mortality in patients with New York Heart Association (NYHA) class II, III, or IV heart failure, and they are first choice, along with diuretics, in the management of hypertensive patients who have heart failure or left ventricular systolic dysfunction. In addition, they blunt diuretic-induced hypokalemia and hypomagnesemia.
- ACE inhibitors do not alter lipid levels or cause glucose intolerance. Thus, they are advisable in patients with hyperlipidemia and/or diabetes mellitus. They decrease diabetic proteinuria and appear to preserve nephron life in patients with diabetes. Hyperkalemia may occur in patients with renal failure and in diabetic patients with hyporeninemic hypoaldosteronism, however, and caution is necessary.

Contraindications

- Renal artery stenosis of a solitary kidney or severe bilateral renal artery stenosis
- Severe anemia
- Aortic stenosis
- Hypertrophic and restrictive cardiomyopathy

- Hypertensive, hypertrophic "cardiomyopathy" of the elderly with impaired ventricular relaxation
- Severe carotid artery stenosis
- Hypertensive patients with concomitant angina
- Uric acid renal calculi
- Pregnancy and breastfeeding
- Porphyria
- Relative contraindications: patients with collagen vascular diseases or concomitant use of immunosuppressives, because neutropenia and rare agranulocytosis observed with ACE inhibitors appear to occur mainly in this subset of patients.

Adverse Effects

These include hyperkalemia in patients with renal failure, pruritus and rash in about 10% of patients, and loss of taste in approximately 7% of patients. A rare but important adverse effect is angioedema of the face, mouth, or larynx, which may occur in approximately 0.2% of treated patients and can be fatal. Mouth ulcers, neurologic dysfunction, gastrointestinal disturbances, and proteinuria occur in about 1% of patients with preexisting renal disease; neutropenia and agranulocytosis are rare and occur mainly in patients with serious intercurrent illness, particularly immunologic disturbances, altered immune response, or collagen vascular disease. Cough occurs in about 20% of treated patients; wheezing, myalgia, muscle cramps, hair loss, impotence or decreased libido, hepatitis or occurrence of antinuclear antibodies, and pemphigus occasionally occur.

Dosage

See Appendix Table C–5.

■ CALCIUM ANTAGONISTS

The BP-lowering effects of calcium antagonists are due to peripheral arteriolar dilatation. Normally, calcium enters the cells through slow calcium channels and binds to the regulatory protein troponin, removing the inhibitory action of tropomyosin, which, in the presence of adenosine triphosphate, allows interaction between myosin and actin, resulting in contraction of the muscle cell. Calcium antagonists inhibit calcium entry into cells by blocking voltage-dependent calcium channels, thereby inhibiting contractility of vascular smooth muscle, thus producing vasodilatation.

The dihydropyridine calcium antagonists, i.e., amlodipine, nifedipine, felodipine, nicardipine, and nitrendipine, are more potent vasodilators and more effective antihypertensive agents than verapamil; diltiazem has modest vasodilator properties, and high doses are usually required to achieve adequate lowering of blood pressure. In addition, verapamil and diltiazem have added electrophysiologic effects on the sinoatrial and atrioventricular (AV) nodes and can produce bradycardia, sinus arrest, and AV block in susceptible individuals with disease of the sinus and AV nodes.

Advantages

- Calcium antagonists do not usually lower the blood pressure of normotensive individuals.
- They can be used without a diuretic because they have a mild natriuretic effect; their effectiveness may or may not be enhanced by adding a diuretic.
- Calcium antagonists are useful in hypertensive patients with coexisting angina and peripheral vascular disease or when beta blockers produce adverse effects or are contraindicated.
- They do not cause abnormalities of lipid or glucose metabolism nor influence potassium and uric acid excretion, and they have advantages over diuretics in this subset of patients.
- Nifedipine has shown modest but significant regression and inhibition of progression of atheromatous obstruction of coronary arteries in patients with coronary artery disease.
- Most calcium antagonists prevent left ventricular hypertrophy and cause regression, although some reports show a lack of salutary effects.

Adverse Effects

- Calcium antagonists, particularly amlodipine, cause no serious adverse effects, and their use requires virtually no laboratory monitoring, unlike diuretics and ACE inhibitors.
- Although nifedipine and amlodipine have no electrophysiologic effects, verapamil and diltiazem can occasionally produce bradycardia, sinus arrest, and AV block in susceptible individuals.
- Verapamil has significant negative inotropic activity and can precipitate heart failure.
- Diltiazem has mild negative inotropic activity.
- Although it is relatively safe to combine amlodipine or nifedipine with a beta blocker in the management of hypertension and of hypertension associated with angina, verapamil must not be added to a beta blocker, and diltiazem must be used with caution.
- Nifedipine does not alter digoxin levels; however, verapamil

and diltiazem cause about a 47% increase in digoxin level
and may rarely precipitate bradycardia and AV block.

Dosage

See Appendix Table C–4.

■ VASOPEPTIDASE INHIBITORS

The vasopeptidase inhibitors (VPIs) are a new class of antihypertensive agents (e.g., omapatrilat) that are a welcome addition
to our armamentarium. VPIs cause simultaneous inhibition of the
following:

1. Neutral endopeptidase, which results in enhancement of
   vasodilatory peptides and produces vasodilation, sodium
   excretion, decreased aldosterone, and inhibition of sympathetic activity
2. Angiotensin-converting enzyme

In small clinical trials, the BP-lowering effect of omapatrilat
appears to be equal or superior to that of ACE inhibitors regardless of age or race. Unfortunately, the VPIs available for clinical
trials appear to have a higher incidence of angioedema than ACE
inhibitors (see page 326).

24 | Syncope

Syncope is defined as transient loss of consciousness associated with a loss of postural tone caused by a sudden fall in systolic blood pressure (BP) to <70 mm Hg that interrupts cerebral blood flow for >8 seconds. Syncope is a common problem representing up to 1% of emergency room diagnoses.

■ PHONE CALL

Questions

1. Was there a definite loss of consciousness for a few seconds?
2. What are the vital signs?
3. Did the patient complain of palpitations?
4. Did the patient feel a warning of an impending faint?
5. Did the patient have seizures, incontinence, or tongue biting, indicating epilepsy?
6. Did the patient sustain injuries?
   Injuries do not occur with a simple faint, and they indicate a serious problem.

Orders

1. Obtain an electrocardiogram (ECG) and a long rhythm strip of leads II and V$_1$.
2. If second-degree atrioventricular (AV) block or complete heart block is considered, attach the patient to a cardiac monitor and call the resident.

Inform RN

"Will arrive at the bedside in . . . minutes."

■ ELEVATOR THOUGHTS

What are the causes of syncope?
1. An obvious cardiac cause can be defined by patient history, physical examination, ECG, and Holter monitoring in about 10% of cases (Table 24–1).
2. Vasodepressor, vasovagal syncope (neurocardiogenic syn-

Table 24–1 □ **CARDIAC CAUSES OF SYNCOPE**

Tachyarrhythmias	Sustained and nonsustained ventricular tachycardia
	Torsades de pointes
	Atrial fibrillation
	Supraventricular tachycardia
	Long QT syndrome
	Wolff-Parkinson-White syndrome
	Pacemaker mediated
Bradyarrhythmias	Sinus node dysfunction (sick sinus syndrome)
Carotid sinus syncope	
Obstruction to stroke volume	Aortic stenosis
	Hypertrophic cardiomyopathy
	Tight mitral stenosis
	Atrial myxoma or thrombus
	Cardiac tamponade
	Prosthetic valve dysfunction
	Pulmonary embolism
	Pulmonary hypertension
	Pulmonary stenosis
Others	Mitral valve prolapse
	Inferior myocardial infarction
	Coronary artery spasm
	Aortic dissection

cope) accounts for >30% of cases of syncope and must be excluded by a relevant history (Table 24–2).

3. Unexplained syncope constitutes a large group (30%).
4. Syncope may be the clue to life-threatening cardiac diseases, including the long QT syndrome commonly misdiagnosed in children and adolescents as seizures or simple fainting.
5. Postural hypotension is an important cause of syncope and must be quickly excluded (Fig. 24–1).

■ MAJOR THREAT TO LIFE

- Cardiac conditions, e.g., severe aortic stenosis, obstructive cardiomyopathy, acute inferior infarction, and Mobitz type II or third-degree AV block
- If bodily injury occurred without a warning

■ BEDSIDE

Quick Look Test

Does the patient look well (comfortable), sick (uncomfortable or distressed), or critical (about to die)?

Table 24–2 □ NONCARDIAC* CAUSES OF SYNCOPE

1. Vasodepressor (vasovagal) or neurocardiogenic causes (>30%)
2. Postural hypotension (10%)
   A. Decreased preload
      (1) Venous pooling, caused by extensive varicose veins, postexercise vasodilation, venous angioma in the leg
      (2) Drugs: nitrates, diuretics, and angiotensin-converting enzyme inhibitors
      (3) Decreased blood volume: blood loss
      (4) Dehydration: vomiting, diarrhea, excessive sweating, and Addison's disease
   B. Drugs
      (1) Alpha blockers
      (2) Ganglion blockers
      (3) Bromocriptine
      (4) L-Dopa
      (5) Nifedipine
   C. Neurogenic decrease of autonomic activity
      (1) Bedrest
      (2) Neuropathies and diabetes
      (3) Shy-Drager syndrome
      (4) Idiopathic causes
3. Cerebrovascular disease
   A. Transient ischemic attack
   B. Subclavian steal
   C. Basilar artery migraine
   D. Cervical arthritis, atlanto-occipital dislocation, compression of the vertebral artery
4. Situational causes
   A. Cough, sneeze, micturition, and defecation
5. Other causes
   A. Drugs or alcohol
   B. Hypoglycemia
   C. Hypoxemia
   D. Hypoventilation
   E. Hysterical reaction
6. Unexplained

*No electrical or structural heart disease.

Selective History and Selective Physical Examination

A detailed relevant history should verify or exclude the simple faint. Many attacks over several years or since childhood indicate a diagnosis of fainting spells, but the long QT syndrome should be excluded by the assessment of an ECG. Verify the presence or absence of a subtle warning that lasts a few seconds. Conditions such as sick sinus syndrome may or may not give a few seconds' warning.

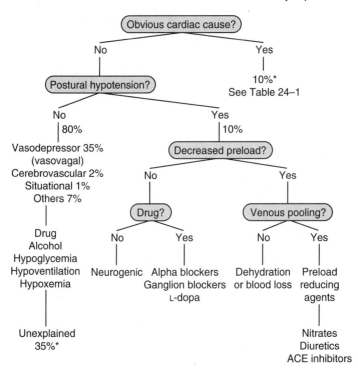

Figure 24-1 □ Algorithm for the assessment of syncope. *Approximate incidence. ACE = angiotensin-converting enzymes. (Redrawn from Khan, M Gabriel: Heart Disease Diagnosis and Therapy: A Practical Approach. Baltimore, Williams & Wilkins, 1996, p 530.)

1. Assess BP with the patient recumbent for >3 minutes and then on standing to elicit postural hypotension.
2. Listen for bruits over the subclavian and carotid arteries.
3. Perform a full cardiovascular examination (see Chapters 3 and 4).
4. Assess for aortic stenosis, hypertrophic cardiomyopathy, mitral stenosis, mitral valve prolapse, and prosthetic heart valve.
5. Assess for tachyarrhythmias and bradyarrhythmias.
6. Assess for pulmonary embolism, which may present with syncope.
7. Vasodepressor or vasovagal syncope and all known causes of syncope should be methodically excluded (see Table 24–1 and Fig. 24–1).
8. Dizziness is often a feature of presyncope and has several

causes that are difficult to determine. Figure 24–2 indicates steps to consider.

Neurocardiogenic Syncope. A good history identifies a faint and can prevent expensive and time-consuming investigations. Look for *gradual onset–gradual offset syncope.* A simple faint never occurs with the patient in the recumbent position. Precipitating circumstances of simple faint include exhaustion; hunger; prolonged standing or sitting in a hot, crowded room; sudden, severe pain or trauma; venipuncture; fright; and sudden emotional stress. There is virtually always a warning period spanning seconds to minutes. One or more of the following heralds the faint: weakness, nausea, abdominal discomfort, diaphoresis, unsteadi-

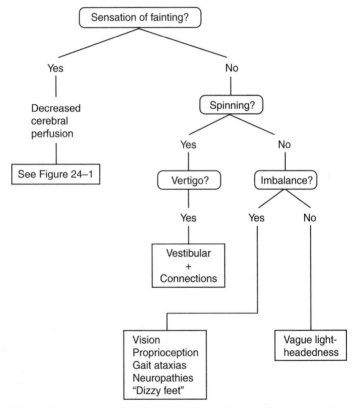

Figure 24–2 □ Algorithm for evaluating patients with dizziness. (Redrawn from Khan, M Gabriel: Heart Disease Diagnosis and Therapy: A Practical Approach. Baltimore: Williams & Wilkins, 1996, p 533.)

ness, and blurring of vision. Vertigo is not a symptom associated with a faint.

A combination of vasodepressor and vasovagal (bradycardic) features results in the faint; the vasodepressor component, with sudden reduction in BP, plays an important role in loss of consciousness. Bradycardia plays a secondary role. Marked vasodilatation causes temporary but profound hypotension. The marked vasodilatation is caused by the inhibition of sympathetic vasoconstrictor activity at the very moment when arteriolar vasoconstriction is necessary to combat the marked fall in BP. An increase in myocardial contractility occurs 2 to 4 minutes before the onset of syncope. Return of consciousness occurs in a few seconds to 1 minute if the individual remains supine with the legs elevated.

The exclusion of epilepsy is straightforward; i.e., look for *abrupt onset–gradual offset*. The aura, if any, in epilepsy is transient but tells a story; convulsive movements occur with loss of consciousness. Injuries, including lip and tongue biting, and incontinence with a prolonged postictal state, are hallmarks.

Long QT Syndrome. Children and young adults with mysterious fainting episodes or "blackouts" are often misdiagnosed as having epilepsy or simple fainting and can end up with an unexplained sudden death. The average age of patients with these preventable deaths is between 8 and 16 years, although risk continues through adulthood. These blackouts are usually caused by torsades de pointes, which is transient and reverts back to normal rhythm.

Look for *abrupt onset–abrupt offset syncope*. Episodes are precipitated by acute stress, anger or fright, the sound of a siren, thunder, telephone ringing or a clock alarm, and vigorous exertion. A family history positive for fainting spells or unexplained sudden death is often present. This condition is diagnosable only by an ECG, a simple, inexpensive test. Once the diagnosis is made, the whole family should be screened. Congenital deafness and long QT is a rare form of the syndrome.

Postural Hypotension. Several cardiac medications may cause postural hypotension, in particular in elderly patients. Perform the following:

1. Check the BP with the patient recumbent for at least 3 minutes and then standing; a reduction in systolic BP of ≥ 20 mm Hg represents orthostatic hypotension.
2. Check for evidence of a decrease in preload. Preload-reducing agents include nitrates, angiotensin-converting enzyme (ACE) inhibitors, and alpha$_1$ blockers. Blood loss and dehydration are obvious causes; a hidden cause of the latter is Addison's disease.
3. Inquire about the use of medications that cause arterial dilatation, in particular alpha$_1$-adrenergic blockers such as pra-

zosin and labetalol, ganglion-blocking drugs, L-dopa, bromocriptine, and rarely, nifedipine.
4. If drug use is excluded, postural hypotension may be caused by autonomic imbalance or neurologic diseases. Neuropathy, especially due to diabetes, Shy-Drager syndrome, and other neurologic problems, must be excluded (see Fig. 24–1).

■ DIAGNOSTIC TESTING

Routine Investigations

- Complete blood count, electrolytes, and creatinine
- ECG with rhythm strip

Other Investigations

Head-up Tilt Testing. Although commonly done in tertiary hospitals, it is not necessary for confirming the diagnosis of neurocardiogenic syncope. Tilt testing causes minor degrees of asystole, but this can be occasionally prolonged and can cause cerebral damage, **and several deaths have been reported. It is illogical to perform this test to verify the diagnosis of a benign condition that can be obtained from a skillful history.** For example, there is a case report of a surgeon who had a syncopal episode while performing surgery, and during a tilt test he had a stroke. A $60 million lawsuit is pending.

Tilt testing has a small role in patients with no detectable heart disease and "truly unexplained" syncope (see Fig. 24–1).

In truly unexplained syncope, head-up tilt testing and electrophysiologic (EP) evaluation are complementary and can identify the underlying cause in approximately 74% of patients presenting with unexplained syncope.

Nonetheless, the tilt test precipitates hypotension that can be dangerous in patients with ischemic heart disease (IHD), cerebrovascular disease, aortic stenosis, and hypertrophic and dilated cardiomyopathy. Because cortical damage, prolonged cardiac arrest, and several deaths have occurred, causing many lawsuits in the United States, the test must not be considered noninvasive. Isoproterenol infusion is not innocuous and has the disadvantage of dosing difficulties. In Europe, nitrolingual spray is used instead of isoproterenol. Most important, a positive tilt test should not be used as an indication for electrical pacing, because without pacing syncope may not recur over the next year or two. The natural history of unexplained syncope poses several difficulties in assessing the results of poorly run clinical trials.

Electrophysiologic Studies. An EP study is useful in revealing a cardiac cause in approximately 12% of patients with unexplained syncope; >21% of patients with negative studies are subsequently diagnosed as having intermittent high-degree AV block or sinus node disease. An EP study is not a sensitive test to expose symptomatic bradycardia.

■ MANAGEMENT

1. Orthostatic hypotension
   - Review underlying causes outlined previously.
   - Autonomic neuropathies and autonomic failure may respond to increased sodium intake or **fludrocortisone (Florinef) 0.1 to 0.2 mg daily,** and in some, a trial of clonidine patch. The management of orthostatic hypotension caused by autonomic failure can be managed, in properly selected patients, with midodrine (Amatine), a selective postsynaptic alpha$_1$-adrenergic agonist. Salutary effects are caused by an increase in arterial and venous tone; venous pooling is prevented.
   - **Dosage: Initially, 2.5 mg three times daily with monitoring of supine blood pressure, then increased in 2.5-mg increments at weekly intervals to a maximum of 10 mg 3 times daily.**
   - Caution is needed because midodrine may cause supine hypertension that can precipitate heart failure, myocardial ischemia, infarction, or stroke in susceptible individuals. Urinary retention is an important adverse effect in elderly men. The drug is contraindicated in patients with significant coronary heart disease, heart failure, renal failure, urinary retention, thyrotoxicosis, and pheochromocytoma; care is necessary when decreasing the dose and increasing the dosing interval in patients with renal dysfunction.
2. Transient ischemic attack (TIA)
   Syncope occurs in approximately 7% of individuals with TIA and is more common with vertebral artery–basilar artery TIA. Associated symptoms include vertigo, diplopia, ataxia, and loss of postural tone in the legs. A drop attack (no loss of consciousness) is more common than syncope. Treatment with **enteric-coated aspirin 325 mg once daily** is advisable.
3. Cardiac causes
   The major cause of cardiac syncope is a decrease in cardiac output due to reduced heart rate or ineffectual cardiac contractions secondary to arrhythmia. Obvious cardiac causes of syncope are listed in Table 24–1.
   - **Tachyarrhythmia.** Sustained rapid ventricular tachycardia (VT) (with a duration >30 seconds) or symptomatic nonsustained VT commonly causes presyncope or syn-

cope. If VT is not apparent on the ECG rhythm strip or Holter monitoring, EP testing is advisable; discuss the management with your resident.

Amiodarone has a role in patients with structural heart disease, especially IHD or cardiomyopathy, and with severely impaired ventricular function, with Holter monitoring manifesting sustained monomorphic VT or EP-initiated sustained VT.

Atrial fibrillation or other supraventricular tachycardia with fast ventricular rates may cause syncope, especially in elderly patients, or when rapid rates supervene in patients with Wolff-Parkinson-White syndrome.

Torsades de pointes is usually caused by class 1A agents, e.g., quinidine and procainamide, and class 3 agents, e.g., sotalol and amiodarone. Noncardiac drugs that cause torsades de pointes include erythromycin, pentamidine, trimethoprim-sulfamethoxazole, tricyclic antidepressants, astemizole, terfenadine, ketoconazole, itraconazole, and phenothiazines. Torsades de pointes is a bradydependent arrhythmia; thus, acceleration of the heart rate with isoproterenol or by pacing is effective. Intravenous magnesium sulfate usually terminates the attacks (see Chapter 19).

- **Aortic stenosis and hypertrophic cardiomyopathy.** Syncope in aortic stenosis is typically exertional; if the aortic stenosis is not treated immediately, average survival is 1 to 3 years. Valve surgery is the treatment of choice. With hypertrophic cardiomyopathy, syncope may be precipitated by exercise but may occur with normal activities or at rest.

- **Acute myocardial infarction (MI).** Approximately 64% of patients with acute inferior MI have significant bradycardia and hypotension that predispose to presyncope or syncope. Avoid the use of diuretics and ACE inhibitors during the first 24 hours except if congestive heart failure requires their use.

- **Sick sinus syndrome.** Severe bradycardia, 30 to 40 beats/min, sinus arrest, and bradyarrhythmias or tachyarrhythmias may cause lightheadedness, dizziness, confusion, memory loss, or syncope. One or more of these associated symptoms usually produces a 1- to 10-second warning before syncope; syncope can occur without warning, however, in these patients, and injuries can occur. The ECG may be normal or show evidence of previous infarction, bradycardia, or sinus arrest. Repeated 48-hour Holter monitoring gives approximately a 70% chance of detecting a significant arrhythmia. Discontinue verapamil, diltiazem, digitalis, beta blockers, class 1 antiarrhythmic agents, and amiodarone, which can cause severe bradycardia, AV block, and asystole in susceptible individuals (see Chapter 19).

- **AV block, Stokes-Adams attacks, or Mobitz type II, or third-degree AV block.** These may suddenly cause transient asystole or ventricular fibrillation. The unconscious patient appears very pale and, on arousal, becomes flushed as blood rushes to the head. Cardiac pacing should be instituted (see Chapters 5 and 19).

- **Long QT syndrome.** Syncope in children and young adults with a positive family history may be caused by long QT syndrome. The ECG is the only means of diagnosis; a QT interval of >0.48 second is diagnostic, between 0.46 and 0.48 second is suspicious, and between 0.42 and 0.46 second often results in misdiagnosis (see Table 5–1 for rate-adjusted QT, and pages 68–70). The QT interval is influenced by heart rate, age, and sex and must be analyzed carefully in individuals with unexplained blackouts. At ages 1 to 15 years, the QT is considered prolonged in males if it is >0.45 second and in females if it is >0.47 second; the normal interval in males is <0.43 second and in females is <0.45 second.

    Life-threatening arrhythmias may be precipitated by sudden intense sympathetic stimulation. Acute adrenergic arousal is the trigger in >60% of this form of syncope.

    Beta blockers have been proven useful in management. **Propranolol 80 to 160 mg daily** or a beta blocker without agonist activity is preferred. If recurrent syncopal attacks are uncontrolled by beta blockers, combined pacing and beta-blocker therapy may be required; excision of the left stellate ganglion or implanted defibrillators are considered for cases not controlled by beta blockers.

- **Carotid sinus syncope.** The history of syncope occurring with sudden turning of the head, shaving, or a tight shirt collar should alert the physician. Episodes may occur in clusters or with dizzy spells. Carotid sinus massage should be done with resuscitative equipment standing nearby. Do not attempt carotid massage without discussing it first with your resident and staff physicians; complications are TIA, rare hemiplegia, and asystole. There is a high spontaneous remission rate. Pacing is rarely required.

4. Unexplained syncope

    Approximately 30% of syncopal attacks occur without a defined cause (see Fig. 24–1). If symptoms are bothersome and structural heart disease has been excluded, a trial of increased sodium intake and elevation of the legs higher than the hip at the first sign of the prodome should suffice for the patient.

5. No structural heart disease and neurocardiogenic syncope. **Reconditioning** is the cornerstone of therapy in this benign condition. Exercises such as the proper use of the muscle pump in the legs done daily, or standing upright against a wall for 30 minutes daily for a few weeks then 15 minutes 3 days weekly strengthen the autonomic system.

Such patients often respond to increased salt intake and a trial of **Florinef 0.1 mg daily.** Beta blockers have been shown to prevent neurocardiogenic syncope in 50 to 75% of patients. **Atenolol (25 mg to a maximum of 50 mg), metoprolol (SR) 50 to 100 mg,** or **nadolol (20 mg)** is effective. **The combination of beta blocker with Florinef is superior to use of either drug alone.** Tilt testing can predict the salutary response to beta-blocker therapy, but it is an expensive, time-consuming, and potentially dangerous tool that is overused in the management of this benign medical condition. The test has caused cerebral damage and death in several individuals.

Disopyramide (SR) 100 to 150 mg twice daily may be given a trial in patients who have failed to respond to beta blockers, but caution is necessary with the use of all antiarrhythmic agents.

Study Section: Syncope

■ NEUROCARDIOGENIC SYNCOPE

This may present as
- Vasodepressor syncope: a profound fall in peripheral vascular resistance and marked reduction in BP occurs, but the heart rate usually remains >60 beats/min.
- Vasovagal syncope: predominently cardioinhibitory; a fall in blood pressure occurs, but there is marked vagal-induced bradycardia of <60 beats/min.
- A combination of vasodepressor and vasovagal features: The vasodepressor component with marked reduction in blood pressure appears to play an important role in loss of consciousness. Bradycardia plays a secondary role. These features explain the poor response to atropine. In his classic 1932 paper, Thomas Lewis stated that "While raising the pulse rate up to, and beyond normal levels during the attack, leaves the blood pressure below normal and the patient still pale and not fully conscious." Abboud noted that 60 years later,

Sra and coworkers can make the same statement with respect to pacing. Thus, the marked vasodilatation causes temporary, but profound, hypotension, with systolic BP <65 mm Hg and produces syncope even when the heart rate is 60 to 80 beats/min. The marked vasodilatation is caused by the inhibition of sympathetic vasoconstrictor activity at the very moment when arteriolar vasoconstriction is necessary to combat the marked fall in BP. In the majority of patients, the onset of bradycardia is consistently preceded by hypotension. Sra and coworkers have shown that an increase in myocardial contractility and a decrease in left ventricular (LV) systolic dimensions occur 2 to 4 minutes before the onset of syncope.

The constant findings in vasodepressor syncope are

1. A sudden marked fall in total peripheral resistance, resulting in a drastic fall in BP
2. Decreased cerebral perfusion causing loss of consciousness
3. Loss of consciousness usually occurs within 10 seconds of onset of diminished perfusion
4. Return of consciousness in seconds to minutes if the individual remains flat with the legs elevated
5. Injuries are most uncommon with neurocardiogenic syncope
6. Bradycardia of <55 beats/min is not a feature

The exclusion of epilepsy is relatively easy, but occasionally, syncope may be confused with akinetic seizures. Bradycardia in association with seizures has been described. The aura, if any, in epilepsy is transient but tells a story; convulsive movements occur with loss of consciousness. Injuries, including lip- and tongue-biting, and incontinence with a prolonged postictal state also occur.

In most patients with neurocardiogenic syncope, the diagnosis can be made by a careful assessment of a relevant history and a physical examination. If symptoms are bothersome and structural heart disease has been excluded, a trial of increased sodium intake and an explanation to the patient to elevate the legs higher than the hips at the first sign of the prodome should suffice.

Tilt testing is overused in the workup of these patients, who have a benign ailment that should respond to increased salt intake and repositioning during prodrome, followed, if needed, by beta-blocker therapy. Tilt testing causes minor degrees of asystole, but this can be occasionally prolonged and can cause cerebral damage. **Several deaths have been reported.** Diagnosis, in the majority of cases, can be made clinically because of the prodromal symptoms, occurrence in the upright or seated position, and absence of confusion after syncope. The cost per patient is approximately $4700 for Holter monitoring, echocardiogram, stress testing, and unnecessary electroencephalography, computed tomography scanning, and tilt testing.

Because cardiac sympathetic overstimulation, vigorous left ventricular contraction, and stimulation of intramyocardial mechano-receptors (C fibers) appear to be important mechanisms in the genesis of unexplained syncope without structural heart disease, beta blockers or disopyramide has proven successful in some patients with disabling syncope. **Atenolol (25 mg) or metoprolol (100 mg) daily** may produce a salutary response. The use of timolol, a noncardioselective beta blocker with greater vasoconstrictive properties than selective agents, should be tested in clinical trials.

Fitzpatrick and Sutton described 40 patients who had syncope associated with injuries because these patients had no prodrome. Tilt testing showed mostly vasovagal syncope with a profound bradycardia; some patients had other forms of bradycardias. Dual-chamber pacing appeared to prevent syncope during a 2-year followup. However, these patients were above age 65 and may have had undetected sinoatrial or AV node disease. It is unusual for patients with neurocardiogenic syncope and hence prodrome to sustain injuries. In patients who experience no prodrome and hence sustain injuries, a full workup is necessary. If electrophysiologic (EP) studies are negative, prognosis is usually good, but some patients may have undetected sinoatrial or AV node disease. If injuries continue to occur, a subcutaneous monitoring device, an implantable "loop recorder" as described by Krahn and colleagues, may provide helpful information. In 14 patients with previous syncopal episodes and negative head-up tilt test results, the recorder revealed sinus arrest in three, complete heart block in two, supraventricular tachycardia in one, ventricular tachycardia in one, vasodepressor syncope in two, and a psychogenic cause in one. These authors and others have concluded that an implantable loop recorder is useful for making a diagnosis when episodes are too infrequent for standard monitoring techniques (Fig. 24–3).

■ POSTURAL (ORTHOSTATIC) HYPOTENSION

Several cardiac medications may cause orthostatic hypotension, particularly in the elderly. Assess the following:

- Check the blood pressure with the patient recumbent for at least 3 minutes and then on standing; a reduction in systolic BP of ≥20 mm Hg represents orthostatic hypotension.

Figure 24–3 □ Algorithm for the management of unexplained syncope. *Use is abused: may not assist further with therapeutic strategies and is not without dangers of cortical damage. EP = electrophysiologic. (Redrawn from Khan, M Gabriel: Heart Disease Diagnosis and Therapy: A Practical Approach. Baltimore, Williams & Wilkins, 1996, p 542.)

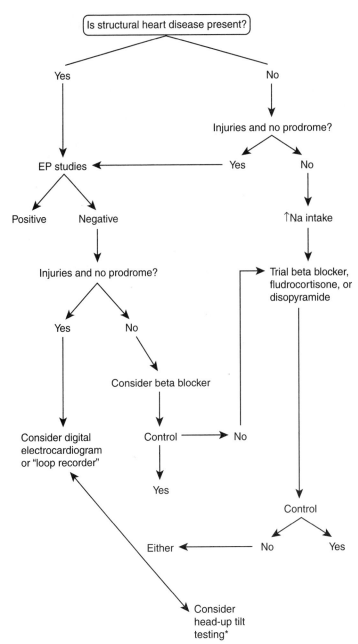

Figure 24–3 □ *See legend on opposite page*

- Check for evidence of a decrease in preload, which may manifest itself by venous pooling that may occur on sudden standing after vigorous exercise or because of extensive varicose veins. Preload-reducing agents, particularly nitrates, ACE inhibitors, or alpha$_1$ blockers, may be implicated. Blood loss and dehydration are obvious causes of decreased preload; an occult cause of dehydration is Addison's disease.
- If conditions causing a decrease in preload are not present, inquire about the use of medications that cause arterial dilatation, particularly alpha$_1$-adrenergic blockers such as prazosin and labetalol, ganglion-blocking drugs, L-dopa, bromocriptine, and, rarely, ACE inhibitors and calcium antagonists.
- If drug use is excluded, postural hypotension may be caused by autonomic imbalance or neurologic diseases. Complete bedrest and a lack of leg exercise, plus a decrease in autonomic activity, commonly result in postural hypotension. Neuropathy, especially due to diabetes, Shy-Drager syndrome, and other neurologic problems, must be excluded.

Standing from a recumbent or sitting position causes immediate pooling of blood in the lower limbs and a consequent fall in blood pressure that normally triggers a baroreceptor response and sympathetically mediated vasoconstriction and an increase in heart rate. As indicated earlier, conditions that impair baroreceptor function and decrease sympathetically mediated alpha$_1$ vasoconstriction may precipitate postural hypotension.

Orthostatic hypotension as a consequence of autonomic neuropathies and autonomic failure is difficult to treat successfully. It may respond to increased sodium intake or **fludrocortisone (Florinef), 0.1 to 0.2 mg daily.** Florinef, however, can cause migraine. The management of orthostatic hypotension caused by autonomic failure can be successfully managed in properly selected patients with midodrine (Amatine), a selective peripherally acting postsynaptic alpha$_1$-adrenergic agonist. Salutary effects are caused by an increase in arterial and venous tone; venous pooling is prevented. **Initial midodrine dosage: 2.5 mg 3 times daily** with monitoring of supine blood pressure, **then increased in 2.5-mg increments at weekly intervals to a maximum of 10 mg 3 times daily.** Caution is needed because the action of midodrine is identical to that of other alpha-adrenergic receptor stimulants such as methoxamine or phenylephrine; an increase in total systemic resistance may cause supine hypertension that can precipitate heart failure, myocardial ischemia, infarction, or stroke in susceptible individuals. Supine hypertension is more common during the initiation of midodrine therapy and may cause headaches and pounding in the ears. Reflex bradycardia may occur, and caution is needed when the drug is combined with agents that cause bradycardia (digoxin, beta blockers, diltiazem, and verapamil). Urinary retention is an important adverse effect in elderly men. The drug is contraindicated in patients with significant coronary heart disease, heart failure, renal failure, urinary retention, thyrotoxicosis, and pheochromocytoma. Midodrine is renally excreted, and care is necessary to decrease the dose and increase the dosing interval in patients with renal dysfunction.

In patients who are not responsive to midodrine, fludrocortisone, or a clonidine patch and have sustained injuries, atrial pacing with a heart rate of 100 beats/min may afford some amelioration if combined with increased salt intake, fludrocortisone, elevation of the head of the bed during sleep, and full-length leotards to enhance venous return. Instruct the patient to change posture slowly and to engage in calf muscle flexion prior to standing.

A release of histamine, prostaglandin D, and other vasodilators from mast cell proliferation (mastocytosis) causes vasodilatation and is a rare cause of postural hypotension.

■ UNEXPLAINED SYNCOPE

Approximately 30% of syncopal attacks occur without a readily defined cause. From 10 to 25% of total electrophysiologic studies in several large EP laboratories in the United States are done to resolve the diagnosis of unexplained syncope. An algorithm for the management of unexplained syncope is given in Figure 24–3.

A provocative EP study is useful in revealing a cardiac cause in approximately 12% of patients with unexplained syncope. Approximately 21% of these patients with negative studies are subsequently diagnosed as having intermittent high-degree AV block or sinus node disease. **Caution is necessary because an EP study is not a sensitive test to expose symptomatic bradycardia.**

EP studies have been shown to initiate sustained monomorphic ventricular tachycardia (VT) in approximately 18% of patients and nonsustained VT in approximately 23%. Nonsustained VT, especially if lasting for only a few seconds, carries a minimal risk in patients with syncope and requires no arrhythmia therapy. Patients with syncope and sustained monomorphic VT do not appear to benefit from antiarrhythmic therapy, and the incidence of syncope is not reduced except when amiodarone is used as therapy.

EP studies appear to be justifiable in patients who have a high probability of induction of sustained monomorphic VT.

- Post-MI patients with unexplained syncope
- Left ventricular ejection fraction <30%
- Left ventricular aneurysm
- Complex ventricular ectopy on Holter monitoring

The exact incidence of sudden death is unknown but appears to be low in patients with syncope unresolved by extended Holter monitoring and EP testing.

In patients with structural heart disease, especially ischemic heart disease or cardiomyopathy, and severely impaired ventricular function, in whom Holter monitoring manifests sustained monomorphic VT or EP-initiated sustained VT, amiodarone therapy is advisable. Holter monitoring documentation of sustained VT is a strong predictor of EP-induced sustained monomorphic VT, but the use of EP testing is of dubious value in these patients.

25 | Cardiac Arrest

Within 4 minutes of cardiac arrest, irreversible anoxic brain damage occurs.

■ BASIC LIFE SUPPORT

- Prove that the patient is **unconscious.**
- Confirm that the patient is **not breathing.**
- Confirm that there is no pulse in the large arteries, i.e., **pulselessness.**

The ABC Steps of Cardiopulmonary Resuscitation (CPR)

A: Airway. If the patient is unresponsive, use the head tilt/chin lift maneuver to open the airway (Fig. 25–1).

B: Breathing. Place your ear over the victim's mouth and nose; if you do not hear or feel air escaping, the victim is not breathing. Pinch the nose with the thumb and index finger of your hand that rests on the forehead. Take a deep breath, seal your lips around the mouth, give two full breaths, 1 to 1.5 seconds per breath, and allow the chest to deflate fully between each breath.

C: Circulation. Check the carotid pulse using the hand that held the victim's chin. If no pulse is present, start chest compression with straight, locked elbows and depress the lower half of the sternum 1.5 to 2 in. The compression rate should be about 90 to 100/min. Count "one and, two and, three and, four and, and five." At the end of compressions, two full breaths are given.

One or two rescuers: 15 compressions to 2 ventilations
When the airway is secured with a cuffed endotracheal tube, use 5 compressions to 1 ventilation.

■ ADVANCED CARDIAC LIFE SUPPORT

Oxygen administered via a bag-valve mask or an endotracheal tube should be started as soon as possible.

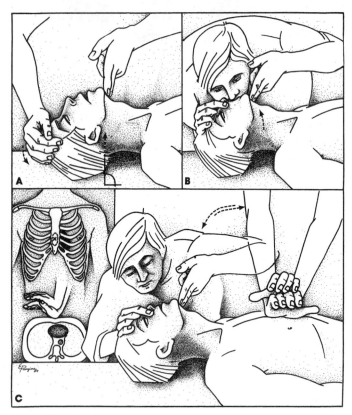

Figure 25–1 □ The ABCs of cardiopulmonary resuscitation. *A*, The airway is opened using the head tilt/chin lift technique. *B*, Breathing: the victim's nostrils are pinched closed and the rescuer breathes twice into the victim's mouth. *C*, Circulation: if no pulse is present, external chest compression is instituted at approximately 100/min, 15 compressions to 2 ventilations. (From Khan, M Gabriel: Cardiac Drug Therapy, 5th ed. London, WB Saunders Co, 2000, p 297.)

Defibrillation

Immediate defibrillation carries the only hope of survival of cardiac arrest victims.

1. Apply gel to paddles and turn on the defibrillator power (nonsynchronized).
2. Set energy at 200 joules, place one paddle over the right second intercostal space, and place the second paddle to the left of the left nipple and centered over the midaxillary line

(lead V_6 position for electrocardiograph [ECG]; in the United Kingdom, leads V_4 to V_5 ECG electrode position is used for this paddle). Apply firm arm pressure with each paddle.

3. Ensure that you or other personnel are not touching the patient. Depress both paddle discharge buttons simultaneously. If ventricular fibrillation (VF) persists, repeat countershock as soon as possible. If no pulse is present, resume basic life support; see Table 25–1 for further cardiac arrest protocols.

Ventricular Asystole

Ventricular asystole indicates a poor prognosis.

1. Because VF may masquerade as asystole, rotate the monitoring electrodes from their original position to ensure that VF is not present; defibrillation may be tried. Continue basic life support if the pulse is not present.

2. Begin a trial of **atropine 1 mg every 3 minutes to a maximum of 0.04 mg/kg and epinephrine 1 mg IV push.** If no

Table 25–1 □ **MANAGEMENT OF VENTRICULAR FIBRILLATION OR PULSELESS VENTRICULAR TACHYCARDIA**

Apply quick look paddles or press analyze*: If VF is confirmed, switch to DF nonsynchronized.

Immediate:	Check pulse, rhythm	
1st shock	200 joules (J)	VF: CPR; recharge DF
2nd shock	300 J	VF persists: recharge DF
3rd shock	360 J	CPR
	Epinephrine 1 mg IV bolus	IV line, intubate
4th shock	360 J	VF: CPR, for 1 min
	Vasopressin 40 U IV	(allow drug action)
5th shock	360 J	VF
	Epinephrine† 1 mg IV	VF persists, assess pH
6th shock	360 J	VF: CPR
	Lidocaine 100 mg IV	allow 2 min
7th shock	360 J	VF: arrest > 10 min
	NaHCO₃ 50 mEq IV bolus	pH < 7.1
8th shock	360 J	VF: CPR or bretylium 5
	Lidocaine 50–75 mg IV bolus	mg/kg, allow 2–4 min
9th shock	360 J	Conversion successful
	Lidocaine 50 mg IV + simultaneous infusion 2 mg/min	

*Semiautomated external defibrillator.
†Repeat every 3 to 5 minutes.
VF = ventricular fibrillation; DF = defibrillator; CPR = cardiopulmonary resuscitation; IV = intravenous.

response, repeat atropine 2 mg IV push. If electromechanical dissociation is caused by irreversible myocardial damage, pacing is usually ineffective. Epinephrine may be tried every 5 minutes for three doses.

Drug Therapy

- **Epinephrine (Adrenaline).** Epinephrine should be administered if the third shock fails to defibrillate. (See Appendix G.)
  Dosage: 1 mg of a 1:10,000 solution IV bolus repeated every 3 to 5 minutes. Adrenaline 1 mg can be instilled directly into the tracheobronchial tree via an endotracheal tube.
- **Vasopressin.** Vasopressin is a powerful vasoconstrictor that duplicates the positive effects but not the adverse effects of epinephrine; it is an adrenergic agent equivalent to epinephrine **only** for VF/VT. The drug requires only one dose because it has a half-life of 10 to 20 minutes, versus 3 to 5 minutes for epinephrine.
  Dosage: 40 U IV, one dose only.
- **Atropine**
  Dosage: For asystole, 1 mg IV bolus repeated every 3 to 5 minutes to a maximum of 0.04 mg /kg. For severe bradycardia, 0.5 mg every 5 minutes to a maximum of 2 mg.
- **Lidocaine (Lignocaine).** Lidocaine is used if the fourth shock fails to defibrillate.
  Dosage: 1.0 to 1.5 mg/kg IV bolus, and after about 1 minute of basic life support, a 360-joule shock is applied. If successful defibrillation is achieved, give a **50-mg bolus of lidocaine** and start immediate **infusion of 2 mg/min.**
- **Bretylium.** Bretylium is no longer recommended, and the drug is not available.
- **Sodium bicarbonate.** This drug is no longer recommended for routine use during cardiac arrest. In some situations, after about 10 minutes of CPR and after a seventh shock fails to result in defibrillation, a **50-mEq bolus** (1 mEq/kg) may be tried.
- **Calcium chloride.** This drug is no longer recommended during cardiac arrest, except for asystole caused by verapamil and in the management of hyperkalemia causing arrest. Calcium chloride is of no value in the management of electromechanical dissociation.
  Dosage: 2.5 to 5 ml of 10% calcium chloride or calcium gluconate IV bolus.

See Appendix G, Adult Emergency Cardiac Care Algorithms.

Deep venous thrombosis (DVT) is a common problem encountered on surgical and medical wards.

The incidence of venous thromboembolism in the United States is approximately 600,000 cases annually. Approximately 30% of patients undergoing major general surgery develop DVT. High-risk procedures such as implantation of a knee or hip prosthesis have an incidence of 55% and 60%, respectively, with proximal DVT occurring in about 20% of each group.

Because pulmonary embolism occurs commonly in patients with thrombosis of the femoral and iliac veins, this situation is considered serious and life threatening. Below-the-knee DVT that fails to extend above the knee rarely embolizes, but the incidence of postphlebitic syndrome is 30 to 40% with calf vein thrombosis. **Thus, the diagnosis and management of DVT both above and below the knee are important.**

Venous occlusion causes chronic passive congestion, and the muscle tissue becomes swollen with edema; a variable inflammatory response and perivascular hemorrhage may occur.

Inciting factors are
- Venous stasis
- Endothelial injury
- Hypercogulability

Venous thrombi are typically fibrin-rich clots that develop in areas of relative stasis, recirculating eddies, valve sinuses, and the left atrium. The clot consists of large fibrin strands and red blood cells. Thus, agents that prevent thrombin generation and fibrin formation prevent the formation of such thrombi or their propagation. It is not surprising that aspirin inhibition of platelet aggregation is only modestly protective against venous thromboembolism and left atrial thrombi and embolism.

The majority of postoperative DVT occurs in the legs, i.e., the soleus sinuses and the large veins draining the gastrocnemius muscles, with extension of the thrombosis to the femoral vein within a few days in some patients.

■ PHONE CALL

Questions

1. Why is the patient in the hospital?
2. Did the patient have recent surgery or immobilization?

3. Is the patient short of breath, suggesting pulmonary embolism?

Orders

1. Elevate the painful leg above the level of the hip.
2. If the patient is short of breath, have heparin at the bedside ready for intravenous (IV) use.

Inform RN

"Will arrive at the bedside in . . . minutes."

■ ELEVATOR THOUGHTS

What are the symptoms of DVT?

Because DVT in the lower limbs is often unrecognized, is difficult to diagnose, and can cause serious complications that include pulmonary embolism and postphlebitic syndrome, rapid and accurate diagnosis is essential.

- Most DVTs are silent.
- Patients with minimal symptoms, i.e., mild pain and tenderness with or without minimal leg swelling, may have large thrombi. DVT occurring in the lower limbs often presents difficulties in diagnosis based on the history and physical examination.
- In patients with symptoms, <33% have the typical features—calf pain, venous distention, edema, or pain on forced dorsiflexion of the foot (Homans' sign). See Table 26–1 for differential diagnosis of DVT.

Table 26–1 □ DIFFERENTIAL DIAGNOSIS OF DEEP VENOUS THROMBOSIS

1. Superficial thrombophlebitis
2. Muscle or tendon tear, muscle cramps
3. Popliteal inflammatory cysts (Baker's cysts)
4. Cellulitis (without lymphangitis)
5. Internal derangement of the knee
6. Postphlebitic syndrome
7. Cutaneous vasculitis
8. Lymphedema

■ MAJOR THREAT TO LIFE

- Chest pain and acute shortness of breath caused by pulmonary embolism (see Chapter 16).

■ BEDSIDE

Quick Look Test

Does the patient look well (comfortable) or sick (uncomfortable or distressed)?

Selective History and Selective Physical Examination

Clinical Features Assisting the Diagnosis of DVT

- The setting in which pain occurred
- The certainty with which an alternative diagnosis can be excluded (see Table 26–1)

If calf pain, tenderness, swelling, and unilateral edema are present in a setting common to DVT occurrence and if an alternative diagnosis cannot be made, the clinical probability of DVT is high; this **probability from clinical assessment (PCA)** is a key in the algorithmic approach to the diagnosis of venous thromboembolism (VTE) (Fig. 26–1; see Fig. 16–1*).

Situations Commonly Associated With DVT. The presence of one or more of these risk factors supports the diagnosis:

- Prolonged anesthesia associated with surgery
- Surgery or injury to the lower extremities or pelvis, including soft tissue injury
- Orthopedic surgery, in particular of the hip or of the knee
- Bedrest, in particular sudden immobilization for >2 days
- Congestive heart failure
- Malignancy
- History of thromboembolic disease or proven previous DVT
- Obesity
- Pregnancy
- Hypercoagulable diathesis
- Travel on an aircraft for >8 hours or steady driving for >12 hours
- Use of oral contraceptives or estrogens

---

*NOTE: Figures 26–1 and 16–1 give an algorithmic approach for the diagnosis of two difficult clinical problems. Algorithms do not cover all scenarios and are open to criticism. Nevertheless, these two algorithms should **provoke thought** and thus assist with the resolution of these two difficult diagnostic problems.

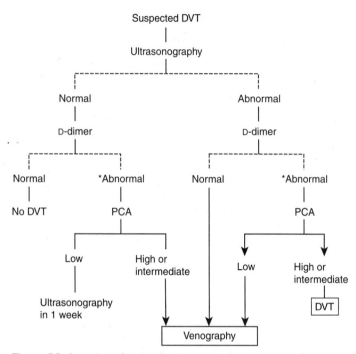

Figure 26–1 □ Algorithm for the diagnosis of deep venous thrombosis (DVT). PCA = probability from clinical assessment. (See Fig. 16–1.)
* = exclude myocardial infarction, congestive heart failure, pneumonia, cancer, post surgery.

- Dehydration
- Tenderness deep in the calf muscle and unilateral pedal edema

■ DIAGNOSTIC TESTING

1. **D-Dimer measured by enzyme-linked immunosorbent assay (ELISA)** is highly sensitive but not specific for the diagnosis of VTE (see Chapter 16). A normal D-dimer provides reassurance in >90% of cases that pulmonary embolism or DVT is not present and with normal ultrasonography can completely rule out VTE (see Fig. 26–1). A rapid automated ELISA that yields a negative predictive value of 99% is available; latex tests are unreliable. **A value of 500 ng/ml (500 μg/L) is abnormal and can be observed with pneumonia, myocardial infarction, congestive heart failure, or cancer or postsurgically (see page 249).**

2. **Ultrasonography.** Compression ultrasonography carried out by highly experienced staff is accurate in detecting above-the-knee thrombosis in symptomatic patients with suspected DVT, but an incomplete obstruction and small clots may not be detected. A meta-analysis indicates **93% sensitivity and 98% specificity in symptomatic patients.** In **asymptomatic patients, however, the sensitivity is only 59%.** Most important, **this test does not adequately visualize the deep veins of the calf or pelvis** (see page 251). Therefore, patients with normal ultrasonography, abnormal D-dimer, and a high or intermediate PCA should have venography; those with low PCA can wait 1 week for repeat ultrasonography.

3. **Venography.** Venography is the investigation of choice for patients with indeterminate diagnosis from ultrasound, D-dimer, and PCA. Venography detects thrombi in the calf veins and proximal thrombi in the iliac, femoral, and popliteal veins.

Adverse Effects. Contrast medium induces thrombosis of the peripheral veins in 2% of patients; hyperosmolality and high volume of the contrast agent may cause pulmonary edema in patients with left ventricular dysfunction. Pretreatment with furosemide is advisable in high-risk patients. Allergic reactions may occur, and patients with a positive allergy history have twice the incidence of reactions of those without a positive allergy history. Serious reactions may occur on initial exposure to the contrast agent, however, or after a prior uneventful test. Thus, medications and skilled personnel should be readily available to deal with these rare, life-threatening possibilities. **A combination of noninvasive tests** in association with the PCA provides diagnostic answers for this difficult clinical problem.

■ MANAGEMENT

Virtually all patients with proven DVT are treated with heparin IV; oral anticoagulants are usually started 24 to 48 hours after the activated partial thromboplastin time (PTT) is in the desired range. Heparin must be given for at least 12 hours before the administration of warfarin. (See discussion under Oral Anticoagulants.) The risk of recurrent VTE increases by 15 times in patients in whom adequate intensity of anticoagulation is not achieved in the first 24 hours.

The goals of therapy are
- To prevent pulmonary embolism
- To restore venous patency and valvular function, thus preventing postphlebitic syndrome

After verifying a normal prothrombin time (PT) or International Normalized Ratio (INR), activated PTT (APTT), and platelets, start heparin IV or low-molecular-weight heparins (LMWHs).

Heparin

Check for contraindications to heparin administration.

Dosage. IV bolus at 80 U/kg, usually 5000 to 7500 U, then a continuous infusion initiated at 18 U/kg/hr, about 1200 U/hr, and not exceeding 1600 U/hr (set up as suggested in Table 26–2). A 40-U/ml solution is commonly used. A more dilute solution, 20,000 U of heparin to 1 L of 0.9% saline (20 U/ml) is recommended in noncardiac patients and in patients in whom the extra fluid volume is required or not harmful. The physician should specify the rate of flow (e.g., 30 ml/hr) and the dose (1200 U/hr). Start the infusion at 1200 U/hr. Check the PTT 6 hours after the bolus injection, and then increase or decrease the infusion (see Table 26–2) to maintain the activated PTT 1.5 to 2.3 times the mean control range that corresponds to a PTT of 52 to 80 seconds and a plasma heparin level of 0.2 to 0.4 U/ml (maximum of 0.5 U/ml by protamine titration). The U.S. pharmaceutical units may be approximately 12% more potent than the international units used elsewhere. If either massive DVT or thromboembolism is suspected, the PTT should be determined 1 hour after the bolus dose. If the PTT is near the control value, another bolus of heparin

Table 26–2 □ CONTINUOUS-INFUSION HEPARIN

Rate (ml/hr)	Units/hr	Units/24 hr
1. 21	840	20,160
2. 25	1000	24,000
3. 28	1120	26,880
4. 30	1200	28,800
5. 32	1280	30,720
6. 34	1360	32,640
7. 36	1440	34,560
8. 38	1520	36,480
9. 40	1600	38,400
10. 42	1680	40,320
11. 44	1760	42,240
12. 46	1840	44,160
13. 48	1920	46,080
14. 50	2000	48,000

From Khan, M Gabriel: Cardiac Drug Therapy, 5th ed. London, WB Saunders Co., 2000, p 366.

Heparin (20,000 U) in 500 ml of 5% dextrose in water. If noncardiac, dilute in 0.9% saline; 1 ml = 40 U.

For each heparin order, specify both the rate of flow and the dose in units per hour. Start with no. 4, 1200 U/hr, and adjust to maintain activated partial thromboplastin time at 1.5 to 2.5 times control value (usual therapeutic range, 60–80 seconds).

should be administered, because this patient may have a more rapid heparin clearance.

Another method, body weight–based dosing of IV heparin, is given in Table 26–3. Check platelet count daily.

Action.   The anticoagulant activity of heparin requires a cofactor, antithrombin III. Heparin binds to lysine sites on antithrombin III and converts the cofactor from a slow inhibitor to a very rapid inhibitor of thrombin. The heparin–antithrombin III complex inactivates thrombin and factor X, as well several coagulation enzymes. The principal anticoagulant effect of heparin–antithrombin III appears to be caused by inhibition of thrombin-induced activation of factor V and factor VIII. Almost 20 times more heparin is required to initiate fibrin-bound thrombin than to inactivate free thrombin. Thus, the prevention of the extension of venous thrombosis requires much higher concentrations of heparin than the prevention of thrombus formation.

Also, heparin inhibits some aspects of platelet function and increases the permeability of vessel walls. Heparin is poorly absorbed from the gut and must be given parenterally. Heparin bound to endothelial cells is internalized and depolymerized, and desulfation occurs in mononuclear phagocytes. The elimination route of heparin remains uncertain. The agent has an apparent half-life of approximately 30 and 60 minutes after 25- and 75-U/kg IV bolus, respectively.

Adverse Effects.   Heparin-induced thrombocytopenia (HIT) occurs in up to 4% of patients between day 6 and day 12 of heparin administration. It is believed to be the result of immune sensitization to a heparin–platelet complex. This complication is associated with life-threatening arterial or venous thrombosis. In up to 80% of patients who develop HIT, serious complications, including limb amputation, pulmonary embolism, or death, occur. The incidence of HIT is increasing, and HIT is the leading cause of death from drug reaction in North America. Platelet counts should be assessed in patients administered heparin IV for >3 days. In patients with HIT, platelet counts are commonly 80,000, with a range of 20,000 to 150,000. Osteoporosis may occur after 5 months of therapy. Alopecia is a rare adverse effect.

Interactions.   High-dose nitroglycerin IV may increase the required dose of heparin, possibly because of an alteration in the antithrombin III molecule.

Contraindications.   These are hemophilia and other hemorrhagic disorders, peptic ulceration, severe uncontrolled hypertension, severe hepatic disease, cerebral aneurysm, recent opththalmic surgery, and pregnancy.

Table 26-3 □ BODY WEIGHT-BASED DOSING OF IV HEPARIN*

APPT (sec)‡	Dose Change (U/kg/hr)	Additional Action	Next APTT (hr)
<35 [<1.2 × mean normal]	+4	Rebolus with 80 U/kg	6
35–45 [1.2–1.5 × mean normal]	+2	Rebolus with 40 U/kg	6
46–70† [1.5–2.3 × mean normal]	0	0	6§
71–90 [2.3–3.0 × mean normal]	−2	0	6
>90 [>3 × mean normal]	−3	Stop infusion 1 h	6

From Hyers TM, Agnelli G, Hull RD: Antithrombotic therapy for venous thromembolic disease. Chest 1998; 114(5 Suppl):561S–578S.
*Initial dosing, loading 80 U/kg, maintenance infusion†: 18 U/kg/hr (APTT in 6 hr).
†Heparin, 25,000 U in 250 ml D₅W. Infusion at rate dictated by body weight through an infusion apparatus calibrated for low flow rates.
‡The therapeutic range in seconds should correspond to a plasma heparin level of 0.2 to 0.4 U/ml by protamine sulfate or 0.3 to 0.6 U/ml by amidolytic assay. When APTT is checked at 6 hr or longer, steady-state kinetics can be assumed.
§During the first 24 hr, repeat APTT every 6 hr. Thereafter, monitor APTT once every morning unless it is outside the therapeutic range.
This table gives heparin 25,000 U in 250 ml (1 ml = 100 U). A high concentration may be harmful if the infusion pump becomes defective.
The suggested dose changes given in the table are appropriate.

Low-Molecular-Weight Heparins

LMWHs are obtained by enzymatic or chemical depolymerization of unfractionated heparin. A predictable anticoagulant effect is achieved for 24 hours because of a longer half-life than unfractionated (UF) heparin and almost complete bioavailability following subcutaneous injection. **Several randomized trials have proved that LMWHs are as effective and safe as UF heparin for the management of DVT in outpatients, which greatly reduces costs and represents a major breakthough.**

Therapy is as follows.

- **Enoxaparin (Lovenox):** for acute DVT. **Dosage: 1 mg/kg every 12 hours;** continue for 5 to 10 days (average 7 days). Warfarin should be commenced preferably after 24 hours of heparin; then, when an INR of 2 to 3 is achieved for at least 2 days, heparin can be discontinued.
- **Dalteparin (Fragmin). Dosage: 120 U/kg every 12 hours.**
- **Tinzaparin (Logiparin). Dosage: 175 U/kg once daily.**

Oral Anticoagulants

Coumarins induce anticoagulation by inhibiting vitamin K epoxide reductase, which causes an accumulation of hepatic and circulating vitamin K epoxide and a depletion of vitamin KH_2, limiting the carboxylation and biologic function of vitamin K–dependent coagulant proteins (prothrombin and factors VII, IX, and X) and anticoagulant proteins (protein C and protein S).

Warfarin, a 4-hydroxycoumarin compound, has some anticoagulant effect within 12 to 24 hours, but peak activity occurs in approximately 72 hours, because it takes time to impair the biologic function of coagulant protein and to clear circulating clotting factors.

Because the half-life of factor VII is about 6 hours and that of factors II, IX, and X is several days, peak warfarin effect is delayed (72 to 96 hours). Protein C has a half-life as short as factor VII, and with depletion during the first 24 to 48 hours of anticoagulant therapy, there is a theoretically heightened risk of thrombosis in the first 12 hours of therapy. Therefore, for optimal salutary effects, **heparin should be administered for 24 hours before giving warfarin.**

Because protein C has a short half-life, a 5-day overlap of heparin IV and warfarin is necessary to prevent a potentially thrombogenic effect, which can be caused by low levels of protein C during the period when the levels of factors II and X are normal (during the first 4 days of warfarin therapy).

Adverse Effects. Bleeding is common with a prothrombin ratio of >2.5 or an INR of >4; if the INR is >3 with an International Sensitivity Index (ISI) of 2.3, search for an underlying cause of bleeding. The risk of bleeding is increased in patients older than 65 years and those who have occult gastrointestinal (GI) lesions, renal failure, anemia from other causes, a history of cerebral vascular disease, or ingestion of aspirin or nonsteroidal anti-inflammatory drugs. Rarely, skin necrosis occurs due to extensive thrombosis of capillaries and venules in subcutaneous tissue. The pathogenesis of this unusual complication, which occurs between day 3 and day 7 of therapy, is undetermined but appears to be linked to the decrease in biologic activity of protein C caused by coumarins.

Contraindications. These are peptic ulcer or recent GI bleeding, pregnancy, severe and uncontrolled hypertension, and bacterial endocarditis.

Interactions. See Table 26–4. **An important interaction occurs with acetaminophen,** a drug that is often used and was claimed to be safe when used with anticoagulants. Patients on oral anticoagulants must not ingest >3000 mg acetaminophen/week because the INR may be significantly elevated; for patients who take >9100 mg/week, the increased odds of having an INR >6 is more than 10-fold. Thus, patients who take the drug on a regular basis must be warned and the **INR must be closely monitored.**

Monitoring of Oral Anticoagulant Effect. The laboratory-determined INR is the PT ratio that reflects the result that would have been obtained if the World Health Organization reference thromboplastin had been used to perform the test in that laboratory.

$$INR = \left(\frac{Patient\ PT}{Control\ PT} \right) \times ISI$$

The INR is based, therefore, on two contributing factors: the PT ratio and the ISI. The ISI is a measure of the responsiveness of a given thromboplastin to reduction in the vitamin K–dependent coagulation factors. All reagent manufacturers should provide the laboratory with the ISI value.

Rabbit-brain thromboplastins have an ISI of 2.0 to 2.6, and the INR should be determined with the consistent use of sensitive thromboplastins with similar ISI values. An INR of 2 to 3, the desired range of anticoagulation for most clinical situations, using a thromboplastin with an ISI of 2.3, gives a corresponding prothrombin ratio of 1.4 to 1.6. This is considered a moderate-intensity regimen that is adequate for the treatment of DVT.

Warfarin

DVT that extends to the midthigh but is noniliofemoral, occurring in patients in whom the precipitating factors are removed

Table 26–4 □ ORAL ANTICOAGULANTS—DRUG INTERACTIONS

Drugs That May Enhance Anticoagulant Response

Acetaminophen
Alcohol
Allopurinol
Aminoglycosides
Amiodarone
Ampicillin
Anabolic steroids
Aspirin
Cephalosporins
Chloral hydrate
Chloramphenicol
Chlorpromazine
Chlorpropamide
Chlortetracycline
Cimetidine
Ciprofloxacin
Clofibrate (fibrates)
Co-trimoxazole
Danazol
Dextrothyroxine
Diazoxide
Dipyridamole
Disulfiram
Erythromycin
Ethacrynic acid
Fenclofenac
Fenoprofen
Fibrates
Flufenamic acid
Fluvoxamine
Liquid paraffin
Mefenamic acid
Methotrexate
Metronidazole
Monoamine oxidase inhibitors
Nalidixic acid
Naproxen
Neomycin
Omeprazole
Penicillin (large doses IV)
Phenformin
Phenylbutazone
Phenytoin
Propylthiouracil
Propafenone
Quinidine
Sulfinpyrazone
Sulfonamides
Tetracyclines
Tolbutamide
Tricyclic antidepressants
Trimethoprim sulfate
Verapamil

Drugs That May Decrease Anticoagulant Response

Antacids
Antihistamines
Barbiturates
Carbamazepine
Cholestyramine
Colestipol
Corticosteroids
Cyclophosphamide
Dichloralphenazone
Disopyramide
Glutethimide
Griseofulvin
Mercaptopurine
Oral contraceptives
Pheneturide
Phenobarbitone
Phenytoin
Primidone
Rifampicin
Vitamins K_1 and K_2

Modified from Khan, M Gabriel: Cardiac Drug Therapy, 5th ed. London, WB Saunders Co., 2000, p 364.

and early mobilization is attained, can be treated with early administration of oral anticoagulants. Warfarin is begun 12 hours after the start of heparin, at which time the diagnosis is usually confirmed by venography and the therapeutic level of heparin has been well maintained. Warfarin may take from 24 to 96 hours to achieve anticoagulation and the biologic activity of protein C is markedly limited within the first 24 hours of warfarin therapy, resulting in an enhanced early thrombogenic state. Therefore, it is necessary to overlap the heparin and warfarin for 5 days to prevent the potentially thrombogenic effect caused by the presence of nearly normal levels of factors II and X during the first 3 or 4 days of warfarin therapy. **Discontinue heparin when the INR is 2.5 to 3; a target of 3 is necessary because concomitant heparin therapy prolongs the INR by an additional 0.5.**

A study reported in the *New England Journal of Medicine* (1999; 340:901) indicates that in patients **with idiopathic VTE, anticoagulants must be continued beyond 3 months; but how much longer these patients must be treated is not known.** In a study of 102 patients reported in the *New England Journal of Medicine* (June 1995), 6 months of oral anticoagulation was compared with a 6-week course of therapy. Recurrence of thromboembolism at 2-year followup occurred in 9.5% of patients treated for 6 months vs. 18% of those treated for 6 weeks.

The following are guidelines for warfarin anticoagulant therapy suggested by recent studies:
- Duration of 4 to 6 months for patients with a first episode of idiopathic DVT
- Duration of 6 months for patients with persistent antiphospholipid antibodies (lupus anticoagulant, anticardiolipin antibody), and perhaps for factor V Leiden
- Duration of 3 months for postoperative patients without other risk factors
- Duration of 6 months for pulmonary embolism
- Duration of 6 to 12 months in patients with persistent risk factors and recurrent VTE
- For patients with the rare deficiencies of antithrombin III, protein C, or protein S, several years' rather than lifelong therapy has been suggested.
- Lifelong therapy only in rare cases.

Dosage: 2.5 to 5 mg daily for 2 days; a rapid loading of warfarin is no longer recommended because in rare cases this may precipitate gangrene of the limbs; the third and daily dose is titrated to maintain the INR at 3.

When the INR is in the desired range of 3, overlap heparin for an additional 2 full days; thus, heparin is given for a total of 5 days. A study has indicated that 9 to 10 days of heparin therapy is not superior to 5 days of heparin with overlapping warfarin in patients with *submassive* venous thrombosis. The short course of heparin reduces the length of hospital stay and is an important patient cost consideration; also, the incidence of HIT is reduced. The short course is not recommended for iliac vein thrombosis or major pulmonary embolism.

The warfarin dose should be given at bedtime; this allows the physician or the nurse to alter the dose, based on the result

of the PT ratio or INR obtained during the day. This is an especially useful strategy for office-based physicians.

Patients with a stable anticoagulant response should be maintained with an estimation of INR or PT every 3 weeks, and more frequently in patients with an INR often outside the target of 2 to 3. In a randomized trial, the incidence of bleeding in patients with an INR of 2.5 to 4.5 was 22%, vs. 4% in those with a target INR of 2.

Thrombolytic Therapy

Acute massive pulmonary embolism and iliac or iliofemoral vein thrombosis, the latter of <14 days' duration, can be managed with thrombolytic therapy. Complete lysis of thrombi occurs in ≤70% of patients treated with streptokinase. The risk of intracranial bleeding, however, has removed some of the enthusiasm for thrombolytic therapy.

Therapy is as follows:

- Streptokinase

    Dosage: Loading dose, 250,000 U IV over 30 minutes; maintenance infusion, 100,000 U/hr for 48 to 72 hours in patients with iliofemoral vein thrombosis. In patients with pulmonary embolism, the infusion is continued from 12 to 24 hours. After the infusion, the PTT should be maintained at 1.5 to 2 times the control with the use of heparin (see Table 26–2). Contraindications for streptokinase or thrombolytic therapy are given in Chapter 7.

- Urokinase. Although it is more expensive than streptokinase, urokinase is nonantigenic, and IV therapy is given for a much shorter duration.

    Dosage: IV bolus of 4000 U/kg over 10 minutes and continuous infusion of 4000 U/kg/hr. Continue the infusion as long as there is continued improvement. Discontinue the infusion if no improvement is observed in 24 hours or if there is no clot resolution over a 24-hour period.

Hypercoagulability and Thromboembolism

Congenital and, more commonly, acquired abnormalities are associated with a high incidence of thrombotic complications and must be clarified by careful history and physical and laboratory investigations in patients. A high index of suspicion is required in patients with the following associated abnormalities:

- A first episode of DVT at age <45 years or arterial thrombosis at age <30 years
- Thrombosis occurring in the absence of usual trigger factors
- Recurrent thromboses
- Skin necrosis if the patient is on warfarin

- Thrombosis of an unusual site, i.e., cerebral or mesenteric veins
- A strong family history

In these clinical settings, inherited deficiency of anticoagulant factors (antithrombin III, protein C, protein S, and abnormal factor V) or an acquired deficiency caused by lupus anticoagulant or antiphospholipid syndrome should be evaluated.

Congenital hypercoagulable disorders are rare. The prevalence of deficiency of antithrombin III, protein C, and protein S is about 5%. These hereditary defects are implicated in <12% of patients presenting with DVT below age 45 years, and in <5% of patients presenting above age 50 years.

Congenital Hypercoagulability Associations

- Antithrombin III deficiency: in the homozygous setting, death occurs in infancy due to overwhelming thrombosis. The heterozygote state may present in the third decade of life or later. An increase in the PTT to 1.5 to 2 times the control, observed after a bolus and infusion of heparin over 6 hours, excludes significant antithrombin III deficiency so that assay of antithrombin III is not required.
- Protein C deficiency: presents as purpura fulminans neonatalis; rarely, thrombotic tendency is manifest in the late teens and early adulthood. Protein C is a vitamin K–dependent protein. Patients presenting as young adults with recurrent DVT, with spontaneous abortions, or with coumarin skin necrosis require protein C assay. Some patients with thrombotic disease have poor anticoagulant responses to activated protein C (APC). It appears that APC resistance is about 10 times more common than antithrombin III, protein C, or protein S deficiencies. Factor V is the cofactor responsible for hereditary APC resistance.
- Protein S deficiency: a rare vitamin K–dependent protein deficiency with manifestations similar to protein C deficiency. Patients with these hereditary defects who have two or more spontaneous thromboembolic episodes are usually administered oral anticoagulant therapy for life.
- Factor V Leiden (a mutation in coagulation factor V that results in resistance to APC) is not rare, but extended anticoagulation beyond 6 months appears unnecessary.

Acquired Hypercoagulability Associations

- Street drugs that increase platelet count and adhesiveness
- Individuals with blood group A appear to have elevated prothrombin and factor VIII and a significant decrease in antithrombin III activity. These abnormalities are mainly observed in the subtype A_1, which represents <5% of the total population.
- Birth control pills or estrogen therapy

- Surgical treatment, which usually triggers an increase in factor VIII, a decrease in protein C, and increased adhesiveness.
- Several cancers, in particular pancreatic, stomach, large intestine, and prostate, induce clotting by increasing coagulability, which is believed to be related to a decrease in platelet antithrombin, an increase in fibrinogen, and a decrease in antithrombin III activity.
- Lupus erythematosus: a lupus anticoagulant, the presence of which can be detected in the laboratory, is present in up to 10% of cases, but its role in thrombus formation is unclear. The presence of lupus anticoagulant should be suspected in patients with unexplained activated PTT, systemic lupus erythematosus, or recurrent fetal loss.
- Antiphospholipid syndrome

Most patients suspected of having a hypercoagulable state should be referred to a hematologist for further evaluation and advice.

Screening Tests for Hypercoagulability
- Complete blood count, platelets, PTT, PT
- Antithrombin III
- Protein C
- Free protein S
- Resistance to activated protein C
- If abnormality in test, screen the family (parents, siblings, and children); low levels in a family member confirm the inherited defect
- Factor V Leiden
- Antiphospholipid antibodies (lupus anticoagulant, anticardiolipin antibody)
- Homocysteine for hyperhomocysteinemia

If the patient is pregnant, repeat the tests after the puerperium, because pregnancy decreases free protein S and can increase protein C.

27 | Evaluation and Treatment of Patients With Murmurs

The trainee or physician who is called to evaluate a patient with a loud murmur and distress must consider the following:
1. The most common causes of loud murmurs
2. The pathophysiology that evokes a life-threatening scenario. The most common diagnoses that must be considered are
   - **Severe aortic stenosis:** This can cause syncope, unstable angina, congestive heart failure (CHF), or sudden death
   - **Severe acute aortic regurgitation** caused by endocarditis or aortic dissection
   - **Severe mitral stenosis:** The soft diastolic murmur is overshadowed by the louder murmur of the often-associated mitral regurgitation. With tight stenosis, a fast heart rate caused by simple sinus tachycardia or atrial fibrillation severely impedes left ventricular (LV) filling and results in fulminant pulmonary edema. This can be life threatening in the pregnant patient and can be easily prevented by the use of a beta blocker.
   - **Severe mitral regurgitation** precipitated by infective endocarditis, acute myocardial infarction (MI), and ruptured chordae or flail mitral leaflet in patients with myxomatous mitral valve prolapse

■ AORTIC STENOSIS

Rheumatic aortic stenosis is now uncommon, except in Asia, Africa, the Middle East, and Latin America. The patient's age at the time of diagnosis usually gives a reasonable assessment of the underlying disease. Diagnosis before age 30 is typical of congenital aortic stenosis. In patients above age 70, calcific aortic sclerosis due to degenerative calcification is common, and significant stenosis develops in up to 5% of these individuals. A bicuspid valve occurs in 2 to 3% of the population, with a male to female ratio of 4:1, and is predisposed to degenerative calcification. Between the ages of 30 and 70, calcification of a bicuspid valve is the most common cause of aortic stenosis, and much less frequently, cases of rheumatic valvular disease are encountered.

Physical Signs

1. A systolic crescendo–decrescendo murmur is best heard at the left sternal border, the second right interspace, or occasionally at the apex, with radiation to the neck.
2. The timing of the peak intensity of the murmur is a more reliable sign of severity of aortic stenosis than is the intensity of the murmur. Severe stenosis is indicated by a murmur that peaks late in systole.
3. The longer the murmur, the greater the gradient.
4. The intensity of the murmur, in the absence of significant aortic regurgitation, is usually grade 3 or greater, except if cardiac output is low, as with heart failure; then, even a grade 2 murmur may be in keeping with severe stenosis. Aortic regurgitation increases flow across the aortic valve and may produce a loud systolic murmur without stenosis.
5. The patient has an absent or very soft aortic component of the aortic second sound (A_2). With increased calcification, mobility of the valve leaflets is reduced; thus, the closing sound of the aortic valve becomes soft or even lost. The soft pulmonary second heart sound (P_2) produces a soft, single second heart sound (S_2). Paradoxical splitting of S_2 may occur, but it is uncommon.
6. An S_4 gallop is usually present and is highly significant in patients below age 50.
7. A thrill is commonly present over the base of the heart or the carotid arteries; this indicates a murmur of grade 4 or louder and may relate to the severity of aortic stenosis if aortic regurgitation is absent.
8. A thrusting, forceful apex beat of left ventricular hypertrophy (LVH) is heard; the apex beat is usually not displaced, except in patients with concomitant aortic regurgitation or with terminal LV dilatation.
9. The carotid or brachial pulse in patients below age 65 shows a typical delayed upstroke. In the elderly, loss of elasticity in arteries often masks this important sign. The decreased elasticity increases the rate of rise of the carotid upstroke, and this may mislead the clinician into thinking that the stenosis is mild when it is severe.

Diagnostic Testing

Electrocardiography.   The ECG in patients with moderate to severe stenosis often shows features of LVH.
- S wave in lead V_1, plus an R wave in leads V_5 or V_6 or >35 mm
- S wave in lead V_3, plus an R wave in lead aVL >20 mm
- Left atrial enlargement

- ST-T change typical of LV strain: The ascending limb of the T wave is steeper than the descending limb in leads V_5 and V_6, with a lesser change in V_4.
- Left bundle branch block

Although some patients with LVH caused by aortic stenosis may not manifest ECG signs of LVH, the ECG remains an important test in those who do show LVH. The presence of LVH on ECG in the absence of significant hypertension is in keeping with severe aortic stenosis.

Echocardiography. The severity of aortic stenosis can be determined by continuous-wave Doppler echocardiography. This technique agrees with data obtained from catheterization in up to 85% of cases.

1. Mild aortic stenosis is indicated by
   - Mean aortic valve pressure gradient ≤20 mm Hg
   - Valve area >1.5 cm^2
2. Moderate stenosis is indicated by
   - Mean pressure gradient of 21 to 39 mm Hg
   - Valve area of >0.9 to 1.4 cm^2
3. Moderate to severe aortic stenosis is indicated by
   - Mean aortic valve pressure gradient >40 mm Hg (range in several clinical studies is 40 to 120 mm Hg)
   - Valve area of 0.8 to 0.9 is a gray area, and symptoms dictate clinical severity.
   - Valve area <0.75 cm^2 in an average-sized adult, 0.4 cm^2/m^2 of body surface area, indicates severe or critical stenosis.
   - Doppler peak systolic pressure gradient >50 mm Hg in the presence of a normal cardiac output
   - Maximal instantaneous Doppler gradient >60 mm Hg (range: 64–165 mm Hg)
   - Peak systolic flow velocity >4 m/sec (range often observed: 4–7 m/sec)

In patients with congenital aortic stenosis, the peak instantaneous valve pressure gradient is used for determining the severity of stenosis.

Management

Surgery

Mechanical obstruction to LV outflow due to significant aortic stenosis is a pressure overload situation that leads to progressive LVH, LV strain, and finally heart failure or sudden death. Symptoms due to obstruction of outflow are usually the main indications for valve replacement in patients with moderate or severe aortic stenosis. In the majority of these patients, the valve area is <1.0 cm^2 and the peak systolic gradient is >60 mm Hg. Fortunately, the hypertrophied myocardium often retains mechanical efficiency, and once the valve is replaced, significant improvement in ventricular systolic performance occurs in the majority of patients. Thus, heart failure is not a contraindication to valve replacement. Patients with LV failure due to severe aortic stenosis and followed for >1 year because of intercurrent illness contraindicating surgery usually regain adequate LV function with later valve replacement, but there are exceptions to these findings. Because the 1-year mortality is >50% in patients with heart failure, surgery should be done promptly. Indications for valve replacement are

- LV failure
- Shortness of breath
- Angina
- Presyncope or syncope not due to preload-reducing agents or other causes of syncope

If valve replacement caused no mortality or morbidity, then there would be no problem with advising surgery for moderate or severe aortic stenosis in asymptomatic patients. In some institutions, in the minimally symptomatic patient without coronary artery disease and other problems, mortality is 1 to 3%. The presence of ischemic heart disease, peripheral vascular disease, cerebral vascular disease, pulmonary disease, renal disease, and diabetes greatly increases the mortality and morbidity of surgery (5–7%).

Patients with chest pain or those above age 35 require coronary angiography to assess the degree of atheromatous coronary stenosis and suitability for coronary artery bypass surgery (CABS).

■ AORTIC REGURGITATION

Since the mid 1970s there has been a major change in the pattern of underlying conditions associated with diseases causing aortic regurgitation. Whereas rheumatic fever and syphilis caused 70% and 20% of cases, respectively, they now account for <30% and 1%, respectively. With the fall in prevalence of these diseases, bicuspid valve, endocarditis, and diseases causing aortic root dilatation have emerged as the common causes.

Diagnostic Hallmarks

With chronic aortic regurgitation, the left ventricle tolerates regurgitant volume overload and compensates adequately; an asymptomatic period of 10 to 30 years is not uncommon. Many patients with a moderate degree of aortic regurgitation deny shortness of breath on walking 3 to 5 miles and/or climbing three flights of stairs. Complaints of shortness of breath on exertion, fatigue, palpitations, and dizziness are generally associated with moderate or severe regurgitation over a prolonged period or severe regurgitation of recent onset. Rarely, angina with diaphoresis occurs as the diastolic blood pressure (BP) falls, frequently at night, causing a decrease in coronary perfusion. Symptoms and signs of heart failure at rest are late manifestations.

Physical Signs

The hallmarks on physical examination include

- Typical collapsing pulse: water-hammer (or Corrigan's) pulse or a bounding pulse. The underlying mechanism is a rapid rise in upstroke followed by an abrupt collapse due to a quick diastolic runoff from the arterial tree. (Indeed, all conditions that cause a brisk runoff produce a collapsing or bounding pulse.) the collapsing quality is detected by the examiner's placing his or her fingers or palm closed firmly over the radial pulse with the patient's entire limb extended to the ceiling. Pulsus bisferiens, a double peak to the pulse, may be observed with the combination of aortic regurgitation and significant aortic stenosis.
- The patient's head often bobs with each cardiac pulsation.
- The blood pressure reveals a wide pulse pressure due to an increase in systolic BP and a diastolic BP that is often <50 mm Hg. Occasionally, Korotkoff sounds persist to zero with diastolic arterial BP still >60 mm Hg.
- Arterial neck pulsations are usually prominent.
- Quincke's sign: Exerting mild pressure on the nail beds brings out intermittent flushing.
- Finger pulsations: collapsing pulsations in the finger pads or tips
- Traube's sign: pistol-shot sounds over the femorals
- Duroziez's sign: Compression of the femoral artery proximal to the stethoscope produces a systolic murmur and a diastolic murmur with distal compression.

The apex beat is virtually always displaced downward and outward to the left, indicating LV enlargement in patients with moderate or severe aortic regurgitation. A diastolic thrill may be palpated in the second right interspace or third interspace at the left sternal border, where the murmur of aortic regurgitation is most prominent.

Hallmarks on auscultation include

- Typical high-pitched blowing, early decrescendo murmur begins immediately after A_2. The early decrescendo murmur beginning immediately after A_2 is unmistakable to the trained ear and is best heard with the diaphragm pressed firmly against the chest, with the patient leaning forward and the breath held in deep expiration. The examiner should then listen to the murmur with the patient breathing normally and in the recumbent position in order to train the ear for detection of the softest diastolic murmur.

- The degree of aortic regurgitation correlates best with the duration of the murmur and may be pandiastolic with severe regurgitation.
- Perforation of an aortic cusp may change the quality of the murmur to one that resembles the cooing of a dove.
- A mid- or late diastolic rumble at the apex, the Austin Flint murmur, may be heard as the regurgitant jet hits the anterior mitral leaflet, as it opens and closes during diastole. The leaflet's shuddering can be heard with the stethoscope or observed with the help of Doppler echocardiography.
- The A_2 sound may be increased, decreased, or normal, and the accompanying aortic systolic murmur and thrill may represent flow rather than stenosis.

Diagnostic Testing

Electrocardiography. The ECG commonly shows nonspecific ST-T wave changes, and with LVH, the pattern of LVH with volume overload is often present.

Echocardiography
- Detection of the type of aortic valve abnormality and underlying disease, e.g., aortic regurgitation due to bicuspid valve or vegetations caused by endocarditis
- Left ventricular chamber dimensions: estimates of LV volume and ventricular function measurements (LV end-systolic dimensions, LV end-diastolic dimensions, fractional shortening, or ejection fraction (EF))
- Dilatation of the aortic root
- Aortic dissection
- Other valve disease
- Other associated states, e.g., perivalvular abscesses in infective endocarditis

Color flow Doppler provides accurate quantification of aortic regurgitation. The degree of aortic regurgitation can be assessed by measuring the width of the aortic regurgitant jet. The measurement is assessed just under the aortic valve in the LV outflow tract as a fraction of the LV outflow tract.

- Mild regurgitation: Width of the jet is up to one-third of the LV outflow tract.
- Moderate regurgitation: Width of the jet is between one-third and two-thirds of the LV outflow tract.
- Severe regurgitation: Width of the jet is greater than two-thirds of the LV outflow tract.

Management

Mild aortic regurgitation does not require special therapy.

Vasodilators. For asymptomatic patients only, with moderate to severe aortic regurgitation and normal LV function, **nifedipine extended-release 30 to 60 mg daily** or an angiotensin-converting enzyme (ACE) inhibitor is recommended by the American College of Cardiology–American Heart Association. The unloading effect of nifedipine is capable of reversing LV dilation and hypertrophy and may prevent the development of LV dysfunction. In a randomized study, after 6 years of followup, 34% of the digoxin-treated group required valve surgery because of the development of LV dysfunction vs. 15% in the nifedipine plus digoxin group. Short-term vasodilator therapy may be used in patients with severe aortic regurgitation and severe LV dysfunction in preparation for surgery but not in those who are undoubtedly surgical candidates.

Surgery. Surgery is offered for symptomatic patients if LV function is mildly impaired, exercise capacity is reduced, or LV dimensions are "highly abnormal" or show significant deterioration. The following echocardiographic or catheter dimensions may be used to help serve in decision making regarding timing for valve surgery. No single estimation should be accepted for making decisions. Marked changes or rate of change at 3- or 6-month visits should guide the physician.

- LV end-systolic dimension (LVESD) between 45 and 55 mm. A dimension >50 mm, or EF below normal for the particular laboratory, usually indicates LV dysfunction and, as outlined previously, one does not wait for more ominous signals.
- LV end-diastolic dimension >66 mm
- LV end-systolic volume index >60 ml/m^2; >90 ml/m^2 indicates severe LV dysfunction.
- LV end-diastolic volume index 140 to 150 ml/m^2; >180 ml/m^2 indicates severe LV dysfunction.
- EF <50% or fractional shortening <35%: Fractional shortening <25% indicates severe LV dysfunction. An EF of <45% represents moderately severe LV dysfunction, and an EF of <35% indicates severe dysfunction.

Preparations for surgery include attention to dental work under antibiotic cover. Coronary angiography is necessary in patients above age 35 or in those with angina. Elective valve surgery has a 3 to 6% oprative mortality, and emergency surgery has >10% mortality. The 5-year survival for patients receiving valve implants ranges from 60 to 85%.

■ MITRAL STENOSIS

Mitral stenosis is almost always due to previous rheumatic fever. It takes 2 or more years following the rheumatic episode for sufficient fibrosis and thickening of the valve to produce the typical murmur. Most patients remain asymptomatic for 15 to 20 years following an episode of rheumatic fever, which is subclinical in over 50%.

Over the past 30 years, the problem of rheumatic valve disease has shown a marked decline in North America, the United Kingdom, and Europe. However, the disease is still endemic in much of Asia, Africa, the Middle East, Latin America, and the West Indies. Indeed, in these countries, significant mitral stenosis may emerge within a few years of the initial acute rheumatic fever and result in symptomatic disease in juveniles and young adults.

Diagnostic Hallmarks

1. **Mild mitral stenosis,** valve area 1.6 to 2.0 cm², may cause mild dyspnea on moderate to severe exertion, but the patient is usually able to do all normal chores and lifestyle is not altered. Symptoms progress slowly, if at all, over the next 5 to 10 years. Some patients with mild mitral stenosis may reduce activities and tolerate symptoms for several years. However, infection, pregnancy, or tachycardias, including atrial fibrillation, may precipitate severe dyspnea.

2. **Moderately severe mitral stenosis,** valve area 1 to 1.5 cm², usually causes symptoms that affect or interfere with daily living. Dyspnea due to progressive pulmonary venous hypertension becomes bothersome. Breathlessness is precipitated by moderate activity such as walking 100 yards briskly, walking up an incline, or even running slowly for 20 yards. Pulmonary infection or atrial fibrillation often precipitates pulmonary congestion, emergency room visits, or hospitalization. Cough, shortness of breath, wheeze, and hemoptysis may mimic bronchitis for several months because the subtle signs of mitral stenosis can be missed by the untrained auscultator. Palpitations are usually due to atrial fibrillation, and some patients may present with a very rapid tachycardia or systemic embolization.

3. **Severe mitral stenosis,** valve area <1 cm² and valve area index <1 cm²/m², usually causes symptoms on mild exertion. The patient presents with one or more of the following symptoms: progressive dyspnea, palpitations, marked fatigue, and occasionally cough, hemoptysis, hoarseness, or chest pain. Progression may be rapid with increasing edema, orthopnea, paroxysmal nocturnal dyspnea, and marked breathlessness. However, some patients tolerate dyspnea and are able to continue work that is not strenuous, at their own pace, for 3 to 12 months prior to interventional therapy. Fortunately, with mitral stenosis, patients with the most

bothersome symptoms benefit the most from mitral valvotomy.

Some patients present with progressive symptoms and signs of low cardiac output and right-sided heart failure with only mild pulmonary congestive features as a result of reactive hyperplasia of pulmonary arterioles and pulmonary arterial hypertension, a scenario appropriately termed "protected" mitral stenosis. At the other extreme, some patients present with florid pulmonary edema associated with only passive pulmonary arterial hypertension and mild or absent right-sided heart failure, which is considered "unprotected" mitral stenosis. A mixture of protected and unprotected mitral stenosis is commonly observed.

Physical Signs

- On inspection, a malar flush is common in the presence of long-standing, moderately severe mitral stenosis.
- A lower left parasternal lift or heave due to right ventricular hypertrophy may be present.
- The apex beat is tapping in quality but usually is not displaced.
- A diastolic thrill localized to the apex beat may be palpated.
- Auscultation reveals a loud slapping S_1 and is so typical that it warns the examiner to search for other signs of mitral stenosis. Immobility of the cusps reduces this valuable sign.
- P_2 is intensified, and this vibration associated with pulmonary valve closure is often palpable with significant pulmonary arterial hypertension.
- An opening snap, a sharp high-pitched sound, is a hallmark of mitral stenosis. The opening snap is best heard with the diaphragm pressed firmly just internal to the apex beat and occurs from 0.04 to 0.14 second after S_2. The opening snap may be heard over a wide area and, with severe mitral stenosis, usually occurs <0.08 second following S_2, audible immediately rather than following a definite gap. The opening snap disappears if the valve becomes heavily calcified and nonpliable.
- The loud slapping S_1 and opening snap produce a particular cadence that alerts the examiner.
- The opening snap is followed by a low-pitched, mid-diastolic rumbling murmur that is associated, if there is sinus rhythm, with presystolic accentuation, best heard with the bell lightly applied over the apex beat. The murmur often is localized to an area the size of a coin and can easily be missed; it is brought out by exercising the patient and listening with the

patient lying on the left side. Occasionally, critical mitral stenosis may cause a marked reduction in transmitral flow, and the murmur may be hardly audible. There is evidence that in these cases, the disease and contracted chordae increase the impedance to ventricular filling so that the reduced mitral valve area is no longer the limiting factor.

- The severity of mitral stenosis correlates best with the length of the murmur rather than the intensity.

Diagnostic Testing

Chest X-Ray

- Straightening of the left heart border due to left atrial enlargement
- Larger-than-normal double density, seen through the right half of the cardiac silhouette, indicating left atrial enlargement
- Elevation of the left main stem bronchus caused by distention of the left atrium with widening of the angle between the two main bronchi
- Redistribution: restriction of lower lobe vessels and dilatation of the upper lobe vessels
- If heart failure is present, signs of interstitial edema are present: Kerley B lines due to lymphatic engorgement and fibrosis, perihilar haze, and eventually frank pulmonary edema is observed.
- Fluoroscopy is no longer commonly done, but it shows posterior displacement of the barium-filled esophagus.
- The heart size on posteroanterior x-ray is generally normal or near-normal, and the lateral film should be assessed for right ventricular enlargement: "creeping up the sternum."

Electrocardiography

- Signs of left atrial enlargement are common with moderate and severe mitral stenosis: broad bifid P waves in lead II and, more specifically, an increase in the P terminal force (PTF_1) ≥ 40 msec/mm, measured in lead V_1 (area subtended by the terminal negative portion of a biphasic P wave). When the PTF_1 is >40 msec/mm, 95% of individuals had left atrial size >4 cm; when the PTF_1 is ≥ 60 msec/mm, 75% had left atrial size >6 cm.
- Right axis deviation 90 to 150 degrees reflects severe mitral stenosis.
- Right ventricular hypertrophy may be present with severe stenosis but does not correlate well with the degree of pulmonary hypertension.

- Atrial fibrillation is common with moderate long-standing rheumatic disease, with the left atrial size exceeding 4.5 cm, and is characteristically coarse in appearance.

Electrocardiographic stress testing is of value in selected patients who are suspected of denying symptoms with the presence of a moderate degree of stenosis; functional capacity can be assessed.

Echocardiography
- The mitral diastolic gradient can be defined.
- Excellent quantification of mitral valve orifice area
- Left atrial enlargement is uniformly present, and the size can be accurately determined.
- The degree of calcification of the mitral valve leaflets can be verified.
- Decreased posterior leaflet movement is often observed.
- The degree of right ventricular enlargement can be documented.
- Left ventricular size is expected to be small.
- Right ventricular systolic pressures reflect the degree of pulmonary hypertension.
- The degree of concomitant mitral regurgitation can be assessed.

Management

Medical Therapy

All patients should receive prophylaxis for the prevention of rheumatic fever for at least 25 years from the acute episode and up to age 45, whichever is the longer. Although pure mitral stenosis is rarely the site of endocarditis, trivial mitral regurgitation is often present, and endocarditis prophylaxis should be strongly enforced. Moderate mitral stenosis, valve orifice area 1 to 1.5 cm^2, is usually mildly symptomatic. Salt restriction is advisable. Potassium-sparing diuretics such as Moduretic (Moduret) ameliorate shortness of breath and prevent potassium and magnesium loss. If palpitations are bothersome or runs of supraventricular tachycardia or atrial fibrillation are documented, a small dose of a beta-blocking drug is useful: **metoprolol 25 to 50 mg twice daily, atenolol 25 to 50 mg daily,** or an equivalent dose of another beta blocker should suffice. Digoxin is not indicated for patients with sinus rhythm or heart failure with pulmonary congestion, except as prophylaxis against fast ventricular rates and pulmonary edema if atrial fibrillation develops.

Chest infections must be vigorously treated because hypoxemia increases pulmonary hypertension and may precipitate right-sided heart failure. Also, tachycardia may precipitate pulmonary edema, particularly during pregnancy, and a small dose of a beta blocker can prevent this crisis.

Severe mitral stenosis, valve area corrected for body surface area (valve area index) <1 cm^2/m^2, usually requires interventional therapy within 3 to 6 months to abolish symptoms or decrease complications and/or progressive increase in pulmonary vascular resistance.

Interventional Management

Balloon valvuloplasty or surgery to relieve valvular obstruction is indicated for most symptomatic patients who have moderate to severe mitral stenosis, valve orifice <1 cm^2, as determined by Doppler echocardiography. The results of this technique correlate sufficiently well with catheterization data. Cardiac catheterization is not required in patients below age 40 in whom ischemic heart disease is not present or suspected and who have typical clinical features of mitral stenosis that are confirmed by Doppler echocardiography.

Mild mitral stenosis, valve area 1.6 to 2.0 cm^2, often remains minimally symptomatic for 5 to 10 years or more.

Moderately severe mitral stenosis, valve area 1 to 1.5 cm^2, usually does not require intervention, but decisions must be individualized. In the following patients, intervention may be required:

- For symptomatic young patients engaged in strenuous activity
- If atrial fibrillation supervenes
- To allow pregnancy in a patient who manifested pulmonary edema in a previous pregnancy

Elective procedures are sometimes performed in women who anticipate pregnancy, but relief of obstruction may be required during the second and third trimesters of pregnancy, because the valve orifice is no longer large enough to permit the necessary increase in cardiac output to occur without an unacceptable rise in left atrial and pulmonary venous pressures. Interventional therapy may take the form of

- Surgical closed commissurotomy
- Surgical open commissurotomy
- Balloon valvuloplasty
- Valve replacement

Mitral Balloon Valvuloplasty.   Percutaneous mitral balloon valvuloplasty appears to give hemodynamic results that are comparable with surgical closed commissurotomy. The valve area is increased 100% from 1 to 2 cm^2 in up to 77% of cases. A mortality of up to 2.7% has been reported by the Valvuloplasty Registry. An iatrogenic atrial septal defect (ASD) has been reported to occur in 20 to 87% of patients, depending on criteria used for defining the ASD, which takes up to 6 months to close. The defect, however, is usually small, the magnitude of the shunt being less than 2:1, and only a few of these ASDs are clinically significant. The procedure should be done only by highly trained and experienced operators. In such hands, the procedure is first choice in appropriately selected patients for relief of severe mitral stenosis.

A multicenter study of 4832 patients in China and 600 patients in India indicates that mitral balloon valvuloplasty is an effective and safe procedure that can be performed worldwide. The reported restenosis rate of approximately 12% at 3 years is similar to that after closed surgical commissurotomy.

Transesophageal echocardiography (TEE) has a role in obtaining information needed for the selection of patients for balloon valvuloplasty: e.g., calcification, thickening, mobility, and subvalvular fibrosis. Atrial or appendage thrombus is best visualized with TEE. The technique is also of value in assessing the magnitude of the ASD following the procedure.

■ MITRAL REGURGITATION

Although mitral stenosis is nearly always due to rheumatic disease, mitral regurgitation is a common valvular lesion that is caused by a number of conditions that alter the mitral valve apparatus: valve leaflets, annulus, chordae, and papillary muscles.

1. **Acute mitral regurgitation** commonly occurs during acute MI, which causes papillary muscle dysfunction, and less commonly, chordal or papillary muscle rupture
2. **Chronic mitral regurgitation:** Causes include
   - Degenerative, ~ 60%, mainly myxomatous mitral prolapse in the Americas
   - Ischemic heart disease ~ 20%
   - Rheumatic ~ 10%
   - Endocarditis ~ 5%

Diagnostic Hallmarks

- Patients may tolerate a mild to moderate degree of mitral regurgitation for 5 to 20 or more years without the appearance of heart failure. Chronic volume overload, however, causes slow progressive dilatation and mild hypertrophy of the left ventricle. Characteristically, a loud holosystolic murmur is heard maximal at the apex with radiation to the axilla, accompanied by an S_3 gallop if regurgitation is moderate to severe. In patients with posterior papillary muscle dysfunction causing mitral regurgitation, however, the murmur radiates anteriorly and is best heard at the left sternal border without radiation to the axilla.

- Mild to moderate shortness of breath indicates pulmonary congestion or LV dysfunction and should be managed with afterload-reducing agents, particularly angiotensin-converting enzyme (ACE) inhibitors, to encourage forward flow at the expense of regurgitation; small doses are advisable: **enalapril or lisinopril, 5 to 10 mg daily,** or equivalent doses of other ACE inhibitors.

- If concomitant ischemic heart disease with angina is present and LV dysfunction is not present, amlodipine is preferred to ACE inhibitors. Also, digoxin and the judicious use of diuretics in combination with amlodipine may cause some beneficial effects prior to consideration of early valve repair or valve replacement. Calcium antagonists should not be used in patients with LV dysfunction because heart failure may be precipitated.

- Atrial fibrillation with a rapid ventricular response is managed with digoxin, a beta blocker, and anticoagulants to prevent embolization.

- Progressive dyspnea is a late stage and heart failure should be anticipated and prevented by timely surgical intervention.

Management

Surgery

The timing of valve surgery, whether it is repair or valve replacement for chronic mitral regurgitation, remains a problem in decision making, as with that of aortic regurgitation. Patients with mitral valve prolapse and acute complications are often suitable for valve repair.

1. There is an increasing tendency to attempt valve reconstruction. It is advisable to repair as many valves as possible and as often as feasible, but success depends on the skill of the surgeon. For mitral stenosis and regurgitation, many valves are beyond repair and require replacement.
2. Surgery should be considered in patients who have moderately severe mitral regurgitation prior to the development of

severe pulmonary arterial hypertension and prior to a fall in EF to <50%. The interpretation of EF has to be adjusted downward to take into account the low impedance to retrograde flow resulting from mitral regurgitation. A patient with severe mitral regurgitation and an EF of <40% has a prohibitively high surgical mortality and fares better with afterload reduction and digoxin because of the problems of assessing EF in the presence of mitral regurgitation. Important parameters of LV function that indicate surgery include end-systolic volume index >50 ml/m² and LV end-systolic dimension (ESD) >45 mm.

3. If surgery is done prior to an EF of <45% and an ESD >55 mm, patient survival, functional class, and LV systolic function should show significant improvement. If mitral regurgitation is moderately severe and LV dysfunction is present, it is hazardous to procrastinate. Early surgery is preferable. It is probably safe to wait until end-systolic diameter reaches 45 mm, but not >50 mm. When the end-systolic diameter is <40 mm in an asymptomatic patient deemed to have severe mitral regurgitation by other parameters, close observation without surgery and the use of nifedipine or an ACE inhibitor is considered sound decision making. Clear answers will become available in these difficult clinical situations, only when the results of further large clinical trials are available.

4. In patients with predominant posterior leaflet prolapse, repair of the posterior leaflet followed by insertion of a nonflexible ring, as recommended by Carpentier, appears to be successful in preventing postoperative systolic anterior motion of the mitral valve.

5. The tricuspid valve is also often severely incompetent; tricuspid annuloplasty is advisable in such cases.

6. Intraoperative TEE is of considerable value in assessing valve repair. The surgeon ensures excellent coapting edges and lines of closure; if the geometry is ideal, saline is pumped into the ventricle.

■ MITRAL VALVE PROLAPSE

Mitral valve prolapse is said to be a common condition affecting an estimated 5% of the U.S. population. The incidence of mitral valve prolapse has been exaggerated because of the inclusion of a large number of patients with a normal variant of mitral valve closure but with correct coaptation; leaflets may billow only slightly into the left atrium with normal coaptation. Also, the appearance may result from the saddle shape of the normal mitral ring.

The minor variant with a click, without a murmur, and with nondiagnostic echocardiographic features commonly labeled mitral valve prolapse is subject to interpretation, and this "normal variant" disappears after age 40. Probably because of the inclusion of normal variants with billowing leaflets without true prolapse, the incidence of mitral valve prolapse is reported to be as high as 30% from ages 10 to 20, 15% at age 30, 10% at age 50, 3% at age 70, and <1% at age 80. Below age 40, the female to male ratio is 3:1, but at age 70, both men and women have about equal incidence. The incidence of significant mitral valve prolapse in adults is about 6% in women and 3% in men.

Genuine mitral valve prolapse has a familial incidence of about 33% as noted in first-degree relatives.

Causes of mitral valve prolapse:

- In developed countries, the common underlying process is a degenerative nonrheumatic condition of unknown etiology described as a dyscollagenosis or myxomatous degeneration of the mitral valve. The anterior and posterior leaflets become elongated, thickened, voluminous, and grossly redundant. The chordae become thin and elongated and have a propensity to rupture. A mural endocardial fibrous plaque is often observed beneath the posterior leaflet in patients who die suddenly from mitral valve prolapse. The mitral valve annulus is often dilated in patients with significant regurgitation, and in those patients who die suddenly, calcification and fibrosis of the annulus appears to be a common finding.
- Myxomatous changes and mitral valve prolapse are associated with Marfan and Ehlers-Danlos syndromes and with osteogenesis imperfecta.
- Rheumatic heart disease, where this disease is still endemic. A dilated annulus allows elongation of chordae with, sometimes, prolapse of the anterior leaflet, but marked billowing or redundancy of leaflets is unusual.
- Papillary muscle dysfunction due to ischemic heart disease

Diagnostic Hallmarks

The majority of patients are asymptomatic. Dyspnea is rather vague, often occurs at rest, and is commonly out of proportion with the degree of mitral regurgitation, which is usually asymptomatic in >80% of patients. Extreme fatigue, dizziness, anxiety, panic disorders, palpitations, presyncope, syncope, and chest pain may occur without a satisfactory explanation. Psychogenic factors play a role in the varied symptomatology.

Physical Signs

One or multiple mid- or late systolic clicks of nonejection type may be constant or intermittent, changing with posture or maneuvers, but do not prove the existence of mitral valve prolapse. The timing of clicks may be misinterpreted as gallop sounds, but apart from their timing, clicks can be differentiated from an S_3 by the high-pitched quality and by being most audible with a diaphragm. In some patients, the click is followed by a murmur; in others, only a murmur is present. The murmur has typical features:

- A typical late systolic murmur is unmistakable and confirms the diagnosis.
- The murmur is usually crescendo–decrescendo, the auscultator gets the impression that the murmur is occurring synchronously with S_2, and the murmur often extends through A_2.
- A whoop, a short honking sound, or a sound of other musical quality may highlight the murmur, which changes in intensity depending on LV volume and blood pressure.
- The late systolic murmur or click is heard earlier and made louder by the following maneuvers that reduce LV volume: standing, tilting upright, Valsalva, and tachycardia. Amyl nitrite decreases ventricular volume and blood pressure; therefore, the murmur is heard earlier but is made softer.
- The murmur or clicks are heard later and are softer with maneuvers that increase LV volume or decrease blood pressure: squatting, bradycardia, beta-blocking agents. Thus, the physician should listen to the patient lying, standing, and squatting because the murmur may be heard only on standing. With more severe mitral regurgitation, the murmur lasts longer and may become pansystolic.
- When chordal rupture occurs, the murmur changes in quality and radiation.
- The posterior mitral leaflet often has three scallops; rupture of the chordae to the middle scallop of the posterior leaflet is the most common chordal rupture. The resulting murmur radiates anteriorly and is maximal at the lower left sternal border and radiates toward the upper right sternal edge. The crescendo–decrescendo quality may simulate an aortic systolic murmur. However, the late timing of the murmur of mitral valve prolapse differentiates the murmur from the early timing of aortic valvular murmurs.
- Chordal rupture of the anterior leaflet causes the murmur to radiate to the posterior axilla.

- The flail mitral valve produces a loud murmur, the intensity of which is characteristically accentuated over the spine and may be heard from the occiput to the sacral spine.
- The mitral regurgitant jet can be identified by TEE; it moves in a counterclockwise direction with flail anterior leaflet involvement and in a clockwise direction with posterior leaflet involvement.

Approximately 15% of patients with mitral valve prolapse have skeletal abnormalities: "straight back," pectus excavatum or pectus carinatum, scoliosis, or some features of Marfan syndrome.

Complications

1. **Severe mitral regurgitation** occurs in approximately 10% of patients with true mitral valve prolapse and is 5 times more common in men above age 45 than in women. Although mitral valve prolapse occurs most commonly in women, severe mitral regurgitation requiring surgery occurs in about 5% of men and <1.5% of women. Chordal rupture is a common occurrence in patients with severe mitral regurgitation.

2. **Arrhythmias** commonly occur and include ventricular premature beats (VPCs), atrial ectopics, paroxysmal supraventricular tachycardia, and occasionally atrial fibrillation. Lethal arrhythmias have been reported.

3. **Sudden death,** although rare, may occur in healthy young active individuals and is unexplained. Patients with mitral valve prolapse who die suddenly appear to have the following clinical and morphologic hallmarks:
   - Women ages 21 to 51 may not have significant mitral regurgitation.
   - Dilated mitral valve annulus
   - Elongated anterior mitral valve leaflet
   - Abnormal elongated posterior mitral leaflet; often there is herniation of the posterior leaflet above the anterior leaflet
   - A fibrous endocardial plaque under the posterior mitral valve leaflet is a common finding
   - Significant, moderate to severe prolapse of the mitral valve
   - Raptured chordae
   - Mitral regurgitant murmur (50%)
   - A click (only 25–37%)
   - Arrhythmia (>50%); VPCs (~33%)

4. **Endocarditis:** The exact incidence of endocarditis in patients with true mitral valve prolapse is unknown but is estimated to be in the range of 1 in 6000 in all patients with mitral valve prolapse and about 1 in 2000 of those patients with mitral regurgitation.

5. **Systemic embolization:** Transient ischemic attacks, stroke, retinal arteriolar occlusions, and amaurosis fugax are rare complications of mitral valve prolapse due to embolization of bland emboli; the exact incidence has not been accurately assessed.

APPENDICES

APPENDIX A
Infusion Pump Charts

Table A–1 □ DOBUTAMINE INFUSION PUMP CHART
(dobutamine 2 amps [500 mg] in 500 ml [1000 µg/ml])

Weight (kg)	40	45	50	55	60	65	70	75	80	85	90	95	100	105
Dosage (µg/kg/min)								Rate (ml/hr)						
1.0	2	3	3	3	4	4	4	5	5	5	5	6	6	6
1.5	4	4	5	5	5	6	6	7	7	8	8	9	9	9
2.0	5	5	6	7	7	8	8	9	10	10	11	11	12	13
2.5	6	7	8	8	9	10	11	11	12	13	14	14	15	16
3.0	7	8	9	10	11	12	13	14	14	15	16	17	18	19
3.5	8	9	11	12	13	14	15	16	17	18	19	20	21	22
4.0	10	11	12	13	14	16	17	18	19	20	22	23	24	25
4.5	11	12	14	15	16	18	19	20	22	23	24	26	27	28
5.0	12	14	15	17	18	20	21	23	24	26	27	29	30	32
5.5	13	15	17	18	20	21	23	25	26	28	30	31	33	35
6.0	14	16	18	20	22	23	25	27	29	31	32	34	36	38
7.0	17	19	21	23	25	27	29	32	34	36	38	40	42	44
8.0	19	22	24	26	29	31	34	36	38	41	43	46	48	50
9.0	22	24	27	30	32	35	38	41	43	46	49	51	54	57
10.0	24	27	30	33	36	39	42	45	48	51	54	57	60	63
12.5	30	34	38	41	45	49	53	56	60	64	68	71	75	79
15.0	36	41	45	50	54	59	63	69	72	77	81	86	90	95
20.0	48	54	60	66	72	78	84	90	96	102	108	114	120	126

From Khan, M Gabriel: Cardiac Drug Therapy, 5th ed. London, WB Saunders Co., 2000.
The above rates apply only for a 1000 mg/L concentration of dobutamine. If a different concentration must be used, appropriate adjustments in rates should be made. Usual dose range: 2.5–10 µg/kg/min.

Table A–2 □ DOPAMINE INFUSION PUMP CHART
(dopamine 400 mg in 500 ml [800 μg/ml])

Weight (kg)	40	50	60	70	80	90	100
Dosage (μg/kg/min)				Rate [ml/hr [pump] or drops/min [microdrip]]*			
1.0	3	4	5	5	6	7	8
1.5	5	6	7	8	9	10	11
2.0	6	8	9	11	12	14	15
2.5	8	9	11	13	15	17	19
3.0	9	11	14	16	18	20	23
3.5	11	13	16	18	21	24	26
4.0	12	15	18	21	24	27	30
4.5	14	17	20	24	27	30	34
5.0	15	19	23	26	30	34	38
6.0	18	23	27	32	36	41	45
7.0	21	26	32	37	42	47	53
8.0	24	30	36	42	48	54	60
9.0	27	34	41	47	54	61	68
10.0	30	38	45	53	60	68	75
12.0	36	45	54	63	72	81	90
15.0	45	56	68	79	90	101	113
20.0	60	75	90	105	120	135	150
25.0	75	94	113	131	150	169	188

From Khan, M Gabriel: Cardiac Drug Therapy, 5th ed. London, WB Saunders Co., 2000.

The above rates apply only for an 800 mg/L concentration of dopamine. If a different concentration must be used, appropriate adjustments in rates should be made. Start at 1 μg/kg/min; ideal dose range: 5–7.5 μg/kg/min. Maximum suggested: 10 μg/kg/min.

Dopamine should be given via a central line.

*Use chart for (1) pump (ml/hr) or (2) microdrip (drops/min).

Example: 60 kg patient at 2.0 μg/kg/min: pump, set pump at 9 ml/hr; microdrip, run solution at 9 drops/min.

Table A–3 □ **CONTINUOUS-INFUSION HEPARIN**

Rate (ml/hr)	Units/hr	Units/24 hr
1. 21	840	20,160
2. 25	1000	24,000
3. 28	1120	26,880
4. 30	1200	28,800
5. 32	1280	30,720
6. 34	1360	32,640
7. 36	1440	34,560
8. 38	1520	36,480
9. 40	1600	38,400
10. 42	1680	40,320
11. 44	1760	42,240
12. 46	1840	44,160
13. 48	1920	46,080
14. 50	2000	48,000

From Khan, M Gabriel: Cardiac Drug Therapy, 5th ed. London, WB Saunders Co., 2000, p 366.

Heparin (20,000 U) in 500 ml of 5% dextrose in water. If noncardiac, dilute in 0.9% saline; 1 ml = 40 U.

For each heparin order, specify both the rate of flow and the dose in units per hour. Start with no. 4, 1200 U/hr, and adjust to maintain activated partial thromboplastin time at 1.5 to 2.5 times control value (usual therapeutic range, 60–85 seconds). (See page 362.)

Table A–4 □ **NITROGLYCERIN INFUSION PUMP CHART**
(50 mg in 500 ml 5% dextrose in water = 100 μg/ml)

Dose (μg/min)	Infusion Rate (ml/hr)
5	3
10	6
15	9
20	12
25	15
30	18
35	21
40	24
45	27
50	30
60	36
70	42
80	48
90	54
100	60
120	72
140	84
160	96
200	120
250	150

From Khan, M Gabriel: Cardiac Drug Therapy, 5th ed. London, WB Saunders Co., 2000.

Increase by 5 μg/min every 5 minutes until relief of chest pain.

Decrease rate if systolic blood pressure <95 mm Hg or falls to 20 mm Hg below the baseline, or if diastolic blood pressure <65 mm Hg.

Table A–5 □ NITROPRUSSIDE INFUSION PUMP CHART
(nitroprusside 50 mg [1 vial] in 100 ml [500 μg/ml])

Weight (kg)	40	50	60	70	80	90	100
Dosage (μg/kg/min)	Rate (ml/hr)						
0.2	1	1	1	2	2	2	2
0.5	2	3	4	4	5	5	6
0.8	4	5	6	7	8	9	10
1.0	5	6	7	8	10	11	12
1.2	6	7	9	10	12	13	14
1.5	7	9	11	13	14	16	18
1.8	9	11	13	15	17	19	22
2.0	10	12	14	17	19	22	24
2.2	11	13	16	18	21	24	26
2.5	12	15	18	21	24	27	30
2.8	13	17	20	23	27	30	34
3.0	14	18	22	25	29	32	36
3.2	15	19	23	27	31	35	38
3.5	17	21	25	29	34	38	42
3.8	18	23	27	32	36	41	46
4.0	19	24	29	34	38	43	48
4.5	22	27	32	38	43	49	54
5.0	24	30	36	42	48	54	60
6.0	29	36	43	50	58	65	72

From Khan, M Gabriel: Cardiac Drug Therapy, 5th ed. London, WB Saunders Co., 2000.

The above rates apply only for a 500 mg/L concentration of nitroprusside. If a different concentration must be used, appropriate adjustments in rates should be made. Start at 0.2 μg/kg/min. Increase slowly. Average dose, 3 μg/kg/min. Usual dose range, 0.5–5.0 μg/kg/min.

APPENDIX B
SI Units Conversion Table

"SI units" is the abbreviation for Le Système International d'Unités. SI units are based on the metric system.

This book gives conventional units because the vast majority of physicians and hospitals in the United States have not converted to SI units and it is unlikely that this will occur during the next decade. SI units and a conversion table for commonly measured laboratory parameters appropriate to cardiovascular disorders are provided here.

Table B–1 □ CONVENTIONAL AND SI UNITS

Laboratory Tests	Conventional	Conversion Factor	SI
Albumin	4–6 g/dl	10	40–60 g/L
Alkaline phosphatase	30–120 U/L	0.0167	0.5–2 μ/kat/L
Amylase (serum)	0–130 U/L	0.0167	0.217 μ/kat/L
Aspartate transaminase (AST)			
Female	9–25 U/L	0.0167	0.15–0.42 μ/kat/L
Male	10–40 U/L	0.0167	0.17–0.67 μ/kat/L
Bicarbonate	22–26 mEq/L	1	22–66 mmol/L
Bilirubin			
Total	0.0–1 mg/dl	17.1	0–17 μmol/L
Direct	0.0–0.4 mg/dl	17.1	0–7 μmol/L
Calcium	8.5–10.5 mEq/L	1	2.1–2.6 mmol/L
Chloride	100–108 mEq/L	1	100–108 mmol/L
Cholesterol	<200 mg/dl	0.0259	<5.2 mmol/L
HDL	34–70 mg/dl		0.88–1.8 mmol/L
LDL	<160 mg/dl, normal		<4 mmol/L
LDL	<130 mg/dl, desirable	0.0259	<3.4 mmol/L
LDL	<100 mg/dl, if CHD		<2.5 mmol/L
Creatinine	0.6–1.4 mg/dl	88.4	55–124 μmol/L
Glucose	70–110 mg/dl	0.0555	3.9–6.1 mmol/L
Creatine kinase (CK)	40–150 U/L	0.0167	0.67–2.5 μ/kat/L
MB fraction in acute MI	>5%	0.01	>0.05
Digoxin	1–2 ng/ml	1.28	1.2–2.6 nmol/L
	<1–2 μg/L		
Ferritin (serum)	18–300 ng/ml	1	18–300 μg/L
Lactic dehydrogenase (LDH)	110–250 U/L	0.01	1.83–4.23 μ/kat/L
Magnesium	1.5–2 mEq/L	0.5	0.8–1 mmol/L
Oxygen (Pao_2) (age-dependent arterial)	5–100 mmHg	0.1333	10–13.3 kPa
$Paco_2$	33–44 mmHg	0.1333	4.4–5.9 kPa
Potassium	3.9–5.2 mEq/L	1	3.9–5.2 mmol/L
Quinidine	2–5 μg/ml		3–5.5 μmol/L
Sodium	135–147 mEq/L	1	135–147 mmol/L
Theophilline	10–20 mg/dl	5.55	55–110 μmol/L
Triglycerides	<200 mg/dl	0.0113	<2.26 mmol/L
Urea	8–18 mg/dl	0.357	3–6.5 mmol/L
Uric acid	2–7 mg/dl	59.48	120–420 μmol/L

Kat = katal; HDL = high-density lipoprotein; LDL = low-density lipoprotein; CHD = coronary heart disease; MI = myocardial infarction.

APPENDIX C

Commonly Used
Cardiovascular Drugs

A large number of cardiovascular drugs are currently available, with a proliferation of similar agents by many pharmaceutical firms. This concise text cannot provide the trade names of all cardiovascular drugs.

The maximum dosage provided in the text is at times less than that suggested by the manufacturer, because in clinical practice a lesser dose suffices and results in fewer adverse effects, especially when medications are combined. Today's practice of cardiovascular medicine often calls for combination drug therapy.

Some drugs have not been listed in the following tables because either they are rarely used or they have been replaced by agents that are more effective and have fewer adverse effects.

It is the final prescription that cures or ameliorates bothersome symptoms. Thus, practicing trainees and clinicians must be well versed in the art and science of cardiovascular prescribing.

Table C–1 □ DRUG THERAPY FOR ACUTE MYOCARDIAL INFARCTION

Drug	Dosage
Aspirin	160–325 mg plain aspirin chewed and swallowed, then 325 mg enteric-coated aspirin daily
Morphine	4–8 mg IV at a rate of 1 mg/min, repeated 2–4 mg at intervals of 10–15 min until pain is relieved
Thrombolytic agents	(see Table C–2)
In selected patients	
Beta blocker*	
Atenolol	5 mg IV over 5 min, 10 min later 5 mg IV over 5 min
Metoprolol	5 mg IV at a rate of 1 mg/min, 5-mg bolus 5 min later, 5-mg bolus 5 min later if needed

*Contraindications: Asthma, systolic BP <100 mm Hg, severe CHF, second- or third-degree AV block. Stop IV if heart rate 50/min, systolic BP <95 mm Hg.
IV = intravenous; BP = blood pressure; CHF = congestive heart failure; AV = atrioventricular.

Table C–2 □ THROMBOLYTIC AGENTS

Drug	Dosage
Streptokinase	1.5 million U in 100 ml 0.9% saline IV infusion over 30–60 min
Anistreplase	30 U in 5 ml sterile water or saline by slow IV bolus over 2–5 min
tPA (alteplase) front loaded	15-mg bolus then 0.75 mg/kg over 30 min (not >50 mg), 0.50 mg/kg over 60 min (not >35 mg); total dose ≤100 mg
Reteplase	Two × 10-unit bolus injections over <2 min, 30 min apart
Tenecteplase (TNK tPA) TNKase	Single-bolus injection over 5 seconds:

	<60 kg	30 mg
	≥60 to <70	35 mg
	≥70 to <80	40 mg
	≥80 to <90	45 mg
	≥90	50 mg

Table C–3 □ DRUGS FOR MAINTENANCE MANAGEMENT OF POST–MYOCARDIAL INFARCTION

Drug	Dosage
ACE inhibitor	
Captopril	3–6 mg test dose, then 12.5–25 mg 3 times daily, maximum 150 mg daily
Enalapril	2.5 mg test dose, then 2.5–10 mg once daily, maximum 15 mg daily
Ramipril	5–10 mg daily
Aspirin	
Enteric coated	81–325 mg daily
Beta blocker	
Metoprolol	50–100 mg twice daily
Propranolol (only in nonsmokers and nondiabetics)	40–80 mg 2 times daily or Inderal LA 80–240 mg once daily
Timolol	5–10 mg twice daily

ACE = angiotensin-converting enzyme.

Commonly Used Cardiovascular Drugs **403**

Table C–4 □ DRUGS FOR THE TREATMENT OF ANGINA PECTORIS

Generic	Trade Name	Supplied As	Dosage
Beta blockers			
Acebutolol	Monitan Sectral	100, 200, 400 mg	100–400 mg twice daily
Atenolol	Tenormin	50, 100 mg	25–50 mg twice daily or 50–100 mg once daily
Metoprolol	Betaloc Lopressor Toprol XL	50, 100 mg	50–200 mg twice daily, 50–200 mg once daily
Nadolol*	Corgard	40, 80 mg	20–160 mg once daily
Timolol*	Blocadren	5, 10 mg	5–10 mg twice daily
Propranolol (in nonsmokers)*	Inderal	20, 40, 80 mg	20–80 mg 3 times daily
	Inderal LA	80, 120, 160 mg	80–240 mg once daily
Calcium antagonists			
Amlodipine	Norvasc	5, 10 mg	2.5–10 mg once daily
Diltiazem**	Cardizem CD	120, 180, 240 mg	120–240 mg once daily
Nifedipine**	Procardia XL Adalat XL	30, 60 mg	30–60 mg once daily
Verapamil**	Covera-HS	180, 240 mg	180–240 mg once daily
Nitrates***			
Isosorbide dinitrate	Isordil	20, 30, 40 mg	20, 30, or 40 mg, 7 A.M., 12 and 4 P.M.
Isosorbide mononitrate	Imdur	60, 120 mg	30–120 mg, 7 A.M. daily
	Ismo	20 mg	20 mg, 7 A.M. and 2 P.M.
Nitroglycerin	Nitrong SR	2.6 mg	2.6 mg, 7 A.M. and 2 P.M.

*Avoid in diabetics; choose a cardioselective agent such as metoprolol or atenolol.

**Do not use short-acting formulation.

***Not later than 4 P.M. so as to avoid nitrate tolerance.

Table C–5 □ ACE INHIBITORS

Generic	Trade Name	Supplied As	Dosage*
Benazepril	Lotensin Cibace/E Cibacène/F	5, 10, 20, 40 mg 10–30 mg once daily	10–30 mg once daily
Captopril	Capoten Lopril, Lopirin/E	12.5, 25, 50, 100 mg	12.5–100 mg twice daily
Cilazapril	Inhibace Vascace/UK	1, 2.5, 5 mg	1.5–5 mg once daily
Enalapril	Vasotec Innovace/UK	2.5, 5, 10, 20 mg	5–30 mg once daily or 5–15 mg twice daily
Fosinopril	Monopril	10, 20 mg	5–40 mg once daily
Lisinopril	Prinivil, Zestril Carace/E	2.5, 5, 10, 20, 40 mg	5–40 mg once daily
Perindopril	Coversyl Acertil/E	2, 4 mg	2–8 mg once daily
Quinapril	Accupril Accupro/E Acuitel/F	5, 10, 20, 40 mg	5–40 mg once daily
Ramipril	Altace	1.25, 2.5, 5, 10 mg	2.5–15 mg once daily
Trandolapril	Gopten Odrik/E	0.5, 1, 2 mg	1–4 mg once daily

* = reduce dose and increase dosing interval with renal failure and in the elderly.
ACE = angiotensin-converting enzyme; E = Europe; F = France; UK = United Kingdom.

Table C–6 □ ANGIOTENSIN II RECEPTOR BLOCKERS*

Generic	Trade Name	Dosage
Candesartan	Atacand, Amias (UK)	2–8 mg once daily, maximum 32 mg (16 mg, UK and C)
Eprosartan	Teveten	200–400 mg twice daily
Irbesartan	Avapro, Aprovel (UK)	75–300 mg once daily
Losartan	Cozaar	50–100 mg once or 50 mg twice daily
Telmisartan	Micardis	20–80 mg once daily (see Chapter 23)
Valsartan	Diovan	40–160 mg once daily; maximum, 320 mg

*Angiotensin II receptor (AT$_1$), blockers (antagonists).
C = Canada; UK = United Kingdom.

Table C–7 □ ANTIHYPERTENSIVE DRUGS

Generic	Trade Name	Supplied As	Dosage
ACE inhibitors	See Table C–5		
Angiotensin II receptor blockers	See Table C–6		
Beta blockers	See Table C–4		
Calcium antagonists	See Table C–4		
Central acting drugs			
Clonidine	Catapres	0.1–0.2 mg	0.1–0.8 mg once daily
Guanfacine	Tenex	1 mg	1–2 mg once daily
Methyldopa	Aldomet	250, 500 mg	250–500 mg 3 times daily
Diuretics			
Hydrochlorothiazide	HydroDIURIL	24, 50 mg	12.5–25 mg, 7 A.M. daily
Indapamide	Lozol Lozide/C	2.5 mg	1.25–2.5 mg, 7 A.M. daily
Furosemide*	Lasix	40, 80 mg	40–80 mg

*If creatinine level is >2.3 mg/dl (203 μmol/L), more effective than thiazides.
ACE = angiotensin-converting enzyme; C = Canada.

Table C–8 □ DRUGS FOR HEART FAILURE

Generic	Supplied As	Dosage
Digoxin (Lanoxin)	0.125, 0.25 mg	0.5 mg twice daily for 2 days, then 0.25 mg preferably at bedtime* daily; age >70 yr or creatinine >1.4 mg/dl (124 μmol/L), give 0.125 mg daily
Torsemide (Demadex)	5, 10, 20, 100 mg	2.5–20 mg once daily
Furosemide (Lasix)	20, 40, 80 mg	40–80 mg once daily, if needed†; 80 mg at 7 A.M. and 2 P.M.
Metolazone‡	1.25, 5 mg	1.25–2.5 mg once daily (monitor serum K$^+$)
ACE inhibitors§		
Captopril (Capoten)	12.5, 25, 50 mg	6.25–12.5 mg three times daily, then 12.5–37.5 mg 3 times daily
Enalapril (Vasotec)	2.5, 5, 10, 20 mg	2.5 mg once daily, then 5–30 mg once daily
Lisinopril Prinivil capace (UK)	2.5, 5, 10, 20 mg	5–35 mg once daily
Angiotensin II receptor blockers	See Table C–6	

*Allows more accurate blood sampling for digoxin levels when needed.
†Severe chronic congestive heart failure (CHF).
‡For refractory CHF.
§For other ACE inhibitors approved for CHF, see Table C–6.
ACE = angiotensin-converting enzyme.

Table C-9 □ USEFUL ANTIARRHYTHMIC AGENTS

Drug	Dosage
For ventricular arrhythmia	
Amiodarone (Cordarone)	200 mg 3 or 4 times daily × 2 weeks; 200 mg twice daily × 6 weeks if arrhythmia controlled, decrease dose by about 400 mg every 4 weeks to maintenance 200 mg daily
Lidocaine	75–100 mg IV bolus with simultaneous IV infusion at 2 mg/ml/min; if recurrence, give further 50–75 mg bolus, then increase to 3 mg/ml/min
Metoprolol	50–150 mg twice daily
Sotalol (Betapace, Sotacor)	80–160 mg twice daily, if needed up to 320 mg daily (maintain normal serum K^+)
For supraventricular tachycardia (SVT)	
Adenosine	6 mg IV over 2 sec into peripheral vein; if recurrence, 2 min later give 12 mg IV bolus
Diltiazem IV	For SVT or slowing the ventricular rate in patients with atrial flutter or atrial fibrillation; bolus IV 20 mg over 2 min (average patient, 0.25 mg/kg); 15 min later if needed, 25 mg (0.35 mg/kg) over 2 min; or treatment as infusion 5–10 mg/hr, maximum 15 mg/hr
Verapamil	2.5–10 mg over 1–2 min, in the absence of LV dysfunction, CHF, or systolic BP <100 mm Hg

LV = left ventricular; CHF = congestive heart failure; BP = blood pressure; IV = intravenous.

Table C-10 □ DRUGS FOR CARDIAC ARREST

Atropine	1 mg every 2–5 min to maximum 3 mg (0.04 mg/kg)
Epinephrine	1 mg repeated every 3–5 min
Vasopressin	40 U IV one dose only
Lidocaine for VF	100-mg IV bolus (1–1.5 mg/kg), simultaneous infusion 2 mg/min
Propranolol for recurrent VF (or metoprolol)	1 mg IV over 2 min, repeat every 5 min to maximum 5 mg 5-mg IV bolus, repeat every 5 min to total 15 mg

VF = ventricular fibrillation

Table C-11 □ DRUGS FOR HYPERLIPIDEMIA*

Generic	Trade Name	Supplied As	Dosage
Statins			
Atorvastatin	Lipitor	Tablet, 10, 20, 40 mg	10–60 mg at night; rarely, 80 mg
Cerivastatin	Baycol	Tablet, 0.2, 0.3, 0.4, 0.8 mg	0.2–0.6 mg at night
Fluvastatin	Lescol	Capsule, 20, 40 mg	20–40 mg at bedtime
Lovastatin	Mevacor	Tablet, 10, 20 mg	10–40 mg after evening meal
Pravastatin	Pravachol	Tablet, 10, 20, 40 mg	10–40 mg at bedtime
Simvastatin	Zocor	5, 10, 20, 40, 80 mg	5–60 mg after evening meal
Resins†			
Choles-tyramine	Questran Light	Powder	4–12 g twice daily
Colestipol	Colestid	Powder	5–10 g twice daily
Fibrates‡			
Bezafibrate	Bezalip	Tablet, 200, 400 mg	200 mg twice daily after food; 400 mg once daily
	Bezalip-Mono	Tablet, 400 mg	400 mg once daily
Fenofibrate	Lipidil Micro	Capsule, 200 mg	200 mg once daily (long acting)
Gemfibrozil	Lopid	Tablet, 300 mg	300–600 mg twice daily before meals
Nicotinic acid‡	Niacin	50, 100, 250, 500 mg	0.5–1 g 3 times daily

*See Table C-12 for American Heart Association guidelines for drug therapy.
†Give other drugs 1 hr before or 4 hr after resins.
‡Do not combine with statins. **Combination not approved by FDA or Health Protection Canada.**

Table C-12 □ AMERICAN HEART ASSOCIATION GUIDELINES: DRUG THERAPY FOR HYPERLIPIDEMIA [TREATMENT DECISIONS BASED ON LDL CHOLESTEROL]

	Initiation Level	LDL Goal
Dietary Therapy		
Without CHD and with fewer than two risk factors	≥160 mg/dl	<160 mg/dl (4.2 mmol/L)
Without CHD and with two or more risk factors	≥130 mg/dl	<130 mg/dl (3.4 mmol/L)
With CHD	>100 mg/dl	≤100 mg/dl (2.6 mmol/L)
	Consideration Level	**LDL Goal**
Drug Treatment		
Without CHD and with fewer than two risk factors	≥190 mg/dl*	<160 mg/dl (4.2 mmol/L)
Without CHD and with two or more risk factors	≥160 mg/dl	<130 mg/dl (3.4 mmol/L)
With CHD	≥130 mg/dl†	≤100 mg/dl (2.6 mmol/L)

From the Expert Panel on Detection, Evaluation, and Treatment of High Blood Cholesterol in Adults (Adult Treatment Panel II). Circulation 1994;89:1339.

*In men <35 years old and premenopausal women with LDL cholesterol levels of 190–219 mg/dl, drug therapy should be delayed except in high-risk patients such as those with diabetes.

†In patients with CHD and LDL cholesterol levels of 100–129 mg/dl, the physician should exercise clinical judgment in deciding whether to initiate drug treatment.

LDL = low-density lipoproteins; CHD = coronary heart disease.

APPENDIX D
Adverse Effects of Cardiac Drugs

Adverse effects of cardiac drugs may be minor, severe, or life threatening. The occurrence of some side effects can be predicted; e.g., edema of the legs is commonly caused by dihydropyridine calcium antagonists. Life-threatening angioedema may occur, albeit rarely, with angiotensin-converting enzyme inhibitors during the treatment of benign, asymptomatic hypertension.

Patients must be warned concerning the risk of severe adverse effects. Most drugs have minor side effects, and it is not necessary to worry the patient with every detail that could decrease compliance.

Table D–1 lists the important adverse effects of commonly used cardiovascular drugs.

Table D–1 □ ADVERSE EFFECTS OF CARDIAC DRUGS

Angiotensin-converting enzyme inhibitors	Angioneurotic edema, cough, hypotension, hyperkalemia, mouth ulcers, neutropenia, pruritic rash, pemphigus, proteinuria, renal failure, taste disturbance, wheeze
Antiarrhythmics	
Adenosine	Chest pain (transient), flushing
Amiodarone	Asystole, hypothyroidism, pulmonary infiltrates, hepatitis, slate-gray skin, torsades de pointes
Flecainide	Proarrhythmias, incessant ventricular tachycardia (VT), ventricular fibrillation (VF) (use severely restricted)
Lidocaine	Sinus arrest, asystole, twitching seizures
Mexiletine	Confusional state, gastric irritation, nausea, nystagmus seizures
Procainamide	Agranulocytosis, congestive heart failure (CHF), lupus
Propafenone	Agranulocytosis, lupus, proarrhythmias, VT (restricted use)
Quinidine	Angioedema, diarrhea, syncope, thrombocytopenia, torsades de pointes, VF
Sotalol	Bradycardia, bronchospasm in asthmatics, CHF, torsades de pointes
Beta blockers	Bradycardia, bronchospasm in asthmatics, CHF, Raynaud's phenomenon
Calcium antagonists	
Diltiazem	Bradycardia, sinus arrest, CHF, hypotension
Dihydropyridine Amlodipine Felodipine Nifedipine	Edema, flushing, hypotension
Verapamil	Bradycardia, asystole, constipation, CHF
Digoxin	Arrhythmias: ventricular premature beats, atrioventricular block, nausea, vomiting, scotomas
Drugs for hyperlipidemia	
Fibrates Bezafibrate Fenofibrate Gemfibrozil	Nausea, abdominal pain, hepatic dysfunction, gallstones, impotence, myositis, skin rash
Resins Cholestyramine Colestipol	Constipation, abdominal pains, gritty, bothersome taste
Statins Fluvastatin Lovastatin Simvastatin	Abdominal cramps, headache, mild hepatic dysfunction, myalgia, rare myositis
Vasodilators Prazosin Hytrin Hydralazine	Syncope, hypotension, palpitation, retrograde ejaculation
Others	
Diuretics	Hypokalemia, hyponatremia
Digoxin	Glucose intolerance, dehydration, pancreatitis
Clonidine	Dry mouth, drowsiness, impotence, rebound hypertension
Methyldopa	Drowsiness, impotence, postural hypotension, rebound hypertension, hepatitis, hemolytic anemia

APPENDIX E
Cardiac Drug Interactions

There are two basic causes of drug interactions. Pharmacodynamic interactions occur between drugs with similar or opposite pharmacologic or adverse effects. Competition may occur at the same receptor site, or the agents may act on the same physiologic system. Thus, hemodynamic effects of an agent may be increased or decreased by another agent. Pharmacokinetic interactions occur when an agent alters the absorption, distribution, metabolism, or elimination of another. Important cardiac drug interactions are summarized in Tables E–1 and E–2.

Table E–1 □ IMPORTANT CARDIAC DRUG INTERACTIONS

Drug	Potential Interactions With
ACE inhibitors	Acebutolol, allopurinol, cyclosporine, and other agents that alter immune response; K^+-sparing diuretics, lithium, nitrates (preload), nonsteroidal anti-inflammatory drugs
Adenosine	Carbamazepine, dipyridamole, theophylline
Amiodarone	Anticoagulants, digoxin, diltiazem, K^+-losing diuretics, sotalol, tricyclic antidepressants, verapamil
Anticoagulants	See Table E–2
Beta blockers	Amiodarone, diltiazem, verapamil
Digoxin	Amiodarone, calcium antagonists (not nifedipine), quinidine, K^+-losing diuretics
Diltiazem	Amiodarone, beta blockers, cyclosporine, digoxin, lithium, quinidine, tissue plasminogen activator
Lidocaine	Beta blockers (hepatic metabolized), phenytoin
Quinidine	Anticoagulants, amiodarone, digoxin, diltiazem, phenytoin, verapamil
Sotalol	Class 1 antiarrhythmics, K^+-losing diuretics, diltiazem, verapamil

Statins
  Atorvastatin
  Fluvastatin
  Lovastatin
  Pravastatin
  Simvastatin
	Niacin, fibrates (gemfibrozil, Lipidil Micro)

Tissue plasminogen activator	Diltiazem; nitroglycerin IV
Verapamil	Amiodarone, beta blockers, cyclosporine, digoxin, lithium, quinidine

ACE = angiotensin-converting enzyme; IV = intravenous.

Table E–2 □ ORAL ANTICOAGULANTS—DRUG INTERACTIONS

Drugs That May Enhance Anticoagulant Response

Acetaminophen
Alcohol
Allopurinol
Aminoglycosides
Amiodarone
Ampicillin
Anabolic steroids
Aspirin
Cephalosporins
Chloral hydrate
Chloramphenicol
Chlorpromazine
Chlorpropamide
Chlortetracycline
Cimetidine
Ciprofloxacin
Clofibrate (fibrates)
Co-trimoxazole
Danazol
Dextrothyroxine
Diazoxide
Dipyridamole
Disulfiram
Erythromycin
Ethacrynic acid
Fenclofenac
Fenoprofen
Fibrates
Flufenamic acid
Fluvoxamine
Liquid paraffin
Mefenamic acid
Methotrexate
Metronidazole
Monoamine oxidase inhibitors
Nalidixic acid
Naproxen
Neomycin
Omeprazole
Penicillin (large doses IV)
Phenformin
Phenylbutazone
Phenytoin
Propylthiouracil
Propafenone
Quinidine
Sulfinpyrazone
Sulfonamides
Tetracyclines
Tolbutamide
Tricyclic antidepressants
Trimethoprim sulfate
Verapamil

Drugs That May Decrease Anticoagulant Response

Antacids
Antihistamines
Barbiturates
Carbamazepine
Cholestyramine
Colestipol
Corticosteroids
Cyclophosphamide
Dichloralphenazone
Disopyramide
Glutethimide
Griseofulvin
Mercaptopurine
Oral contraceptives
Pheneturide
Phenobarbitone
Phenytoin
Primidone
Rifampicin
Vitamins K_1 and K_2

Modified from Khan, M Gabriel: Cardiac Drug Therapy, 5th ed. London, WB Saunders Co., 2000, p 364.

APPENDIX F
Drug Index

The Drug Index gives the generic drug name in lower case; the pharmaceutical trade names begin with a capital letter.

C = Canada when different from US; F = France, G = Germany, I = Italy.

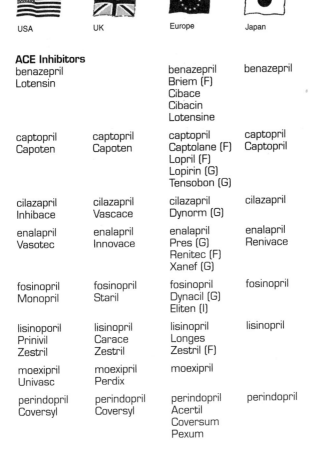

| USA | UK | Europe | Japan |

ACE Inhibitors

USA	UK	Europe	Japan
benazepril		benazepril	benazepril
Lotensin		Briem (F)	
		Cibace	
		Cibacin	
		Lotensine	
captopril	captopril	captopril	captopril
Capoten	Capoten	Captolane (F)	Captopril
		Lopril (F)	
		Lopirin (G)	
		Tensobon (G)	
cilazapril	cilazapril	cilazapril	cilazapril
Inhibace	Vascace	Dynorm (G)	
enalapril	enalapril	enalapril	enalapril
Vasotec	Innovace	Pres (G)	Renivace
		Renitec (F)	
		Xanef (G)	
fosinopril	fosinopril	fosinopril	fosinopril
Monopril	Staril	Dynacil (G)	
		Eliten (I)	
lisinoporil	lisinopril	lisinopril	lisinopril
Prinivil	Carace	Longes	
Zestril	Zestril	Zestril (F)	
moexipril	moexipril	moexipril	
Univasc	Perdix		
perindopril	perindopril	perindopril	perindopril
Coversyl	Coversyl	Acertil	
		Coversum	
		Pexum	

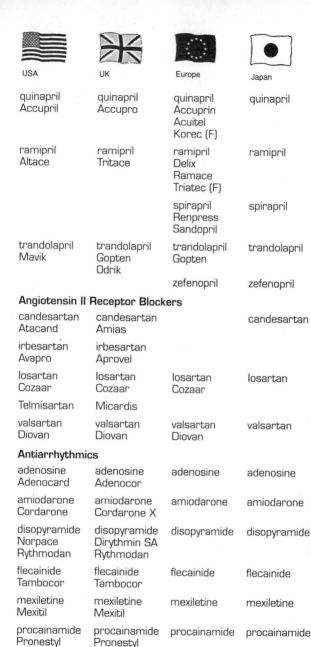 USA	UK	Europe	Japan
quinapril Accupril	quinapril Accupro	quinapril Accuprin Acuitel Korec (F)	quinapril
ramipril Altace	ramipril Tritace	ramipril Delix Ramace Triatec (F)	ramipril
		spirapril Renpress Sandopril	spirapril
trandolapril Mavik	trandolapril Gopten Odrik	trandolapril Gopten	trandolapril
		zefenopril	zefenopril

Angiotensin II Receptor Blockers

candesartan Atacand	candesartan Amias		candesartan
irbesartan Avapro	irbesartan Aprovel		
losartan Cozaar	losartan Cozaar	losartan Cozaar	losartan
Telmisartan	Micardis		
valsartan Diovan	valsartan Diovan	valsartan Diovan	valsartan

Antiarrhythmics

adenosine Adenocard	adenosine Adenocor	adenosine	adenosine
amiodarone Cordarone	amiodarone Cordarone X	amiodarone	amiodarone
disopyramide Norpace Rythmodan	disopyramide Dirythmin SA Rythmodan	disopyramide	disopyramide
flecainide Tambocor	flecainide Tambocor	flecainide	flecainide
mexiletine Mexitil	mexiletine Mexitil	mexiletine	mexiletine
procainamide Pronestyl	procainamide Pronestyl	procainamide	procainamide
propafenone Rythmol	propafenone Arythmol	propafenone Rytmonorm	propafenone
quinidine	quinidine	quinidine	quinidine

416

USA	**UK**	Europe	Japan
sotalol	sotalol	sotalol	sotalol
Betapace	Beta-cardone	Sotacor	
Sotacor	Sotacor		

Anticoagulants

enoxaparin	enoxaparin	enoxaparin	enoxaparin
Lovenox	Clexane		
warfarin	warfarin	warfarin	warfarin
Coumadin	Marevan		

Antiplatelet Agents

abciximab	abciximab		
ReoPro	ReoPro		
aspirin	aspirin	aspirin	aspirin
clopidogrel			
Plavix			
dipyridamole	dipyridamole	dipyridamole	dipyridamole
Persantine	Persantin	Persantin	
	Persantin	Cardoxin	
	Retard		
ebtifibatide			
integrilin			
ticlopidine			ticlopidine
Ticlid			
tirofiban			
Aggrastat			

Beta Blockers

acebutolol	acebutolol	acebutolol	acebutolol
Sectral	Sectral	Prent	
Monitan		Neptall	
		Sectral	
atenolol	atenolol	atenolol	atenolol
Tenormin	Tenormin	Tenormine (F)	
		Tenormin	
		Bêtatop	
betaxolol	betaxolol	betaxolol	betaxolol
Kerlone	Kerlone	Kerlone	
bisoprolol	bisoprolol	bisoprolol	bisoprolol
Zebeta	Emcor		
(Ziac)	Monocor		
carteolol		carteolol	carteolol
Catrol			
carvedilol	carvedilol		carvedilol
Coreg	Eucardic		

USA	UK	Europe	Japan
	celiprolol Celectol	celiprolol Celector Celectol (F)	celiprolol
esmolol Brevibloc	esmolol Brevibloc	esmolol Brevibloc	
labetalol Normodyne Trandate	labetalol Trandate	labetalol Trandate	labetalol
metoprolol Betaloc Lopressor Toprol XL	metoprolol Betaloc Lopresor	metoprolol Lopresor Metohexal Sèloken	metoprolol
nadolol Corgard	nadolol Corgard	nadolol Corgard Solgol (G)	nadolol
oxprenolol Trasicor	oxprenolol Trasicor	oxprenolol Apsolox Trasicor (F)	oxprenolol
propranolol Inderal	propranolol Inderal Inderal-LA	propranolol Angilol Avolacardyl (F) Berkolol Dociton (G) Efektolol	propranolol
sotalol Sotacor Betapace	sotalol Sotacor Beta-Cardone	sotalol Sotacor Sotalex (G) Sotalex (F)	sotalol
timolol Blocadren	timolol Blocadren Betim	timolol Timacor (F) Temserin	timolol

Calcium Antagonists

USA	UK	Europe	Japan
amlodipine Norvasc	amlodipine Istin	amlodipine Amlor (F) Norvasc	amlodipine
diltiazem Cardizem CD	diltiazem Adizem XL Tildiem LA Viazem XL	diltiazem Dilrene (F) Dilzem Herbesser	diltiazem
felodipine Plendil Renedil	felodipine Plendil	felodipine Flodil (F)	felodipine
isradipine DynaCirc	isradipine Prescal	isradipine Flodil (F)	

418

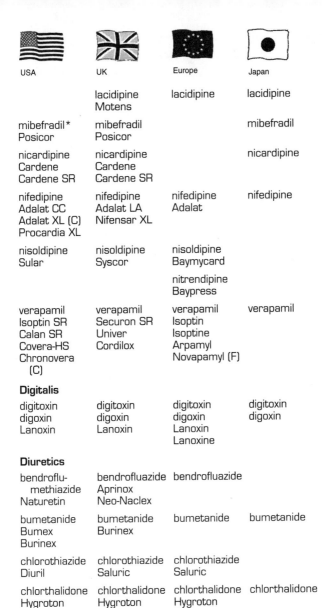

USA	UK	Europe	Japan
	lacidipine Motens	lacidipine	lacidipine
mibefradil* Posicor	mibefradil Posicor		mibefradil
nicardipine Cardene Cardene SR	nicardipine Cardene Cardene SR		nicardipine
nifedipine Adalat CC Adalat XL (C) Procardia XL	nifedipine Adalat LA Nifensar XL	nifedipine Adalat	nifedipine
nisoldipine Sular	nisoldipine Syscor	nisoldipine Baymycard	
		nitrendipine Baypress	
verapamil Isoptin SR Calan SR Covera-HS Chronovera (C)	verapamil Securon SR Univer Cordilox	verapamil Isoptin Isoptine Arpamyl Novapamyl (F)	verapamil

Digitalis

USA	UK	Europe	Japan
digitoxin digoxin Lanoxin	digitoxin digoxin Lanoxin	digitoxin digoxin Lanoxin Lanoxine	digitoxin digoxin

Diuretics

USA	UK	Europe	Japan
bendroflu- methiazide Naturetin	bendrofluazide Aprinox Neo-Naclex	bendrofluazide	
bumetanide Bumex Burinex	bumetanide Burinex	bumetanide	bumetanide
chlorothiazide Diuril	chlorothiazide Saluric	chlorothiazide Saluric	
chlorthalidone Hygroton	chlorthalidone Hygroton Cyclopen- tazide Navidrex	chlorthalidone Hygroton Cyclopen- tazide Navidrex	chlorthalidone
furosemide Lasix	frusemide Lasix	frusemide	furosemide

USA	UK	Europe	Japan
hydrochloro-thiazide	hydrochloro-thiazide	hydrochloro-thiazide	hydrochloro-thiazide
Esidrix	Esidrex		
Hydro Diuril	Hydro Saluric		
indapamide	indapamide	indapamide	indapamide
Lozol	Natramid	Natrillix	
Lozide (C)	Natrilix		
metolazone	metolazone	metolazone	
Zaroxolyn	Metenix	Diulo	
spironolactone	spironolac-tone		
Aldactone	Spiroctan		
torsemide	torasemide		
Demadex	Torem		

Combination Drugs

hydrochlorothi-azide plus amiloride	co-amilozide		hydrochlorothi-azide plus amiloride
Moduretic	Amil-Co		
Moduret (C)	Moduret 25		
	Moduretic		
hydrochlorothi-azide plus trimaterene	hydrochlorothi-azide plus triamterene		hydrochlorothi-azide plus triamterene
Dyazide	Dyazide		

Lipid-lowering Agents

Statins

atorvastatin	atorvastatin	atorvastatin	atorvastatin
Lipitor	Lipitor		
Cerivastatin	Baycol .		
fluvastatin	fluvastatin	fluvastatin	fluvastatin
Lescol	Lescol	Lipur (F)	
lovastatin			
Mevacor			
pravastatin	pravastatin	pravastatin	pravastatin
Pravachol	Lipostat	Elisor	
		Vasten	
simvastatin	simvastatin	simvastatin	simvastatin
Zocor	Zocor	Zocor	
		Lodales	

From Khan, M Gabriel: Cardiac Drug Therapy; 5th ed. London, WB Saunders Co., 2000, pp 421–428.
*Recently withdrawn from market.

APPENDIX G

A Guide to the International ACLS Algorithms*

The ILCOR algorithm presents the actions to take and decisions to face for all people who appear to be in cardic arrest—unconscious, unresponsive, without signs of life. The victim is not breathing normally, and no rescuer can feel a carotid pulse within 10 to 15 seconds. Since 1992 the resuscitation community has examined and reconfirmed the wisdom of most recommendations formulated by international groups through the 1990s. Sophisticated clinical trials provided high-level evidence on which to base several new drugs and interventions. Finally, we have learned that we should continue to place a strong emphasis after 2000 on building a base of critically appraised, international scientific evidence. Evidence-based review opened many eyes; only a small proportion of resuscitation care rests on a base of solid evidence.

---

*From Circulation 2000;102(8) Supplement:I-142–I-165. Copyright (c) 2000 American Heart Association, Inc.

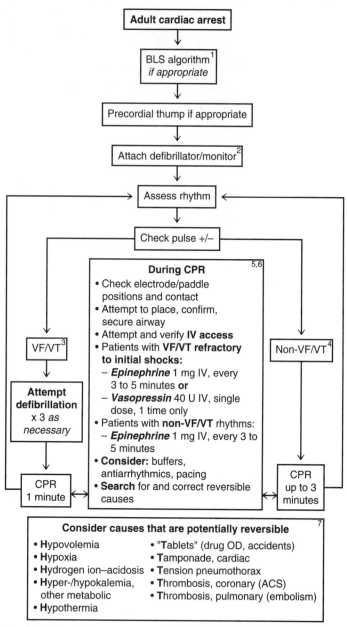

Figure G–1 □ ILCOR Universal/International ACLS algorithm. (From *Circulation* 2000;102[8] Supplement:I-142–I-165. Copyright (c) 2000 American Heart Association, Inc.)

NOTES

1 BLS algorithm. The simple instruction "BLS algorithm" directs the rescuers to start the 6 basic steps of the international BLS algorithm:

1. Check responsiveness
2. Open the airway
3. Check breathing
4. Give 2 effective breaths
5. Assess circulation
6. Compress chest (no signs of circulation detected)

Note that step 6 does not use the term "pulse." In their 1998 BLS guidelines, the European Resuscitation Council and several ILCOR councils dropped a specific reference in their algorithms to "check the carotid pulse." They replaced the pulse check with a direction to "check for signs of circulation," namely, "look for any movement, including swallowing or breathing (more than an occasional gasp)." Their guidelines instruct rescuers to "check for the carotid pulse" as one of the "signs of circulation," but the pulse check does not receive the prominent emphasis that comes from inclusion in the algorithm. By 2000 many locations had confirmed the success of this European approach. Additional evidence had accumulated that the pulse check was not a good diagnostic test for the presence or absence of a beating heart. After international panels of experts reviewed the evidence at the Guidelines 2000 Conference, they also endorsed the approach of omitting the pulse check for lay responders from the International Guidelines 2000.

2 Attach defibrillator/monitor; assess rhythm. Once the responders start the BLS algorithm, they are directed to attach the defibrillator/monitor and assess the rhythm.

3 VF/pulseless VT. If they are using a conventional defibrillator and the monitor displays VF, the rescuers attempt defibrillation, up to 3 times as necessary. If using an AED, the rescuers follow the signal and voice prompts of the device, attempting defibrillation with up to 3 shocks. After 3 shocks they should immediately resume CPR for at least 1 minute. At the end of the minute, they should repeat rhythm assessment and shock when appropriate.

4 Non-VF rhythm. If the conventional defibrillator/monitor displays a non-VF tracing or the AED signals "no shock indicated," the responders should immediately check the pulse to determine whether the nonshockable rhythm is producing a spontaneous circulation. If not, then start CPR; continue CPR for approximately 3 minutes. With a non-VF rhythm the rescuer needs to return and recheck the rhythm for recurrent VF or for spontaneous return of an organized rhythm in a beating heart. At this point the algorithm enters the central column of comments.

5 During CPR: tracheal tube placement; IV access. In this period the rescuers have many tasks to accomplish. The central column includes the major interventions of ACLS: placing and confirming a tracheal tube, starting an IV, giving appropriate medications for the rhythm, and searching for and correcting reversible causes. Note that the ECC Comprehensive Algorithm (Figure 2) conveys this same approach using the memory aid of the Secondary ABCD Survey. In this survey A = advanced airway (tracheal tube placement); B = confirmation of tube location, oxygenation, and ventilation; and C = circulation access via IV line and circulation medications.

6 VF/VT refractory to initial shocks: epinephrine or vasopressin. The

ILCOR Universal Algorithm indicates that response personnel give all cardiac arrest patients a strong vasopressor, either epinephrine IV or vasopressin. This recommendation for vasopressin is one of the more interesting new guidelines. The discussions on adding amiodarone are detailed later in this section.

Consider buffers, antiarrhythmics, pacing, atropine; search for and correct reversible causes. This short phrase covers a multitude of interventions discussed and debated during the Evidence Evaluation Conference and the international Guidelines 2000 Conference: multiple antiarrhythmics, neutralization of acidosis, and transcutaneous pacing. The word "consider" has become an informal code in the resuscitation community interpreted to mean that we lack the evidence that establishes one intervention as superior to another. Whether this means that two interventions are equally effective or equally ineffective is a debate being waged constantly in resuscitation research.

7 Consider causes that are potentially reversible. This guideline applies primarily to non-VF/VT patients. For this group there is often a specific cause of the loss of an effective heartbeat. The International Guidelines 2000 take the innovative step of listing the 10 most common reversible causes of non-VF/VT arrest at the bottom of the algorithm. This is discussed in detail in the section on pulseless electrical activity.

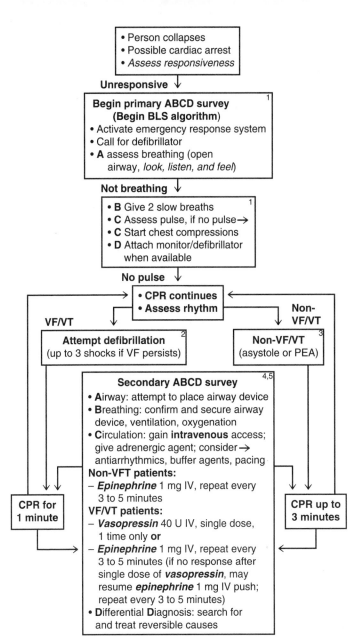

Figure G-2 □ Comprehensive ECC algorithm. (From *Circulation* 2000;102[8] Supplement:I-142–I-165. Copyright (c) 2000 American Heart Association, Inc.)

NOTES

1 Begin Primary ABCD Survey. Unresponsive; not breathing. Boxes 1 and 2 cover the steps of the BLS Algorithm and cover the *Primary ABCD Survey*. The survey is a memory aid and conveys no therapeutic value as stated and displayed. The Primary and Secondary ABCD Surveys are simple mnemonics that assist initial learning. They also provide a useful mental "hook" for later review and recall. Listing more details within the algorithm provides easy review of the steps, especially when the learner has not participated routinely in actual resuscitation attempts.

2 VF/VT: attempt defibrillation (up to 3 shocks if VF persists). Rhythm assessment and continued CPR are the center of the Comprehensive ECC Algorithm. The metaphor of a clock ticking away for a cardiac arrest victim in VF is overused but accurate. With each minute of persistent VF, the probability of survival declines. Two clocks are racing. One is the clock that measures the *therapeutic interval* (from collapse to arrival of the defibrillator). One is the block that measures the *irreversible damage interval* (from cessation of blood flow to the brain to the start of permanent, irreversible brain death).

Here is an observation that will put the racing clocks into perspective. Several experts have observed that great amounts of time and money are spent on the development of new defibrillation waveforms, novel antiarrhythmics, innovative vasopressors, and fresh approaches to ventilation and oxygenation. The total combined effect on survival of these interventions is equivalent to nothing more than cutting the interval from collapse to defibrillatory shock by 2 minutes.

3 Non-VF/VT. The ILCOR recommendation is to consider the non-VF/VT rhythms as one rhythm when the patient is in cardiac arrest. Consider non-VF/VT as either asystole, or PEA. The treatment in the algorithm is the same for both: epinephrine, atropine, transcutaneous pacing. Electrical activity on the monitor screen is a more positive rhythm than asystole. Later in this discussion PEA and asystole are presented in much greater detail.

Both rhythms have a "differential diagnosis" in terms of what entities can produce a PEA and an asystolic rhythm. Responders must aggressively evaluate PEA victims to discover a potential reversible cause. There is a narrow diagnostic interval of just a few minutes at the discovery of PEA. Asystole, on the other hand, is rarely salvaged unless a reversible cause (eg, severe hyperkalemia, overdose of phenothiazine) is found. Only occasionally does asystole respond to epinephrine in higher doses, atropine, or pacing, because the patient is simply destined to die, given the nature of the orginal precipitating event.

4 Secondary ABCD Survey. Use of a vasopressor: epinephrine for non-VF/VT, vasopressin for refractory VF. This section of the algorithm makes the same points about persistent arrest from VF/VT and non-VF/VT as the ILCOR Universal Algorithm. The ECC Comprehensive Algorithm, however, uses the memory aid of the Secondary ABCD Survey, a device repeated in all the cardiac arrest algorithms. The algorithm notes expand on these concepts.

5 Potentially reversible causes. Sudden VF/VT arrests are straightforward in their management. Management consists of early defibrillation, which can succeed independently of other interventions and independently of discovery of the cause of the arrhythmia. With non-VF/VT arrest, however, successful restoration of a spontaneous pulse depends almost entirely on recognizing and treating a potentially reversible cause.

As an aide mémoire, Figure 1 places the following list, referred to as "the 5 H's and 5 T's," in the algorithm layout:

The "5 H's"

- Hypovolemia
- Hypoxia
- Hydrogen ion (acidosis)
- Hyperkalemia/hypokalemia and metabolic disorders
- Hypothermia/hyperthermia

The "5 T's"

- Toxins/tablets (drug overdose, illicit drugs)
- Tamponade, cardiac
- Tension pneumothorax
- Thrombosis, coronary
- Thrombosis, pulmonary

The Comprehensive ECC algorithm expands the table of reversible causes by listing possible therapeutic interventions next to each of the potential causes.

Consider: Is one of the following conditions playing a role?

Hypovolemia (volume infusion)
Hypoxia (oxygen, ventilation)
Hydrogen ion-acidosis (buffer, ventilation)
Hyperkalemia (CaCl plus others)
Hypothermia (see Hypothermia Algorithm in Part 8)
"Tablets" (drug overdoses, accidents)
Tamponade, cardiac (pericardiocentesis)
Tension pneumothorax (decompress-needle decompression)
Thrombosis, coronary (fibrinolytics)
Thrombosis, pulmonary (fibrinolytics, surgical evacuation)

Figure G–3 □ Ventricular fibrillation/pulseless VT algorithm. (From Circulation 2000;102[8] Supplement:I-142–I-165. Copyright (c) 2000 American Heart Association, Inc.)

NOTES

Assume the VF/VT persists after each intervention.

1 Defibrillatory shock waveforms

- Use **monophasic shocks** at listed energy levels (300 J, 300 to 360 J, 360 J) or **Biphasic shocks** at energy levels documented to be clinically equivalent (or superior) to the monophasic shocks.

2A Confirm tube placement with

- Primary physical examination criteria *plus*
- Secondary confirmation device (end-tidal CO_2, end-diastolic diameter) (Class IIa)

2B Secure tracheal tube

- To prevent dislodgment, especially in patients at risk for movement, use purpose-made (commercially available) tracheal tube holders, which are superior to tie-and-tape methods (Class IIb)
- Consider cervical collar and backboard for transport (Class Indeterminate)
- Consider continuous, quantitative end-tidal CO_2 monitor (Class IIa)

2C Confirm oxygenation and ventilation with

- End-tidal CO_2 monitor *and*
- Oxygen saturation monitor

3A *Epinephrine* (Class Indeterminate) 1 mg IV push every 3 to 5 minutes. If this fails, higher doses of epinephrine (up to 0.2 mg/kg) are acceptable but not recommended (there is growing evidence that it may be harmful).

3B *Vasopressin* is recommended only for VF/VT; there is no evidence to support its use in asystole or PEA. There is no evidence about the value of repeat vasopressin doses. There is no evidence about the best approach if there is no response after a single bolus of vasopressin. The following Class Indeterminate action is acceptable, but only on the basis of rational conjecture. If there is no response 5 to 10 minutes after a single IV dose of vasopressin, it is *acceptable* to resume epinephrine 1 mg IV push every 3 to 5 minutes.

4A *Antiarrhythmics* are indeterminate or Class IIb: acceptable; only fair evidence supports possible benefit of antiarrhythmics for shock-refractory VF/VT.

- *Amiodarone* (Class IIb) 300 mg IV push (cardiac arrest dose). If VF/pulseless VT recurs, consider administration of a second dose of 150 mg IV. Maximum cumulative dose: 2.2 g over 24 hours.
- *Lidocaine* (Class Indeterminate) 1.0 to 1.5 mg/kg IV push. Consider repeat in 3 to 5 minutes to a maximum cumulative dose of 3 mg/kg. A single dose of 1.5 mg/kg in cardiac arrest is acceptable.
- *Magnesium sulfate* 1 to 2 g IV in polymorphic VT (torsades de pointes) and suspected hypomagnesemic state.
- *Procainamide* 30 mg/min in refractory VF (maximum total dose: 17 mg/kg) is acceptable but not recommended because prolonged administration time is unsuitable for cardiac arrest.

4B *Sodium bicarbonate* 1 mEq/kg IV is indicated for several conditions known to provoke sudden cardiac arrest. See Notes in the Asystole and PEA Algorithms for details.

Resume defibrillation attempts: use 360-J (or equivalent biphasic) shocks after each medication or after each minute of CPR. Acceptable patterns: CPR-drug-shock (repeat) or CPR-drug-shock-shock-shock (repeat).

```
┌─────────────────────────────────────────────┐
│          Pulseless electrical activity        │
│  (PEA = rhythm on monitor, without detectable pulse) │
└─────────────────────────────────────────────┘
                        ↓
┌─────────────────────────────────────────────┐
│             Primary ABCD survey               │
│       Focus: basic CPR and defibrillation     │
│  • Check responsiveness                       │
│  • Activate emergency response system         │
│  • Call for defibrillator                     │
│  A Airway: open the airway                    │
│  B Breathing: provide positive-pressure ventilations │
│  C Circulation: give chest compressions       │
│  D Defibrillation: assess for and shock VF/pulseless VT │
└─────────────────────────────────────────────┘
                        ↓
┌─────────────────────────────────────────────┐
│            Secondary ABCD survey              │
│   Focus: more advanced assessments and treatments │
│  A Airway: place airway device as soon as possible │
│  B Breathing: confirm airway device placement by exam plus │
│    confirmation device                        │
│  B Breathing: secure airway device; purpose-made tube holders │
│    preferred                                  │
│  B Breathing: confirm effective oxygenation and ventilation │
│  C Circulation: establish IV access           │
│  C Circulation: identify rhythm→ monitor      │
│  C Circulation: administer drugs appropriate for rhythm and │
│    condition                                  │
│  C Circulation: assess for occult blood flow ("pseudo-EMT") │
│  D Differential Diagnosis: search for and treat identified │
│    reversible causes                          │
└─────────────────────────────────────────────┘
                        ↓
┌─────────────────────────────────────────────┐
│          Review for most frequent causes   [1] │
│  • Hypovolemia            • "Tablets" (drug OD, accidents) │
│  • Hypoxia                • Tamponade, cardiac │
│  • Hydrogen ion–acidosis  • Tension pneumothorax │
│  • Hyper-/hypokalemia     • Thrombosis, coronary (ACS) │
│  • Hypothermia            • Thrombosis, pulmonary (embolism) │
└─────────────────────────────────────────────┘
                        ↓
          ┌─────────────────────────────────┐
          │   Epinephrine 1 mg IV push,  [2] │
          │   repeat every 3 to 5 minutes    │
          └─────────────────────────────────┘
                        ↓
      ┌─────────────────────────────────────────┐
      │   Atropine 1 mg IV (if PEA rate is slow), [3] │
      │   repeat every 3 to 5 minutes as needed, to a total │
      │        dose of 0.04 mg/kg                │
      └─────────────────────────────────────────┘
```

Figure G–4 □ Pulseless electrical activity algorithm. (From Circulation 2000;102[8] Supplement:I-142–I-165. Copyright (c) 2000 American Heart Association, Inc.)

NOTES

Both VF/VT and PEA are "rhythms of survival." People in VF/VT can be resuscitated by timely arrival of a defibrillator, and people in PEA can be resuscitated if a reversible cause of PEA is identified and treated appropriately. The PEA algorithm puts great emphasis on searching for specific, reversible causes of PEA. The algorithm features a table of the top 10 causes of PEA, arranged as the "5 H's and 5 T's." If reversible causes are not considered, rescuers will have little chance of recognition and successful treatment. Sodium bicarbonate provides a good example of how the cause of the PEA relates to the therapy. Sodium bicarbonate can vary between being a Class I intervention and being a Class III intervention, depending on the cause.

1 Sodium bicarbonate 1 mEq/kg is used as follows:

Class I (acceptable, supported by definitive evidence)

- If patient has known, preexisting hyperkalemia

Class IIa (acceptable, good evidence supports)

- If known, preexisting bicarbonate-responsive acidosis
- In tricyclic antidepressant overdose
- To alkalinize urine in aspirin or other drug overdoses

Class IIb (acceptable, only fair evidence provides support)

- In intubated and ventilated patients with long arrest interval
- On return of circulation, after long arrest interval

May be harmful (Class III) in hypercarbic acidosis

2 Epinephrine: recommended dose is 1 mg IV push every 3 to 5 minutes (Class Indeterminate).

- If this approach fails, higher doses of epinephrine (up to 0.2 mg/kg) may be used but are not recommended.
- (Although one dose of vasopressin is acceptable for persistent or shock-refractory VF, we currently lack evidence to support routine use of vasopressin in victims of PEA or asystole.)

3 Atropine: the shorter atropine dose interval (every 3 to 5 minutes) is possibly helpful in cardiac arrest.

- *Atropine* 1 mg IV if electrical activity is *slow* (absolute bradycardia = rate <60 bpm) or
- *Relatively slow* (relative bradycardia = rate less than expected, relative to underlying condition)

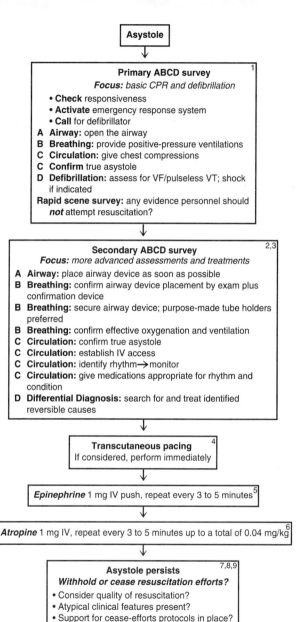

Figure G–5 □ Asystole: The silent heart algorithm. (From Circulation 2000;102[8] Supplement:I-142–I-165. Copyright (c) 2000 American Heart Association, Inc.)

NOTES
1 Scene Survey: DNAR patient?

If Yes: do not start/attempt resuscitation. Any *objective* indicators of DNAR status? Bracelet? Anklet? Written documentation? Family statements? If Yes: do not start/attempt resuscitation.

- Any *clinical* indicators that resuscitation attempts are not indicated, eg, signs of death? If Yes: do not start/attempt resuscitation.

2 Confirm true asystole

- Check lead and cable connections
- Monitor power on?
- Monitor gain up?
- Verify asystole in another lead?

3 Sodium bicarbonate 1 mEq/kg

- Indications for use include the following: overdose of tricyclic antidepressants; to alkalinize urine in overdoses; patients with tracheal intubation plus long arrest intervals; on return of spontaneous circulation if there is a long arrest interval.
- Ineffective or harmful in hypercarbic acidosis.

4 Transcutaneous pacing

- To be effective, must be performed early, combined with drug therapy. Evidence does not support routine use of transcutaneous pacing for asystole.

5 Epinephrine

- Recommended dose is 1 mg IV push every 3 to 5 minutes. If this approach fails, higher doses of epinephrine (up to 0.2 mg/kg) may be used but are not recommended.
- We currently lack evidence to support routine use of vasopressin in treatment of asystole.

6 Atropine

- Use the shorter dosing interval (every 3 to 5 minutes) in asystolic arrest.

7 Review the quality of the resuscitation attempt

- Was there an adequate trial of BLS? of ACLS? Has the team done the following:
  - Achieved tracheal intubation?
  - Performed effective ventilation?
  - Shocked VF if present?
  - Obtained IV access?
  - Given epinephrine IV? atropine IV?
  - Ruled out or corrected reversible causes?
  - Continuously documented asystole >5 to 10 minutes after all of the above have been accomplished?

8 Reviewed for atypical clinical features?

- Not a victim of drowning or hypothermia?
- No reversible therapeutic or illicit drug overdose?

"Yes" to the questions in Notes 7 and 8 means the resuscitation team complies with recommended criteria to terminate resuscitative efforts where the patient lies (Class IIa)

If the response team and patient meet the above criteria, then withhold urgent field-to-hospital transport with continuing CPR-Class III (harmful; no benefit)

9 Withholding or stopping resuscitative efforts out-of-hospital

If criteria in 7 and 8 are fulfilled:

- Field personnel, in jurisdictions where authorized, should start protocols to cease resuscitative efforts or to pronounce death outside the hospital (Class IIa).
- In most US settings, the medical control official must give direct voice-to-voice or on-scene authorization.
- Advance planning for these protocols must occur. The planning should include specific directions for
  - Leaving the body at scene
  - Death certification
  - Transfer to funeral service
  - On-scene family advocate
  - Religious or nondenominational counseling

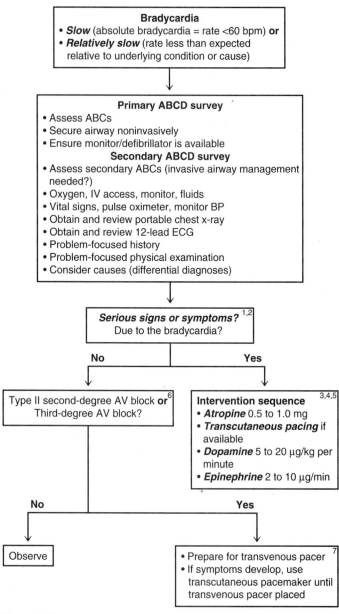

Figure G–6 □ Bradycardia algorithm. (From Circulation 2000;102[8] Supplement:I-142–I-165. Copyright (c) 2000 American Heart Association, Inc.)

NOTES

1 If the patient has *serious signs or symptoms,* make sure they are related to the slow rate.

2 Clinical manifestations include

- Symptoms (chest pain, shortness of breath, decreased level of consciousness)
- Signs (low blood pressure, shock, pulmonary congestion, congestive heart failure)

3 If the patient is symptomatic, do not delay transcutaneous pacing while awaiting IV access or for *atropine* to take effect.

4 *Denervated transplanted hearts* will not respond to *atropine.* Go at once to pacing, *catecholamine* infusion, or both.

5 *Atropine* should be given in repeat doses every 3 to 5 minutes up to a total of 0.03 to 0.04 mg/kg. Use the shorter dosing interval (3 minutes) in severe clinical conditions.

6 Never treat the combination of *third-degree heart block* and *ventricular escape beats* with *lidocaine* (or any agent that suppresses ventricular escape rhythms).

7 Verify patient tolerance and mechanical capture. Use analgesia and sedation as needed.

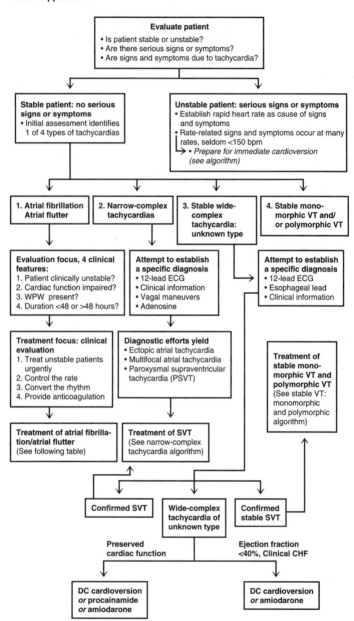

Figure G–7 □ The tachycardia overview algorithm. (From Circulation 2000;102[8] Supplement:I-142–I-165. Copyright (c) 2000 American Heart Association, Inc.)

CONTROL OF RATE AND RHYTHM

Atrial fibrillation/ atrial flutter with • Normal heart • Impaired heart • WPW	1. Control Rate		2. Convert Rhythm	
	Heart Function Preserved	Impaired Heart: EF <40% or CHF	Duration <48 Hours	Duration >48 Hours or Unknown

Normal cardiac function	**Note:** *If AF >48 hours' duration, use agents to convert rhythm with extreme caution in patients not receiving adequate anticoagulation because of possible embolic complications.*
	
	Use only 1 of the following agents [see note below]:
	• Calcium channel blockers [Class I]
	• β-Blockers [Class I]
	• For additional drugs that are Class IIb recommendations, see Guidelines or ACLS text
		[Does not apply]	**Consider**
			• DC cardioversion
			
			Use only 1 of the following agents [see note below]:
			• Amiodarone [Class IIa]
			• Ibutilide [Class IIa]
			• Flecainide [Class IIa]
			• Propafenone [Class IIa]
			• Procainamide [Class IIa]
			• For additional drugs that are Class IIb recommendations, see Guidelines or ACLS text
				• **NO DC cardioversion!**
				• **Note:** *Conversion of AF to NSR with drugs or shock may cause embolization of atrial thrombi unless patient has adequate anticoagulation.*
				• Use antiarrhythmic agents with extreme caution if AF >48 hours' duration *[see note above].*
				
				or
				
				Delayed cardioversion
				Anticoagulation × 3 weeks at proper levels
				• Cardioversion, *then*
				• Anticoagulation × 4 weeks more
				
				or
				
				Early cardioversion
				• Begin IV heparin at once
				• TEE to exclude atrial clot
				   then
				• Cardioversion within 24 hours
				   then
				• Anticoagulation × 4 more weeks

Table continued on following page

CONTROL OF RATE AND RHYTHM *Continued*

Atrial fibrillation/ atrial flutter with • *Normal heart* • *Impaired heart* • *WPW*	1. Control Rate		2. Convert Rhythm	
	Heart Function Preserved	Impaired Heart EF <40% or CHF	Duration <48 Hours	Duration >48 Hours or Unknown
Impaired heart (EF <40% or CHF)	*[Does not apply]*	**Note:** *If AF >48 hours' duration, use agents to convert rhythm with extreme caution in patients not receiving adequate anticoagulation because of possible embolic complications.* *Use only 1 of the following agents [see note below]:* • Digoxin [Class IIb] • Diltiazem [Class IIb] • Amiodarone [Class IIb]	**Consider** • DC cardioversion *or* • Amiodarone [Class IIb]	• **Anticoagulation** as described above, followed by • **DC cardioversion**

WPW

Note: *If AF >48 hours' duration, use agents to convert rhythm with extreme caution in patients not receiving adequate anticoagulation because of possible embolic complications.*

- DC cardioversion

  or

- **Primary antiarrhythmic agents** *Use only 1 of the following agents (see note below):*
  - Amiodarone [Class IIb]
  - Flecainide [Class IIb]
  - Procainamide [Class IIb]
  - Propafenone [Class IIb]
  - Sotalol [Class IIb]

Class III [can be harmful]
- Adenosine
- β-Blockers
- Calcium blockers
- Digoxin

Note: *If AF >48 hours' duration, use agents to convert rhythm with extreme caution in patients not receiving adequate anticoagulation because of possible embolic complications.*

- DC cardioversion

  or

- Amiodarone [Class IIb]

- DC cardioversion

  or

- **Primary antiarrhythmic agents** *Use only 1 of the following agents:*
  - Amiodarone [Class IIb]
  - Flecainide [Class IIb]
  - Procainamide [Class IIb]
  - Propafenone [Class IIb]
  - Sotalol [Class IIb]

Class III [can be harmful]
- Adenosine
- β-Blockers
- Calcium blockers
- Digoxin

- **Anticoagulation** as described above, followed by
- **DC cardioversion**

WPW = Wolff-Parkinson-White syndrome; AF = atrial fibrillation; NSR = normal sinus rhythm; TEE = transesophageal echocardiogram; EF = ejection fraction.

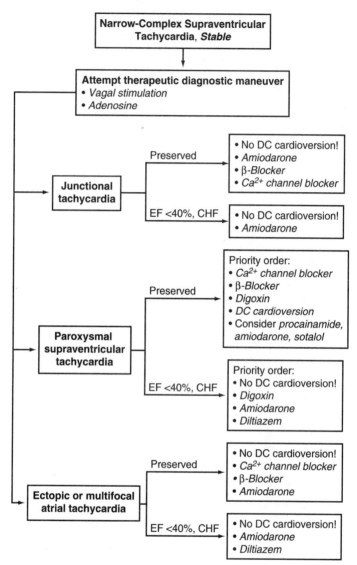

Figure G–8 □ Narrow-complex supraventricular tachycardia algorithm. (From Circulation 2000;102[8] Supplement:I-142–I-165. Copyright (c) 2000 American Heart Association, Inc.)

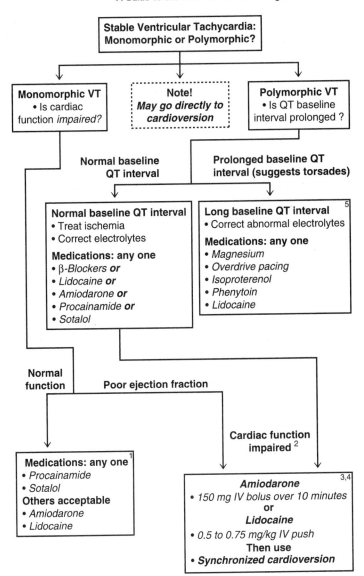

Figure G–9 □ Stable ventricular tachycardia (monomorphic or polymorphic) algorithm. (From Circulation 2000;102[8] Supplement:I-142–I-165. Copyright (c) 2000 American Heart Association, Inc.)

NOTES

1 Monomorphic VF with normal cardiac function

Use just 1 agent (to avoid proarrhythmic effects of combination therapy).

This reduces adverse side effects. Choose 1 agent from these lists:

Top agents

- Procainamide (IIa)
- Sotalol (IIa)

Others acceptable

- Amiodarone (IIb)
- Lidocaine (IIb)

2 Monomorphic or polymorphic VT with impaired cardiac function

If clinical signs are suggestive of impaired LV function (ejection fraction <40% or congestive heart failure) in either long- or normal-QRS tachycardias, use

- Amiodarone (IIb)
- Lidocaine (IIb)

then use

- Synchronized cardioversion

3 Detailed dosing of amiodarone (Class IIb) in patients with impaired cardiac function

- 150 mg IV bolus over 10 minutes (international dose: 5 mg/kg)
- Repeat 150 mg IV (over 10 minutes) every 10 to 15 minutes as needed
- Alternative infusion: 360 mg over 6 hours (1 mg/min over 6 hours), then 540 mg over the remaining 18 hours (0.5 mg/min)
- Maximum total dose: 2.2 g in 24 hours. This means that *all* doses (including those used in resuscitation) should be added together, so the total cumulative dose per 24 hours is limited to 2.2 g
- See guidelines or ECC Handbook Drug Table

4 Detailed dosing of lidocaine (Class Indeterminate) in patients with impaired cardiac function

- 0.5 to 0.75 mg/kg IV push
- Repeat every 5 to 10 minutes
- Then infuse 1 to 4 mg/min
- Maximum total dose: 3 mg/kg (over 1 hour)

5 If rhythm is suggestive of torsades de pointes

- Stop/avoid treatments that prolong QT
- Identify and treat abnormal electrolytes

Medications (all Class Indeterminate):

- Magnesium
- Overdrive pacing (with or without β-blocker)
- Isoproterenol (as temporizing measure to overdrive pacing)
- Phenytoin or lidocaine

```
┌─────────────────────────────┐
│ Tachycardia                 │
│ With serious signs and      │
│ symptoms related to the     │
│ tachycardia                 │
└─────────────────────────────┘
              ↓
┌───────────────────────────────────────────┐
│ If ventricular rate is >150 bpm, prepare   │
│ for immediate cardioversion. May give      │
│ brief trial of medications based on        │
│ specific arrhythmias. Immediate            │
│ cardioversion is generally not needed if   │
│ heart rate is ≤150 bpm.                    │
└───────────────────────────────────────────┘
              ↓
┌─────────────────────────────┐
│ Have available at bedside   │
│ • Oxygen saturation monitor │
│ • Suction device            │
│ • IV line                   │
│ • Intubation equipment      │
└─────────────────────────────┘
              ↓
┌─────────────────────────────────────┐
│ Premedicate whenever possible[1]    │
└─────────────────────────────────────┘
              ↓
```

┌──┐
│   [2,3,4,5,6]   │
│ *Synchronized cardioversion*   │
│ • Ventricular tachycardia ──┐   100 J, 200 J,   │
│ • Paroxysmal supraventricular│ 300 J, 360 J   │
│   tachycardia   │ monophasic energy dose   │
│ • Atrial fibrillation   │ (or clinically equivalent   │
│ • Atrial flutter ────────────┘ biphasic energy dose)   │
└──┘

Steps for synchronized cardioversion

1. Consider sedation.
2. Turn on defibrillator (monophasic or biphasic).
3. Attach monitor leads to the patient ("white to right, red to ribs, what's left over to the left shoulder") and ensure proper display of the patient's rhythm.
4. Engage the synchronization mode by pressing the "sync" control button.
5. Look for markers on R waves indicating sync mode.
6. If necessary, adjust monitor gain until sync markers occur with each R wave.
7. Select appropriate energy level.
8. Position conductor pads on patient (or apply gel to paddles).
9. Position paddle on patient (sternum-apex).
10. Announce to team members: *"Charging defibrillator—stand clear!"*
11. Press "charge" button on apex paddle (right hand).
12. When the defibrillator is charged, begin the final clearing chant. State firmly in a forceful voice the following chant before each shock:
    • *"I'm going to shock on three. One, I am clear."* (Check to make sure you are clear of contact with the patient, the stretcher, and the equipment.)
    • *"Two, you are clear."* (Make a visual check to ensure that no one continues to touch the patient or stretcher. In particular, do not forget about the person providing ventilations. That person's hands should not be touching the ventilatory adjuncts, including the tracheal tube!)
    • *"Three, everybody's clear."* (Check yourself one more time before pressing the "shock" buttons.)
13. Apply 25 lb pressure on both paddles.
14. Press the "discharge" buttons simultaneously.
15. Check the monitor. If tachycardia persists, increase the joules according to the electrical cardioversion algorithm.
16. **Reset the sync mode after each synchronized cardioversion because most defibrillators default back to unsynchronized mode.** This default allows an immediate defibrillation if the cardioversion produces VF.

Figure G–10 □ Synchronized cardioversion algorithm. (From *Circulation* 2000;102[8] Supplement:I-142–I-165. Copyright (c) 2000 American Heart Association, Inc.)

NOTES

1 Effective regimens have included a sedative (eg, *diazepam, midazolam, barbiturates, etomidate, ketamine, methohexital*) with or without an analgesic agent (eg, *fentanyl, morphine, meperidine*). Many experts recommend anesthesia if service is readily available.

2 Both monophasic and biphasic waveforms are acceptable if documented as clinically equivalent to reports of monophasic shock success.

3 Note possible need to resynchronize after each cardioversion.

4 If delays in synchronization occur and clinical condition is critical, go immediately to unsynchronized shocks.

5 Treat polymorphic ventricular tachycardia (irregular form and rate) like ventricular fibrillation: see ventricular fibrillation/pulseless ventricular tachycardia algorithm.

6 Paroxysmal supraventricular tachycardia and atrial flutter often respond to lower energy levels (start with 50 J).

INDEX

Note: Page numbers in *italics* refer to illustrations; page numbers followed by (t) refer to tables.

A

A₂ (aortic second heart sound), 35, *36*
  abnormalities of, 36
  splitting of, from P₂, 36–37, *38*
ABCD's, of cardiopulmonary resuscitation, 353, *354*, 426–427, *428*, 429–430, *431*
Abrupt on- and offset syncope, in long QT syndrome, 341. See also *Electrocardiography, QT interval in, prolonged; Syncope.*
Abrupt onset–gradual offset syncope, 341. See also *Syncope.*
Absent y descent, of jugular venous pulse, 27
Acebutolol, management applications of, in angina, 403(t)
  in hypertension, 323, 331
  in myocardial infarction, 175
  trade names for, 403(t), 417(t)
ACE inhibitors. See *Angiotensin-converting enzyme inhibitors.*
Acetaminophen, interaction of, with oral anticoagulants, 366
Acquired hypercoagulability, 370–371
Acromegaly, cardiovascular complications of, 12
Activated protein C, resistance to, 370
Acute myocardial infarction (AMI). See *Myocardial infarction.*
Adenosine, adverse effects of, 411(t)
  drugs interacting with, 413(t)
  management applications of, in AV nodal reentrant tachycardia, 275

Adenosine *(Continued)*
  in supraventricular tachycardia, 407(t)
  response to, in diagnosis of arrhythmias, 132
  trade names for, 416(t)
Adenosine-thallium scintigraphy, in patient with angina, 202
Advanced cardiac life support, 353–356
  algorithms for, 421–446
    comprehensive ECG, *425*
    in asystole, *433*
    in atrial fibrillation, *438*
    in atrial flutter, *438*
    in bradycardia, *436*
    in cardiac arrest, *422*
    in junctional tachycardia, *442*
    in multifocal atrial tachycardia, *422*
    in paroxysmal supraventricular tachycardia, *422*
    in pulseless electrical activity (EMD), *431*
    in pulseless ventricular tachycardia, *428*
    in supraventricular tachycardia, *442*
    in tachycardia, *438*, *445*
    in ventricular fibrillation, *425*, *428*
    in ventricular tachycardia, *443*
    universal, *422*
AHA (American Heart Association) objectives, of therapy for hyperlipidemia, 409(t). See also *Hyperlipidemia.*
Air, in pleural space, chest pain due to, 154
  management of, 158–159
Airway management, in CPR, 353, *354*